THE NATURAL REMEDY BIBLE

Easy, inexpensive methods of treatment for every day

Did you know ...
- You can relieve a headache by pressing your thumb against the roof of your mouth?
- Foot odor can be treated—and cured—with pine needle extract?
- Cayenne pepper combined with echinacea root can help relieve a toothache?
- Varicose vein ulcerations that refuse to heal respond very well to the effects of brewer's yeast?

Everything you need to know—*naturally.*

JOHN LUST, N.D., is the author of the bestselling *The Herb Book,* a classic credited with launching the herbal renaissance in America. He was encouraged by his father, Benedict Lust, M.D., N.D., who was known as "The Father of Natural Medicine" and wrote many important books in the field.

MICHAEL TIERRA, C.A., N.D., is one of the nation's most respected herbalists, a pioneer in the integration of Eastern and Western principles of herbal medicine. He is the author of several books, including *The Natural Remedy Bible* and *Planetary Herbology.*

Books by Michael Tierra

The Natural Remedy Bible
(with John Lust)

The Way of Herbs

Published by POCKET BOOKS

THE

NATURAL

REMEDY BIBLE

Revised & Updated

Michael Tierra, C.A., O.M.D.
and John Lust, N.D.

POCKET BOOKS

New York   London   Toronto   Sydney   Singapore

*This book is respectfully dedicated to all
people throughout the world.*

*To all those who helped me during the
years of its preparation I extend my
grateful acknowledgment.*

POCKET BOOKS, a division of Simon & Schuster, Inc.
1230 Avenue of the Americas, New York, NY 10020

Copyright © 1990, 2003 by James Charlton Associates

Originally published as a mass market paperback in 1990 by
Pocket Books

ISBN: 0-7434-6642-X

This Pocket Books paperback printing April 2003

10 9 8 7 6 5 4 3 2 1

POCKET and colophon are registered trademarks of
Simon & Schuster, Inc.

For information regarding special discounts for bulk purchases,
please contact Simon & Schuster Special Sales at 1-800-456-6798
or business@simonandschuster.com

Front cover illustration by Peggy Turchette

Printed in the U.S.A.

The information and treatments in this book are not intended to replace the services of a qualified health professional or to serve as a replacement for medical care. They are simply offered to describe the possibilities that exist beyond the normal range of orthodox medicine.

Thus, in describing the various self-treatments of disease in this book, we are aware of the obvious fact that, prior to commencing any course of treatment prescribed in this book, you should consult a qualified healthcare professional. It is our opinion that seeking such consultation is in line with the gentle, non-invasive natural health care described in this book.

Any application of the treatments set forth in this book is at the reader's sole discretion and sole risk.

CONTENTS

PREFACE

From the time *The Herb Book* was published, I wanted to write its companion work—a reference book about herbal remedies, organized according to ailments. Here in the *Natural Remedy Bible,* you will find information about common illnesses and their natural treatments, as well as various combinations of herbal preparations and methods of applying them. The emphasis is on the use of herbs (broadly designed to mean any form of plant material), water, and nutritional substances. This information is presented to help you develop informed self-reliance in the area of your personal health.

My intent is to promote a modified life-style that respects our fundamental relationship with nature and helps us make the most out of life. My earnest wish is that this book will encourage and enable you to follow nature's path to health and happiness.

JOHN B. LUST
Greenwich, Connecticut
May 1985

INTRODUCTION

by John Lust

The words *heal, health,* and *whole* all came from a Germanic ancestral word that means "whole" or "intact." In one sense, the words are still closely connected in meaning: to heal is to make whole. But in another sense, a more profound connection has been largely lost, in practice if not in principle. It is that health is the harmonious functioning of one's whole being—body, mind, and spirit.

In Western cultures, the health care empire is neatly carved up among specialists in physical, mental, and spiritual illnesses. The problem is that people and their problems can't be so neatly divided. In the living human being, body, mind, and spirit are closely interrelated parts that form a single entity. Whatever happens to one part of us intimately affects the other parts also.

Ideally, we should always be well. But how we get well and stay well depends not only on our own nature but also on the environment in which we exist. Each of us has both internal and external physical, mental, and spiritual realities, which are constantly changing. Total health is the harmonious function of all these elements in a complex and dynamic balance.

Health in this sense is the normal condition of human

life. If the body is able to function at all, for example, it automatically tries to repair any damage done to it. Quite literally where there's life there's hope. Most of the history of medicine consists of attempts to promote these natural healing processes with help from magic, prayer, plants, animals, minerals, sunshine, water, exercise, rest, surgery, manipulation, and other materials and methods. Some of the more drastic interventions, though well-intentioned, turned out to be misguided and interfered with healing instead of helping it. The practices of bleeding patients and of cauterizing wounds are two well-known examples from the past. Today, when drastic intervention is the rule rather than the exception, doctors are still finding that time and nature can be better healers than their most current treatments. For example, a fingertip that has been amputated can grow a fingernail and even a fingerprint if it is kept clean and bandaged, but it heals as a stump if it is surgically sewn up. Less dramatic but just as miraculously, a razor nick can disappear without a trace from one morning to the next. Repair and healing are inherent in every living thing.

The basic methods described here apply to all three sectors of healing: preventive, curative, and regenerative. They also have the special advantage that they can be practiced at home.

The emphasis in this book is on the following three methods of treatment:

1. *Botanical Medicine:* Carefully selected use—both internally and externally—of clinically proven medicinal plant materials.
2. *Hydrotherapy:* A series of specialized water treatments, often employing botanicals, adapted indi-

vidually to induce the body to produce healthful reactions.

3. *Nutrition and Diet:* Well-balanced nutritional therapy through a basic natural diet.

Two other forms of treatment are valuable parts of an
overall therapeutic regimen, but they cannot be considered in detail within the scope of this book:

1. *Exercise, Manipulation, and Activity:* Active and passive movement therapy includes general gym-
nastics, physiotherapy, chiropractic adjustment,
massage, walking, sports, baths, and running. Its
purpose is to provide motion the body needs to
increase and maintain health and vigor.

2. *Mental Attitude, Mental Hygiene:* Development of a
positive attitude to establish a generally natural
order of life. Aimed at high-level wellness and
efficiency, taking into consideration psychoso-
matic, ecological, sociological, and environmental relationships.

These are integral parts of a healthful life-style and can
play an important part in the treatment of illness.

True healing, then, is restoration of the internal and
external harmony or balance of the living being through
the use of materials and methods that are compatible with
the nature and function of the being. What are these
materials and methods? They are substances, energies,
forces, and activities associated with humanity's physical,
mental, and spiritual ties to our external environment.

It is because the balance of this relationship has changed per-
ilously in the last hundred years that this book is necessary.

INTRODUCTION

by Michael Tierra

The public has always been interested in books on self-healing. The reasons are the same today as always: distrust of the prevailing medical system and the need for safe, alternative natural treatments for disease, the high cost of contemporary health care, and the unavailability of qualified health practitioners in certain remote areas.

Despite the obvious contributions of Western medical science, mostly in terms of first line emergency care, it has proven to be limited in the treatment of degenerative conditions such as cancer, arthritis, viral diseases, heart conditions, and neurological, metabolic, and dermatologic diseases. This is because of its failure to emphasize the value of prevention over cure. Preventive care, too often overlooked, is an essential aspect of healing and includes such factors as diet, environment, exercise, emotional and other life-style factors as well as individual constitutional differences that predispose one to certain diseases.

Thus there are increasing numbers of people who feel that what Western medicine has to offer is simply not enough. Because of the well-known risks of certain therapies and drugs, what was once held up as the hope to end all disease and suffering has, with the increase of iatrogenic diseases (those caused by doctors), become a major contributor instead.

With the pollution of our air, water, and food supplies, one thing is certain—the health food industry has an assured place in the future of all our lives. Many have already found that health is no longer something that can be taken for granted, nor can we depend upon the dominant medical establishment, with the increasing cost of health care, to consistently have our best interests at heart.

Thus, in our time, increasing numbers of people are seeking help for their ills outside the established medical profession. Despite the attempts to undermine the rise of alternative medical systems, each year there is a significant increase in numbers of patients who are willing to go to great lengths to seek the help of acupuncturists, chiropractors, naturopaths, herbalists, homeopaths, therapeutic massage practitioners, and other practitioners of alternative health systems. Further, the sales of health products continue to increase. Herbs and herbal products are increasing at a growth rate of approximately thirty to fifty percent each year.

The world today is in great need of healing and dedicated healers of all types. Even the World Health Organization (WHO), based in Geneva, Switzerland, found it necessary to acknowledge and endorse traditional folk healers as part of their plan to deliver health care to all of the world's population by the year 2000. This means that it is not only possible but also desirable for Western scientific medicine and folk medicine to work together to provide the best health care for all.

This book is an extension of both the work of John Lust and my own previous efforts begun in *The Way of Herbs* and *Planetary Herbology.* It is our humble offering in a distinguished line of self-healing dating back to the *Complete Herbal* by the seventeenth-century herbalist Nicolas Culpepper.

When confronted with the task of completing a work by such a respected author as the late John Lust, I was faced with possible conflicts between his purely naturopathic and my own somewhat eclectic approach, an approach based on the principles of Traditional Chinese and Ayurvedic medicines. These differences are most evident in John's espousal of raw vegetables and juices and my own approach, which is more in accord with the traditional nutrition of cultures that emphasize the use of cooked foods.

This should pose an interesting diversion especially for those who are familiar with issues surrounding the controversy of the two approaches. Fortunately, throughout this book such differences are few, and when they occur I offer my view alongside John's. Since I have seen the appropriateness of espousing both approaches, I offer my perspectives on the relative value of these methods in the chapter on Diet and Nutrition. Thus the reader will have the opportunity to observe the value of each way according to individual circumstances and conditions.

Once a disciple in search of some absolute vision of truth visited his master and exclaimed, "How can it be that when I use one cure, a portion of the patients are cured and a portion are not, and if I reverse the method there is still a portion who are cured and a portion who are not?" The master gave an understanding smile and simply replied, "Maybe it is in the change!"

It is seldom easy to determine what is or is not good for a patient. No matter how deeply one studies or how well one is trained, there will always be questions. Books like this are intended to engage and empower the patient in the process of his or her own healing.

This returns us to the central issue: healing as a question of balance. While we all have a tendency to fall back into an unconscious mode of behavior, including how we live, what we eat, and so forth, a higher power persists in demanding from us greater conscious awareness of ourselves and the laws of the universe in which we live.

It seems that nature is determined to trick us into evolving awareness. One may notice, for instance, that for nearly every beneficial wild plant there is another unpalatable or poisonous herb growing somewhere nearby that vaguely resembles it. In such ways, mother nature herself favors the evolution of awareness and higher consciousness in her human children.

Similarly, one of the many dangers of living in the jungle of modern civilization is to assume the safety and validity of a pesticide, drug, or medical procedure merely because it is offered in the name of science. Such a naive attitude will always make us vulnerable to error, whether it is slanted toward that which comes from a health food store or that which comes from a drug store.

Thus, this book in itself cannot save us from the necessity of awareness and good judgment. History has proven that it is unwise to completely abandon our personal responsibility for our health to a privileged class of physicians and professionals who stand to profit from our disease. The purpose here is to provide some of the options and tools which might be useful for those who, for whatever reasons, have the inclination and desire to utilize more natural healing alternatives.

PART ONE

THE BASICS

OF NATURAL

HEALING

NATURE AND NEO-NATURE

A Partnership for Life

> The quality of life depends above all on our rela-
> tionships to the rest of Creation—the earth, the
> plants, the animals, and our fellow men.
>
> RENE DUBOS

Through most of human history, the dominant external
reality was primal nature. Unpredictable and uncontrol-
lable, nature held many dangers but also provided food,
shelter, clothing, and medicine. There was no question that
people were intimately connected with their physical environment. A few hundred years ago, that connection
began to weaken rapidly as science and then technology
made people less and less directly dependent on their natural environment, substituting instead dependence on
man-made products and other people's services. But in re-
treating from primal nature, particularly in the last hundred years, we have created for ourselves a new artificial
environment to take nature's place. The resulting blend of
primal nature and human artifacts is what we might call
neo-nature—it is the environment in which we exist
today.

Although primal nature still regularly reminds us—

through volcanic eruptions, earthquakes, hurricanes, and even rained out picnics—that it is the ultimate controlling physical force in our lives, the reality of daily living is dominated by the man-made aspects of neo-nature. This has brought us many benefits, but we also pay a price:

- We are relatively safe from wild animals, but we live under the threat of nuclear disasters.
- We travel far and freely and produce abundantly, but we pollute our environment and deplete our natural resources.
- We eat well and live in comfort, but acquired deficiencies threaten our natural immunity to disease and we suffer epidemic levels of cardiovascular diseases and cancer.
- We perform spectacular medical feats, but we rely more and more on highly specialized skills, sophisticated equipment, and esoteric treatments provided at astronomical cost.

The neo-nature we have created has caused us to retreat too far from primal nature and we have forgotten that human beings were created in nature and must remain in a harmonious relationship with it. This doesn't mean that we all should "go primitive"; it means merely that we must avoid the excesses of our technological enthusiasm and respect the fundamental natural laws to which all of Earth, and we as Earthlings, are subject.

How does all this relate to medicine and healing? The recent history of medicine has been one of retreat from nature as well. For countless centuries, medical remedies were based on plant, animal, and a few mineral substances. Their uses were based on experience, on physiological theories of the time, and in some cases on superstition (such as a superficial resemblance between part of a plant and a bodily part or organ). The results were undoubtedly as diverse as the patients and practitioners themselves, but for our purposes these results are not directly relevant. What is relevant is the general belief during much of this time that whatever effects the substances had were due to "active principles" in their nature. Here is where the science of chemistry enters the picture.

THE SCIENCE OF CHEMISTRY: FUEL FOR OUR FLIGHT FROM NATURE

The discoveries of modern chemistry have affected medicine in three ways:

1. By analyzing substances into their chemical constituents, chemistry focused attention on identifying and extracting the "active principles" in medicine.
2. By creating synthetic versions of natural compounds, it promised a ready source of supply for man-made new "active principles."
3. By creating new chemical substances, it opened new possibilities for medicines and treatments.

A pivotal point in the history of chemistry was the first synthesis of an organic substance—urea—from inorganic materials by Friedrich Woehler, in 1828. Although Woehler himself was concerned more with the chemistry of the process than with its philosophical significance, in retrospect his achievement had profound implications. It—and similar chemical discoveries after it—seemed to suggest that there was, after all, no fundamental distinction between animate and inanimate matter; that life was just a matter of chemistry. This mechanistic view of life gained strength throughout the nineteenth century and still dominates orthodox scientific thinking today.

Medicine, too, found the charms of chemistry irresistible and began its determined retreat from nature in earnest. If complex organic substances were made up of simple compounds, then it should be possible to isolate the "active principle" from a substance and make it into a drug. Even better, having identified the "active principle," one could make it synthetically from basic chemicals. Finally, one could make completely new chemical compounds with medicinal properties and bypass nature altogether.

Thus, the emphasis of medicine changed from supporting the body's power to heal itself—by restoring its internal balance and cleansing impurities from it—to an emphasis on using powerful drugs for aggressive attacks on specific disease-causing invaders or symptoms of illness. Unquestionably, this "allopathic" approach has had its spectacular successes; it has also had some equally spectacular failures. Also, to the extent to which the allopathic approach has come to dominate medical theory and practice in the twentieth century, particularly in the United States, it has institutionalized the view that the individual is helpless in the face of illness and must trust his or her body only to the skilled ministrations of a licensed, orthodox physician. In effect, a medical monopoly has been established. Only recently—and in the face of revolt by the masses—has the orthodox medical establishment "rediscovered" the body's own ability to fight disease and heal itself, as well as the importance of such factors as life-style, nutrition, manipulation, and mental and spiritual outlook for physical well-being.

Even during the rise of allopathic medicine, there were some practitioners—including medical doctors—who never lost sight of the truths that others are only now discovering. Such men as Father Sebastian Kneipp, his disciple and protégé Benedict Lust, M.D., Samuel Hahnemann, M.D., Adolf Just, Nicenz Priessnitz, Johann Schroth, Arnold Rikli, Louis Kuhne, and Henry Lindlahr, M.D., continued and improved the natural healing methods of the past, promoting the "naturopathic" approach as an alternative to allopathic medicine. Today their legacy is being carried on by thousands of doctors of naturopathic medicine, chiropractic physicians, doctors of botanical medicine, nutritionists, physical therapists, and other medical practitioners who are responding to a growing demand for "alternative medicine."

Unfortunately, through most of this century the naturopathic and allopathic approaches have been considered incompatible rivals and their proponents have been generally antagonistic to each other. This may have been inevitable, since significant changes in human affairs rarely occur smoothly; rather, we tend to swing between extremes like a pendulum. But the recent grassroots revival of naturopathy, the art and science of holistic medicine, suggests that it is time to recognize that no one has a monopoly on truth, knowledge, or wisdom. The two sides have much to learn from each other about illness and health. Naturopathic medicine offers its emphasis on a wholesome life-style, with the body/mind/spirit itself as the primary healer of illness and outside medical intervention playing a supporting role. The allopathic system brings its specialized knowledge of the mechanisms of disease and of bodily processes, knowledge that can be objectively applied to understand, assess, and improve the effectiveness of many types of medical procedure. In recognition of the strengths and limitations of each type of medicine and combining the best of the old with the best of the new, a truly eclectic medical system could evolve—to the benefit of everyone.

The natural remedies described in this book represent much of the experience and wisdom accumulated during centuries of naturopathic medicine. As such, they are valuable and useful in themselves. At the same time they are part of the raw material on which to base an eclectic approach to medicine. This book, therefore, is offered in a cooperative rather than a competitive spirit—as a contribution to restoring balance and harmonious functioning to the great body, mind, and spirit of medicine itself.

Like children with new toys, we have used science and technology exuberantly to reshape the environment in which we live. The creation of neo-nature, however, is not a game in which we can change the rules at will; in medicine, as in other aspects of modern civilization, the laws of primal nature cannot be written off as "outmoded." Although it will not be easy to overcome established habits, divisive prejudices, and vested interests, the stakes are too high to justify anything other than mature, open-minded cooperation by all factions toward the common goal of human well-being.

HEALING OURSELVES

You as an individual can do more for your health than anyone else—including your doctor. Consider that 85 percent of our illnesses are self-correcting and run their natural course. And with proper life-styles, for example, perhaps half of us could increase our life span by as much as thirty years.

There's a new attitude in our country with respect to health. We're searching for a better way to take care of ourselves—a way in which we can be in partnership with physicians, seeing them more as teachers than as those we pay to "make us well."

Perhaps by considering the best medical knowledge from both the past and the present, we can gain a new perspective on how important a role we personally play in our individual state of health and happiness.

This compendium of natural methods for treating the ailments listed in this part of the book contains much of the learned and folk wisdom of the past, often as verified or modified by modern discoveries. In the course of hundreds of years, natural healing and herbal medicine have accumulated a considerable burden of erroneous and half-true beliefs that make it easy for their critics to label even serious practitioners as quacks. But true natural medicine has nothing to fear from objective scientific analysis; indeed, modern research in natural healing and herbal medicine is progressing at a rapid pace, often encouraged by members of the scientific community who have had personal experiences with them.

The natural method of healing has been developing for more than two hundred years. It is a traditional, proven, and comprehensive system of medicine based on scientific principles applied to the body, mind, and spirit.

The description of ailments and their symptoms, causes, and natural methods of healing that follow are meant to serve as your guide. Trust your "inner doctor"— your intuition and your instinct; but remember that if there is any uncertainty whatsoever as to the seriousness of a condition, you should not delay in seeking the assistance of a competent physician.

I have also added references to Chinese acupuncture and moxibustion, and homeopathic practices, which are increasingly available throughout the Western countries of the world.

1

SELF-DIAGNOSIS

THE PULSE

The pulse is an expression of our fundamental life energy. To the Western medical doctor as well as those trained in Traditional Chinese, Ayurvedic, or Middle Eastern Tibb or Unani medicine, the pulse can be used as an indicator of the health of specific bodily organs and systems.

TAKING A PULSE

It is customary and convenient to take the pulse on the radial artery of the wrist located on the arm at the base of the thumb. To feel one's own pulse, reach one hand under the arm of the other and position the index finger in the slight hollow at the base of the thumb. Eventually one may want to compare the qualities of the pulse in three positions so that immediately next to the index finger and over the styloid process is where the middle finger will naturally fall and next to it the ring finger. In most people the position of the middle finger is where the pulse will be most apparent.

To take another's pulse, hold their hand as if in a friendly greeting. With the opposite hand, place your index finger in the hollow at the base of their thumb and place the remaining middle and ring fingers similarly, as before. Other areas for taking the pulse include the carotid artery on the side of the neck and on the inside of the ankle.

SPEED

The most obvious and easily determined quality is the number of pulse beats per minute. This is also an indication of overall metabolism: if fast, metabolism is too high, and it would be a sign of yang-heat; if slow, then it is low and would indicate yin-coldness.

To begin, feel the pulse and observe the second hand of a watch, counting the number of beats in fifteen seconds and multiplying this by four. Since the normal resting pulse is approximately 72 beats per minute, a slow pulse would be 60 or below while a fast pulse would be 80 or above.

A pulse less than 60 beats per minute generally indicates hypotension, possibly with accompanying weakness, anemia, low thyroid, a weakened immune system, and poor circulation. A pulse faster than 80 is a sign of hyper-metabolism indicating a tendency toward inflammatory conditions, fever, hyperacidity, anxiety, stress, and possible heart or lung problems.

Exceptions being the rule in nature, those who are more athletically inclined may have a normal slow or so-called athletic pulse. Further, one should consider whether the individual is exhibiting a reaction to recent excitement caused by vigorous exertion, which would naturally increase their normal speed.

DETECTING ALLERGIES WITH THE PULSE

Some have found that it is possible to detect allergic reactions by first establishing the normal mean pulse rate and then measuring it immediately after eating a particular food. If the pulse noticeably increases even a few beats per minute, it may indicate an allergic reaction to that food or substance.

While the rate of speed is a fairly certain pulse measurement, with experience, one may become aware of other more subtle qualities associated with the pulse.

DEPTH, LOCATION, AND OTHER QUALITIES

Feeling the pulse at different locations and depths may indicate specific conditions. If the pulse feels stronger closer to the surface, it is indicative of a more acute or external disease process. If it must be depressed noticeably deeper than usual, then the condition is considered chronic.

A strong pulse on the surface indicates an excess condition, and sweating or purgative therapies would be indicated. If it feels fast, then it is a condition of excess heat or fever. Both of these may be commonly encountered in colds and flus or acute skin problems. In general, a surface pulse indicates the body's outer resistance to disease.

A slow or weak surface pulse indicates coldness and deficiency and must be treated with warming stimulants such as ginger, cinnamon, or garlic taken as a warm tea with honey or barley malt syrup, added to taste.

A pulse that must be depressed deeper than the norm indicates an internal or chronic condition. A deep and fast or strong pulse would indicate internal heat and would point to the use of alternative such as echinacea, red clover or golden seal, and/or purgatives such as rhubarb root and cascara or triphala complex.

A deep, slow pulse indicates internal coldness; if it feels weak and "thready," then it could indicate anemia and low energy and would necessitate the use of blood, chi, or yang tonics. Herbs such as ginger, cinnamon, ginseng, dong quai, or astragalus might be useful.

Another quality commonly encountered when examining a pulse is a soggy or slippery pulse. This has a smooth, gliding quality and indicates fluid retention or phlegm and is treated with expectorants or diuretics. Some expectorants might be yerba santa, grindelia, or mullein, whereas diuretics would include parsley, buchu, uva ursi, and corn silk. A pregnant woman will naturally have a slippery pulse and one should consider this as normal.

One who is nervous and tense will exhibit a tense or bowstring pulse, which is described as feeling like the string of a guitar. A somewhat similar but slightly different quality is a tight pulse, which is a sign of severe pain.

SPECIFIC ORGAN DIAGNOSIS

This is the most subtle method of pulse diagnosis and requires still greater skill and experience. Still, one may notice that a pulse is unusually weaker or stronger in a particular position.

According to Traditional Chinese Medicine, the position of the index finger closest to the thumb indicates the condition of the organs of the upper part of the body, the heart and lungs. The position of the middle finger over the styloid process indicates the condition of the middle of the body including the stomach, spleen, and liver. The position of the ring finger in the hollow immediately above the middle finger, toward the elbow, indicates the condition of the organs of the lower parts of the body, especially the bladder, kidneys, and colon.

There are different depths which indicate different organ processes. The deep position at the base of the thumb of the left hand indicates the condition of the lung while the more surface position of the pulse indicates the colon. The deep position of the left hand, however, indicates the condition of the heart while the more surface position indicates the small intestine.

The middle-deep position of the right hand indicates the condition of the spleen-pancreas and is concerned with the assimilation of food. The middle-surface position indicates the condition of the stomach.

The middle-deep position of the left hand indicates the condition of the liver. The middle-surface position indicates the gall bladder.

The farthest-deep position of the left hand under the ring finger indicates the condition of the kidney-adrenals. The more surface position indicates the bladder.

The farthest-deep position of the right hand indicates the circulatory system while the surface position may indicate the lympatic system or heat regulating system of the body.

BLOOD PRESSURE

Blood pressure is a good indicator of the risk of stroke, heart disease, and kidney problems. It is also an indicator of the function of the adrenal glands. The adrenal glands are the regulators of the hormone system and are an important aspect of the immune system. They secrete the stress hormone, adrenaline, and thus influence blood pressure and indicate one's reaction to stress.

One's standing blood pressure should not be above 140 over 85. The second number indicates the diastolic pressure, which tells of the continual pressure being exerted upon the small blood vessels and arteries of the body. A diastolic pressure over 90 is considered a high-risk stroke or heart attack factor.

In each person there should be a difference in standing blood pressure as opposed to sitting. This difference measures the capacity of the adrenal glands to compensate for stress. There should be a rise of about 5 degrees when going from a sitting to a standing posture. Failure to show an elevation of blood pressure upon rising may indicate a condition of postural hypotension. There may also be associated symptoms of dizziness and adrenal depletion.

High blood pressure complicated by stress requires rest and adjustment of one's life attitudes and priorities. Herbs that are useful include European mistletoe (not American, which can raise blood pressure), hawthorn berries, scullcap, or wood betony. If there is associated internal heat or liver stagnation, then one should also use liver cleansing herbs such as Oregon grape root or dandelion root. Herbal diuretics can be added if there is a problem with mucus or fluid retention.

Chronically low blood pressure may be an indication of low metabolism, hypothyroidism, coldness, and tiredness. Such individuals require more stimulating herbs such as cayenne, ginger, and cinnamon as well as tonics such as Chinese ginseng. Diet should include more warming proteinaceous foods.

Garlic is able to regulate either high or low blood pressure. One or two cloves can be taken daily.

BODY WEIGHT

Body mass is also an indicator of health. There are many individual differences in body size and weight. What is normal for one may be abnormal for another. A lot of serious health problems arise either immediately or later in life if one overly interferes with one's natural weight. Being either over- or underweight can cause chronic health problems.

Indications for the need to lose weight are: feelings of heaviness of the stomach, breasts and buttocks; shortness of breath even with the slightest physical exertion; profuse perspiration even when it is not hot; excessive thirst, especially at night; excessive appetite; a tendency to sluggishness and unsatisfying sleep; strong body odors; general stiffness and achiness; rashes under the breasts, between the buttocks, under the arms; a general lack of enthusiasm for life.

THE HOLISTIC APPROACH TO WEIGHT LOSS

To lose weight, cultivate a discipline of diet and exercise. The general idea is to speed up the metabolism with exercise while following a wholesome, light, reducing diet. Herbal supplements can be very useful to help in the following ways: Herbs that provide low-calorie nutrition and alleviate appetite are: spirulina, wheat, and barley grass. Herbs that detoxify and remove internal organ stagnation: cleavers, chickweed, fennel seeds, senna, rhubarb, triphala complex. Herbs that aid nutrition and assimilation: fennel seeds, sprouted barley, sprouted rice.

Of course, one should reduce general caloric intake, especially avoiding dairy products, fats and oils. Also limit salt, which causes fluid retention, and strong spices that tend to stimulate the appetite.

Crash diets and amphetamine-type weight loss drugs throw the system off tremendously. They usually result in the eventual regaining of the weight that was lost, and because of the imbalance they cause, additional weight could be taken on.

It is important to realize that weight gain is not always a simple case of overeating. Quite often, it is indicative of a general organic and metabolic imbalance. Thus, using herbs such as cleavers, chickweed, and fennel during a weight loss program can do a lot to restore organic function.

HAIR

The hair is nourished and maintained by small capillaries on the scalp; thus, hair luster indicates the condition of the blood and circulatory system. Lusterless hair and chronic dandruff may indicate a lack of protein and B vitamins, weak digestion and poor assimilation of nutrients.

Hair loss can sometimes be effectively treated by the use of a Chinese dermal hammer. This is regularly used in acupuncture but is also commercially available to the general public. It consists of a small hammerlike instrument with tiny needles at one end. Lightly tap on the affected areas of the head with the dermal hammer until it appears slightly reddened. This indicates the presence of more blood and energy to the area. Doing this daily for a few minutes each day has stopped hair loss and stimulated new hair growth.

Of course, inherited tendencies for hair loss will be more difficult to remedy, but this approach is worth a try for at least three months.

One of the best herbs to use to offset premature graying is Ho Shou Wou *(Polygonum multiflorum)*, which counteracts anemia. An herbal wine called Shou Wou Chih can be obtained in most Chinese herb pharmacies. It is an alcoholic extract of Ho Shou Wou and other Chinese tonic herbs good for the blood and liver. One or two tablespoons could be taken daily to offset the effects of eyestrain. This is a very good daily tonic for those who work with computers for extended periods daily. A Western herb with somewhat similar properties is yellow dock *(Rumex crispus)*.

EYES

Dullness of the eyes indicates a general lack of energy. Redness of the whites of the eyes indicates a mild to severe inflammatory tendency. It can also indicate certain nutritional deficiencies such as a lack of vitamin C, zinc, the clotting vitamin K, vitamin E (which helps to maintain the capillary strength), or B-complex vitamins.

The iris of the eye has become the basis of an entire system of diagnosis called iridology. The effectiveness of iridology as a diagnostic tool is dependent upon the sensitivity and expertise of the practitioner.

Of specific value is the outer circle of the iris, which delineates the iris from the whites of the eyes, and the inner circle, which delineates the pupil. If the outer circle becomes whitish and undifferentiated, it denotes a general dulling of the body and senses and a deterioration of vision. The pupil should contract immediately under the influence of direct light. If after reflecting a flashlight the pupil remains dilated or expanded, it may indicate weakness of the brain, brain injury, or drug intoxication.

An eyewash of goldenseal and eyebright tea is very effective for clearing and strengthening the eyes. Triphala tea, which is made by steeping a teaspoon of triphala in a cup of boiling water and then straining the resultant fluid through a fine mesh cloth, is one of the best eyewashes and strengtheners of the eyes. To use any of these teas as an eyewash, purchase a small eyecup in a pharmacy. These eyewashes are also good for many other eye abnormalities, including glaucoma and cataracts.

TONGUE

The tongue, like the pulse, is also widely used by traditional practitioners as an indicator of the overall health of the body. The tissue of the tongue is a continuation of that of the stomach and digestive system, so the tongue is a reliable indication of the condition of the digestive organs. However, Oriental tongue diagnosis, like the pulse, can be used as an indication of the overall condition and health of the body as well as its specific organs.

A pale, flaccid tongue indicates weakness, anemia, and a tendency toward fluid retention. A deep red tongue indicates an inflammatory condition. A white-coated tongue represents an overly alkaline state with coldness, poor digestion, and internal congestion of the digestive system and/or the lungs. A yellow-coated tongue signifies an overly acid state, toxicity, inflammation, and congestion. A red-colored tongue, heavily fissured and smooth, lacking normal papillae or small whitish bumps, is a certain indication of B-complex deficiency.

A trembling tongue indicates general weakness of the nervous system. A stiff, rigid tongue indicates tenseness, while a tongue with tooth marks on the edge tells of fluid retention, possible low energy, and overlaxness.

LIPS, MOUTH, AND NOSE

Chronically chapped lips, especially accompanied by cracks and redness of the corners of the mouth or nose, indicates inflammation and excessive acidity in the digestive system. This may tend to destroy or impair our body's ability to absorb and utilize the B vitamin complex, because such an overly acid condition in the intestines tends to imbalance the favorable bacteria responsible for generating these B vitamins. When one encounters complaints of dry or cracked lips, it is a good idea to avoid sugar in all forms, including fruits.

GUMS AND TEETH

Red, inflamed gums indicate a deficiency of B vitamins, folic acid, vitamin C, calcium, magnesium, and phosphorus. They also point to an overly acidic condition of the digestive system and may be due to an overconsumption of refined carbohydrates such as white sugar. Since this is an indication of the integrity of the immune system as regulated by the adrenal glands, weakening, decayed teeth and chronic gum infections are often a later manifestation of earlier drug, tobacco, or alcohol abuse.

For bleeding gums, one can use the carbonized calyx of the eggplant, called "dentie" by the Japanese macrobiotics. Another alternative is an herbal toothpowder made from the following: equal parts powdered cinnamon bark, bayberry bark, oak bark, alum root and baking soda.

HALITOSIS

Strong-smelling, stale breath indicates poor digestion, acidity and general sluggishness of the passage of food through the stomach and intestines. Internally, the breath may be improved with an increase of dietary fiber and triphala, which will gradually help to cleanse the digestive tract, intestines, and blood. Triphala can be taken once each evening. One should avoid acid-producing foods such as fried foods, coffee, sugar, red meat, and alcohol. Externally, an herbal mouth rinse can be used with a combination of aromatic oils such as thyme, cinnamon, and cloves. A few drops of each should be stirred into a half cup of water.

DIGESTION

Digestive problems associated with bloating, pain and gas are a sign of imbalanced diet and can lead to more chronic digestive disorders such as bowel inflammation and colitis. Chronic problems can be a sign of poor food combinations and possibly a lack of favorable intestinal flora. For this, one might include some fermented foods such as a small amount of acidophilus, or salt-fermented German sauerkraut.

Allergy to dairy products can have a genetic or constitutional base, though it may simply be an indication of a diminished need for dairy, especially as one ages. Another reason for adverse reactions to food can be the combination of heavy grain and protein foods with fruits and fruit juice. For some, raw vegetables are a problem; lightly steaming them will aid assimilation and digestion.

In addition, the Ayurvedic herbal combination called

Hingashtak can be taken during or after meals and if used regularly will aid assimilation, eliminate and prevent gas. Triphala can be used each evening to cleanse the digestive tract.

FLUID RETENTION

The first sign of fluid retention is commonly seen as puffiness under the eyes or around the legs and ankles. This is often an indication of weakness of the adrenal glands and the kidneys. Being attached to the kidneys, the adrenal glands secrete a hormone that regulates the salinity of the blood. Thus excessive salt retention can be a sign of either weakness of the adrenals or excessive salt intake. Sudden fluid retention is another indication of allergic reaction, further pointing to adrenal deficiency.

A tendency to take on fluid weight, especially during middle to late years, may be caused by increased sedentary habits. This is best treated with regular exercise and use of occasional diuretic herbs, such as dandelion leaf or horsetail herb combined with fennel seed. Limiting one's salt intake is another positive step to take.

LUNGS AND BREATHING

Allergies or chronic rhinitis with or without a slight cough may indicate either a low-grade infection or depleted efficiency of the lungs and heart. Allergies generally are a sign of a weakened immune system.

To help clear the sinuses, take one teaspoon of powdered or fresh grated horseradish root with one tablespoon of apple cider vinegar. Chew it until the strong, pungent flavor is dissolved. Another remedy is to take six or seven furry buds of the magnolia tree with a little licorice root and steep them in a cup of boiling water until cool enough to drink. Spicy herbs such as powdered black pepper, ginger and anise seed mixed into a bolus with honey and taken one teaspoon at a time is also a good treatment for warming and drying the system and thus treating colds and allergies.

URINE

Light or colorless urine may indicate a hypometabolic condition, an overly alkaline system and perhaps the need for more protein. Generally vegetarians have a lighter colored urine than those who consume large amounts of meat on a daily basis. These people will have stronger-smelling, darker urine, indicating excessive uric acid. Blood in the urine is a sign of inflammation and could also be a sign of more serious problems warranting evaluation by a doctor.

For men it is common to have a weaker stream of urine in later years. This can be caused by an enlarged prostate gland and is often a natural sign of aging. If there is associated pain during urination or ejaculation, then one would consider a prostate inflammation as likely. Try treating this with formula number 4 or a tea of uva ursi, damiana leaf, saw palmetto berries and echinacea root.

Normal urination, depending upon what is eaten and how much is drunk, takes place four to six times daily. More often is considered frequent and may be a sign of energy deficiency; this can be treated with tonics such as formula number 29. Less than four may be a sign of congestion and stagnation suggesting a yang, overly stimulated, hypermetabolic condition. Try treating this with formula number 2.

Painful urination and cloudiness can be indications of stones or urinary tract infection. This is treated with formula number 3 or a tea of gravel root, parsley, uva ursi and marshmallow root. One should consider eliminating overly acid-forming foods such as sugar, meat, coffee, and alcohol. To relieve kidney stone pain, use a hot ginger fomentation over the middle to lower back. The herbal formula mentioned above should be sipped frequently, at least a cup every one to two hours during an acute attack and three or four times daily over a period of some time necessary to dissolve and eliminate the stones.

STOOLS

Normal stools tend to float and are usually neither too loose nor too hard. This is an indication of a good diet with sufficient fiber. Loose stools may be an indication of weak digestion and poor assimilation. A light or chalky colored stool means a blockage of bile and may be caused by gallstones or high blood cholesterol (often associated with gallstones) or hepatitis.

Triphala is one of the safest and best mild laxatives and is non-habit-forming so that it can be used on a daily basis as needed. A dose of triphala can be taken each evening when treating many acute or chronic disorders. Triphala is also a good liver and blood cleanser and can be used with psyllium seed husks as a bulk-forming, demulcent laxative, if needed.

Loose stools or diarrhea is treated with ginger and cinnamon tea along with half to one teaspoonful of nutmeg powder. Cranesbill root and blackberry root bark taken as a tea or powder are also good for diarrhea. Brown rice is the best diet for the condition; a little boiled milk may be added, as well as a teaspoon of cinnamon and a pinch of nutmeg.

SKIN

Dry skin, eczema, dermatitis, and other skin affections may indicate a need for vitamin A, zinc and B₆ as well as essential fatty acids. Evening primrose or borage seed oil is very useful for such skin problems.

For acne and skin blemishes, including psoriasis, one would use an herbal blood purifying formula such as a combination of equal parts dandelion root, yellow dock root, burdock root and seed, sassafras bark, red clover blossoms, Oregon grape root and one-eighth-part rhubarb root. Again, triphala taken each evening is very useful for this condition.

For psoriasis, eczema and dry skin, one can use chickweed oil made by macerating fresh or dried chickweed in olive oil for a few days and then press-straining through a muslin cloth. This can be applied topically as often as needed.

2

HERBS AND HEALING

There are many ways to prepare and use herbs. To choose the appropriate herb or formula combination is the first step; next is to select the most effective method to administer it.

Herbs are classified as mild, strong, and toxic. In most cases, foodlike mild herbs are more than adequate. Herbs that are classified as strong or toxic are seldom used, even by experienced herbalists.

The special healing properties of herbs are dependent upon their unique chemistry, which is communicated through their flavors, textures, and other qualities. Because of this, they are able to effectively stimulate organic healing processes. Being generally recognized and treated as food by the body, herbs can also be a significant source of important nutrients from which the body is able to repair and heal itself.

One can use either fresh or dried herbs, and quality is a definite consideration. This is influenced by many factors, including where and how an herb is grown, when it is harvested, methods of drying and preparing for use.

An herb that has a fresh appearance, bright color, and distinctive smell is probably of good quality. Assuming they are grown, harvested, and prepared properly, dried herbs will nevertheless lose some of their potency within six months to a year, powdered herbs even sooner. Those that are the least stable are the aromatics. These comprise the majority of known spices along with such well-known herbs as the mints, yarrow, angelica, and generally herbs whose distinctive odor and properties depend upon their volatile oils.*

As stated, most dried herbs, if stored away from moisture, heat, and direct sunlight, are good for at least a year, but special herbal preparations, such as alcoholic tinctures and extracts, can retain potency for up to three to seven years or more in many instances. Syrups, if properly made and stored, keep for a couple of years; tablets, pills, and capsules, because they are in a condensed form, last for two to three years.

Many people do not realize that common weeds or plants found in their place and season are usually superior or at least equal to those that are purchased dried. It does not take much to identify and recognize the healing benefits of common wayside or garden weeds that we invest so much energy in trying to control. It is as if they are crying out for us to use them: dandelion or plantain leaf tea for urinary tract infections; dandelion or chicory root for liver problems; malva leaves for ulcers and fevers; chickweed for fat reduction and skin problems; chamomile for digestive and nervous disorders; yarrow for painful men-

---

*Nevertheless, when nothing else was available, I have seen even dried, lackluster herbs retain enough potency to generate a healing response.

struation. The list of common weeds and medicinal herbs that have faithfully dogged the steps of humankind could go on and on.

Many find it a peaceful, meditative experience to learn to cultivate herbs in the garden or to harvest them in secret places away from harmful pollutants; then there is also the gratification of knowing how to use them for ourselves and others to help speed recovery from occasional ills.

Herbs have many gentle lessons to share about our relationship to life and the nature that is within and without. We achieve inner harmony when we learn to recognize and humbly respect the offerings and gifts of each season. Is it no wonder that to many, just being near herbs can be healing?

How much love and practical healing are transmitted through a cup of herb tea! Down through time, people have used herbal teas as a message of love and caring. Thus herbs are effective not only because of their chemical contents but also in the very ritual of their preparation.

If we want to pick herbs for future use, we can tie them in small bundles and prettily hang them in the house upside down in order to dry them. This should be done in an area that is well ventilated and away from direct sunlight. After a period they will be dry enough so that we can strip the leaves from the stems, store the flower buds (which can be laid out on a screen to dry), chop and break the roots or retain whatever parts may be needed in the future. Our homegrown, dried herbs are then stored in an airtight jar and sequestered in a special place in the cupboard.

The quality of herbs depends upon how and when they are picked. Because our attitude and inner state of being can certainly have an effect on the quality of the herbs we pick, Native Americans and many other traditional people throughout the world offer a prayer or some symbolic offering in order to establish an inner connection with the plant they intend to harvest for medicine.

When an herb is picked makes a big difference. At different seasons the active principles of herbs are concentrated in different parts of the plant. Thus, roots and barks are generally gathered in the late autumn, winter, or early spring. Leaves are picked just before the plant flowers in the late spring; flowers, fruits, and seeds at the peak of their respective seasons.

While gathering we give due respect for the continued growth and survival of the tree or plant. If we are harvesting barks we must decide whether it is better to cut down an entire tree for its bark (perhaps to thin out a specific area of dense growth) or take only a part from its trunk or limbs. Whatever we do in that regard, we should bear in mind that to strip the entire circumference will definitely kill the tree.

For some plants, such as comfrey and others, leaving a piece of the root will promote the growth of another plant. If a plant has gone to seed, we can help its proliferation, in some cases, by sowing the seed in a wider area.

It is generally a good idea to harvest where the plant appears to be thriving, as that is where we will be able to find the strongest plants. Always be sure to leave enough so that the plant can easily recover its growth. The art of "wildcrafting," which is picking wild herbs, actually can be practiced in such a way as to aid the growth of wild plants by judicious thinning and pruning.

Most of the herbs we pick are best dried in a well-ventilated, semi-shaded environment. Leaves and flowers can be tied in small bundles and hung upside down either indoors or under a tree. Another method is to make a screen or curtain and lay the plants out so that they are not touching and can receive the benefit of maximum air circulation. The idea is to dry the herbs as quickly as possible, retaining as much of their color and fragrance as possible. Whatever we choose to do, we should avoid the unconscious tendency to pluck and plunder everything in sight.

MAKING HERB TEA

To make medicinal tea, add an ounce of dried herbs (which is approximately a handful) for each pint of water (which is two cups). Of course, an ounce of a light leaf or flowery herb has a much greater volume than an ounce of heavier roots or barks. Furthermore, fresh-picked herbs that contain more than 50 percent moisture as part of their content will require nearly half to double as much to attain the same degree of concentration.

There are two general methods for brewing herb teas. The first method is an infusion made by steeping the herbs in a covered container for ten to twenty minutes. This is best used when preparing aromatic herbs, whose oils (and flavor) are likely to boil away.

The second is a decoction method made by slowly simmering heavier roots and barks for thirty to forty-five minutes. This extracts the deeper minerals while sacrificing the more superficial volatile elements. It is used for heavier roots or barks.

An even stronger, more concentrated decoction (strong decoction) is used when we need a more concentrated preparation. Make this with twice the amount of water and slowly reduce the liquid to half. This method is the one recommended by practitioners of Traditional Chinese Medicine.

Herbs should be prepared in glass, enamel, or good-quality stainless steel containers. This is because the delicate chemistry of herbs can be altered when prepared in containers made of soluble metals such as aluminum, iron, or copper.

An average adult dose (see Dosage Guideline Table, below) consists of two or three cups of the tea daily. If the problem is severe, it may be better to take a half dosage every two hours in order to keep the herb in constant availability in the blood. These are average dose recommendations and should be adjusted according to weight, height, and sensitivity.

DOSAGE GUIDELINE TABLE

Age	Fraction
1 year and younger	1/10 to 1/8 normal adult dose
2 to 6 years of age	1/10 to 1/8 normal adult dose
7 to 12 years of age	1/3 to 1/2 normal adult dose
13 to 15 years of age	1/2 to 2/3 normal adult dose
16 to 70 years of age	normal adult dose
over 70 years of age	1/2 normal adult dose

Acute conditions generally respond favorably within the first three days. As the acute symptoms diminish in severity, the dose can be gradually lessened, but to prevent reoccurrence, it should be maintained in reduced amounts for another week after all symptoms have vanished.

Chronic conditions associated with deficiencies require a smaller dose taken over a prolonged period. One should allow approximately a month for every year that the disease has been present. This is to give the body sufficient time for regeneration.

HERBAL SOUPS

Tonic herbs are best used with food in the form of soup or porridge. This is done by first preparing a decoction and then using the resultant liquid as a base or stock in which soup or rice is cooked.

A nutritive herb tonic generally has a foodlike, pleasant quality, with a hearty texture and an acrid, pungent, or most typically a sweet flavor. It is these qualities and flavors that are needed for regenerative herbal soups and porridge. Examples of herbs used as nutritive tonics include Chinese ginseng, astragalus membranicus, dong quai *(Angelica sinensis)*, lycii berries *(Lycium chinensis)*, garlic *(Allium sativa)*, iceland moss *(Cetraria islandica)*, ginger *(Zingiberrisoff)*, shiitake mushrooms *(Lentinus edodas)*, reishi mushrooms *(Ganoderma lucidum)*, longnan berries *(Longan arillus)*, and jujube dates *(Zizyphus jujube)*.

The amount of herbs used is in part dependent upon their flavor. One can use more of sweet herbs such as astragalus or jujube dates, for instance, than the bitter dong quai. Generally, about three to nine grains of a selected herb are used for a quart of soup or rice porridge.

Make astragalus herb soup with six to nine grams of astragalus root, four to eight ounces of beef boiled together in water, perhaps with the addition of a little onion, garlic, ginger and a pinch of sea salt and rice. This is good to strengthen vitality and energy and can be taken anywhere from daily to a few times a week. Chinese ginseng can be added to counteract weakness and fatigue.

For women, make dong quai soup by simmering three to six ounces of dong quai root with four to six slices of fresh ginger and two to four ounces of organic lamb or chicken. This is a good blood tonic and useful to help overcome many gynecological disorders including painful menstruation, irregular periods, and discomfort associated with female menopause.

Garlic soup is made by simmering three or four fresh cloves of chopped garlic in a quart of water along with some onions and brown rice. This is good for many diseases including colds, fevers, flus, and respiratory ailments. It is also good for many chronic circulatory problems such as atherosclerosis, arthritis, digestive weakness, and impotence.

Congee or rice porridge is made by cooking one part brown rice in seven to ten parts water or herbal decoction slowly over a period of six to twelve hours (a Crockpot or slow cooker is useful for this). Rice porridge, called congee by the Chinese, is a favorite breakfast and is the best food to serve for those who are weak or unable to assimilate other foods.

A similar herb gruel is made with the powder of slippery elm bark *(Ulmus fulva)*. This remarkable substance was first used by the Native Americans as a source of food. Its mucilaginous quality is very soothing to the throat and all mucous membranes.

To make slippery elm gruel, slowly mix a little warm honey water (or a tonic herb tea), to form the desired consistency. One can add a sprinkle of cinnamon and ginger. This will often stay down when all else fails. It is a very good herb food and remedy for infants and small children with symptoms of nausea and vomiting.

TINCTURES AND EXTRACTS

Herbal tinctures are made by macerating about four ounces of powdered herb in a pint of spirits (use good-quality vodka or brandy) in a widemouthed jar. Let this stand in a warm place for at least two weeks and then press-strain through muslin or linen cloth to extract the liquor.

These tinctures are very convenient for storage and use and have the feature of high bioavailability. The average dose is from five to thirty drops three or more times a day. For those who are alcohol sensitive, steep a single dose of tincture in a little boiling water for a few minutes to allow the alcohol to evaporate. Herb wines are similarly made, only using rice wine (sake), which has a lower alcohol content.

To make ginseng and deer antler liquor, macerate a whole root of good-quality ginseng and one ounce of deer antler in a quart of rice wine. This is taken in teaspoon doses once or twice a day through the winter months. It is good to increase energy and counteract coldness, weakness, fatigue, low libido, and poor memory. It is also good for older folks to use in cold weather to prevent sensitivity to cold and damp, which can aggravate rheumatic pains.

Extracts are made through a process of steam distillation where the water and alcohol is slowly distilled or evaporated with heat. While most tinctures are in a ratio of one part herb to five parts menstruum, extracts are more concentrated, as much as one to one. Adding greater amounts of herbs to strained tinctures is another way to increase the ratio of strength without the volatilizing influence of heat.

Dried extracts are made by concentrating a decoction under low heat until a thick paste is formed at the bottom of the pan. The concentrated extract can then be rolled into pills or spread out on a sheet and allowed to dry in the open air.

Extracts offer the advantage of requiring a much smaller dose and greater bioavailability. There is a danger, however, of losing some of the more balanced aspects of the whole herb and increasing the risks of overdose and side effects.

SYRUPS

Syrups are especially useful for upper respiratory, throat, and lung problems. A cough syrup is simply made by first making a strong decoction of violet leaf tea, for instance, and then adding equal parts honey. This can be taken in spoonful doses for coughs but must be kept refrigerated to prevent spoiling.

A basic syrup is made by slowly cooking one cup of sugar in one cup herbal decoction until it thickens into a syrupy consistency. A syrup having a minimum concentration of 65 percent sugar will keep indefinitely.

A syrup made with vegetable glycerin will also remain stable and not spoil. This is similarly made by adding an equal amount of vegetable glycerin to the finished strong decoction. This is sometimes called a glycerin extract and has a sweet flavor that is quite appealing to children.

For coughs, colds, and minor throat irritations, simply squeeze the juice of a whole fresh lemon into a half cup of honey. This can be freely taken in teaspoonful doses as often as desired.

Another home syrup remedy is made by blending several whole cloves of garlic with honey. This is similarly taken for colds, flus, fevers, and lung inflammations, as well as arthritic and rheumatic complaints. The disadvantage is the strong lingering odor of the garlic which is exuded from the breath afterwards.

HERBAL ELECTUARIES, SUPPOSITORIES, PILLS, AND TABLETS

Herbal electuaries are sweetened combinations of herbs made by blending powdered herbs with enough honey to form a thick paste. Since there is no additional water, this preparation will also last indefinitely. To take it, spoon out a required amount or roll it into a ball. This method is the best to use with children, substituting, if desired, maple syrup or nut butters for the honey.

One delicious East Indian Ayurvedic tonic uses amla fruits *(Emblic myrobalans)*, also known as Indian gooseberries. Being intensely sour, amlas are transformed into a rich sweet-sour-spicy tonic herbal food by cooking them into a thick paste together with small amounts of over forty rare herbs and spices and a base made with raw sugar, honey, and ghee (clarified butter).

The secret of amlas is in their high vitamin C content, which is uniquely bound up with certain harmless food tannins that cause them to retain their high vitamin C content even after exposure to heat and aging.

This revered ancient tonic made from amlas is known as Chyavanprash (Royal Tonic of India) and has a history that goes back some three thousand years, to Vedic times. Legend states that the preparation was given to Lord Chyavan by the gods to rejuvenate his amorous capacity in order to satisfy the desires of a young princess given to him in wedlock. For centuries the Indian people have prepared and used Chyavanprash, not only in times of disease and sickness but also prophylactically, to maintain vitality and well-being, much as the Chinese have used ginseng.

Trikatu is another traditional Ayurvedic electuary commonly made and used by people living near water. It is spicy, hot, and dry in nature and is useful for people with symptoms of coldness with clear fluid discharges.

Trikatu is made by combining equal parts powdered ginger and black pepper and two parts anise seed with enough honey to make a thick pill mass. Other warming and spicy herbs that could be used include cinnamon, cloves, or cardamom.

Trikatu is taken in quarter to half teaspoonful doses two or three times daily for colds, allergies, to dry clear mucus discharges, for coldness and poor circulation as well as weak digestion. It is a very good tonic to use prophylactically through the cold, damp seasons and to prevent and cure diseases usually caused by cold and damp.

Suppositories are made by adding finely powdered herbs to melted cocoa butter. The result is a thick bolus that can be rolled into individual one-inch portions. To create a thicker consistency, dissolve a little beeswax in the melted cocoa butter. Spoon out a little and quickly cool to evaluate the final consistency. More beeswax or cocoa butter can be added to adjust the thickness. While still warm, individually form and wrap the suppositories in tinfoil and store in a cool place.

A suppository to help relieve and shrink hemorrhoids is made with a combination of finely powdered oak bark *(Quercus species)* (and/or witch hazel bark), cranesbill root *(Geranium maculatum)* and yarrow blossoms *(Achillea milli-*

folium). Unwrap and insert a suppository into the rectum once or twice daily.

For vaginal discharge, powdered goldenseal, echinacea, and chaparral can be used. This should be followed with an herbal douche in the morning made with yellow dock root tea.

Vaginal and Rectal Bolus Formula

While complicated, this treatment is useful for a wide variety of chronic and acute genitourinary and intestinal disorders, including cervical dysplasias, tumors, cysts, leukorrhea, trichomoniasis, prolapsed uterus, venereal warts, intestinal problems, hemorrhoids, and various types of local infections. It can also be inserted in the anus for the treatment of swollen prostate and hemorrhoids. The bolus will draw toxins from throughout the pelvic cavity, including the reproductive organs, bowel, and urinary organs.

Use equal parts of the following finely powdered herbs:

squaw vine *(Mitchella repens)*
slippery elm bark *(Ulmus fulva)*
yellow dock root *(Rumex crispus)*
agrimony *(Agrimonia eupatoria)*
marshmallow root *(Althaea officinalis)*
chaparral *(Larrea mexicana)*
goldenseal *(Hydrastis canadensis)*
plantain leaves *(Plantago officinalis)*

HOW TO MAKE THE BOLUS: Be sure the herbs are finely powdered and sifted. Next, procure a good amount of cocoa (or coconut) butter. Melt the cocoa butter in a double boiler or pan under low heat so that it will mix with the powdered herbs. Mix enough of the powdered herb formula with the melted cocoa butter to form a pie-dough consistency. Next, roll it between the hands until it becomes approximately the thickness of one's middle finger, in one-inch-long pieces. Place them in a dish or roll them in tinfoil and put them in the refrigerator to harden.

APPLICATION: Place three of the one-inch-long segments in the vagina before retiring and leave in all night. This is done six days a week. One may need to apply a cloth or pad in the event that when it dissolves it leaks out during the night.

In the morning, wash or douche with a tea made from the following herbs:

6 parts oak bark *(Quercus alba)*
4 parts yellow dock, *(Rumex crispus)*
3 parts plantain *(Plantago species)*
3 parts walnut bark or leaves *(Juglans nigra)*
6 parts comfrey root *(Symphytum officinalis)*
3 parts marshmallow root *(Althea officinalis)*
1 part lobelia *(Lobelia inflata)*

This is used to restore health and tone to the uterus, bowel, or other organs in the pelvic cavity. It can be used for treatment of a prolapsed uterus or hemorrhoids. Simmer two ounces of the combined herbs in four cups of water slowly, until they are reduced to two cups. Strain and allow to cool. Using a bulb syringe available from most pharmacies, lubricate the tip with a little olive oil or another type of oil. Arrange a slant board where you can lie head downward. Inject a cup of the solution into the vagina or rectum and retain it for at least twenty minutes. Apply castor oil over the abdomen and massage the area, gently working on any tender or painful areas to allow for the tea to be absorbed. This program should be followed for two weeks. If there is improvement, continue until all symptoms have abated.

Castor Oil Fomentation

This is useful for the relief of pain, inflammation, and liver detoxification, and to soften and dissolve cysts, warts, bunions, and corns.

Purchase a quart of castor oil from the natural food store or pharmacy (it may need to be ordered specially). Moisten a flannel cloth and apply over the affected area. Then apply a heating pad and leave for approximately thirty minutes.

While one can quickly make pills with honey, another method, good for making throat lozenges as well as pills, is to combine the herbs with a mucilaginous binder such as slippery elm. Slowly add water to make a thick doughy consistency. This can then be rolled or cut into pill size and dried in an open oven or well-ventilated area.

Gelatin capsules provide an efficient method of taking herbs over a long period. Various sizes are available from most health food stores but the size most commonly used is 00 size. Place a mound of herbal powder on a small saucer and then fill the larger part of the capsule by tamping it down; rejoin with its smaller half.

POULTICES, PLASTERS, AND FOMENTATIONS

Many external remedies depend upon their use as counter-irritants. The idea is to create a minor surface irritation in order to draw the congested blood and fluids to the surface and relieve congestion.

While the external application of warm herbal poultices, plasters, or fomentations is commonly used as a counter-irritant to relieve underlying pain and congestion, others having a cooler, anti-inflammatory action are used for the treatment of more inflamed injuries and inflammations, and to promote the healing of burns, tissue, and broken bones.

A healing and cooling poultice of steamed comfrey-plaintain is made by steaming dried or fresh herbs and adding a dash of cayenne pepper before wrapping them in a thin muslin or cheesecloth and finally applying and bandaging the poultice directly to the affected area as hot as possible. This is used to relieve pain and inflammation, to draw out slivers and foreign objects embedded in the flesh, and to promote healing of injuries and fractures. Other cooling poultices include:

- Violet *(Viola tricolor)* or chickweed *(Stellaria media)* poultice for the relief of fever, pain and inflammation.
- Plantain *(Plantago off.)* poultice for venomous bites and stings.
- Grated taro potato poultice for dissolving and drawing out tumors, cysts, and cancers—especially from the breast.
- Grated potato poultice for relieving inflamed and arthritic joints.
- A paste of buckwheat flour and water applied over a swollen joint for drawing out excess fluid from the tissues.
- Grated raw cabbage poultice has a warm energy and is applied to the lower abdomen for promoting

pelvic circulation and dissolving small fibroids and cysts in the pelvic cavity.

For maximum benefit, poultices must be renewed at least twice a day.

A good counterirritant is made by first spreading a thin layer of honey on a gauze or bandage upon which powdered cayenne pepper is generously sprinkled. This is then applied to bruises, injuries, stiff joints, and painful areas of the body to relieve pain and promote circulation. Cayenne or other heating plasters are often available in certain herb and health food stores.

A mustard plaster is made by using powdered mustard seed to which the combination of a small amount of flour and water is added to hold it together. It has similar use as a counterirritant to that of the previously described cayenne plaster.

A fomentation is made by directly applying a cloth wrung out in the hot tea. A ginger fomentation is made with grated fresh ginger root steeped in a basin of hot water until it develops a yellow color. A cloth towel is then dipped into the ginger tea and applied directly over painful sprains, joints, lower back problems, bursitis, and other painful afflictions. As the towel cools, it is repeatedly dipped and reapplied several more times. In between each hot application, the area can be washed with cool water. The application of hot alternating with cold (not ice) causes the tissues to rapidly expand and contract, further stimulating the circulation of blood.

Dr. Christopher's Bone, Flesh, and Cartilage Formula

The following formula is very effective for promoting the healing of bone and open wounds, clearing bone spurs, hernias, severe arthritic pains, congested sinuses, etc.

Make a strong tea of the following:

6 parts oak bark
6 parts comfrey root
3 parts each of marshmallow root, mullein herb,
    walnut bark (or leaves), gravel root
2 parts mugwort or wormwood
1 part each of lobelia and skullcap herb
1 pint glycerin

This can be a long-term treatment, so you should procure the above herbs in bulk quantities. Mix them together in the approximate proportions above.

Soak eight handfuls of the dry herbs in a gallon of distilled water for four to six hours, then simmer them for thirty minutes. Strain and continue simmering the resultant tea down to a half gallon, then add glycerin.

Keep refrigerated.

Next, soak a flannel, cotton, or any other white natural fiber cloth in the solution. Wrap the soaked cloth around the affected area, cover with plastic wrap or comparable product, and fasten with tape. Apply each night for six nights a week until relief occurs, and a week or two longer to be sure the problem has been completely repaired.

Another fomentation made with equal parts comfrey root *(Symphytum off.)*, oak bark, horsetail *(Equisetum species)*, prickly ash bark *(Xanthoxylum americanum)* and a half part each of ginger and cayenne can be used to treat bursitis, back pains, sprains, and painful arthritic and rheumatic problems.

Since these are intended to promote healing over a prolonged period, they are applied and left on each night, covered with plastic to prevent the bed from getting wet.

HERBAL BATHS

Herbal baths are made by straining a pot of herbal tea into the bathwater. One of the best ways to treat infants and small children with fever is with a bath prepared as described using a tea of willow or white poplar bark. For skin problems such as eczema and psoriasis, a chickweed or oatmeal bath is used. (See Part Three.)

HERBAL OILS AND SALVES

Herbal oils can be used both internally and externally. Make ginger sesame seed oil by grating ginger root and squeezing the resultant juice into sesame oil. This can be topically applied to relieve bruises, sprains, injuries, and even burns. A similar oil is made with fresh garlic and olive oil, of which one or two drops can be administered into the ear at night with a wad of cotton.

Chickweed oil is made by macerating fresh chickweed in olive oil and allowing it to stand in a warm place for three to four days. This is then press-strained and bottled for use. It is applied externally to relieve itching, eczema, psoriasis, and other irritating skin ailments.

A salve of chickweed, comfrey, and plantain is made by first making an herbal oil. Begin by simmering one ounce of the combined herbs in a pint of water for twenty minutes. Strain and continue reducing the tea down to a quarter of the volume. Add five ounces of olive oil and continue to simmer until all the water is evaporated. To this add a quarter teaspoon of tincture of benzoin (available at most drug stores) or a half teaspoon of vitamin E as a natural preservative and then dissolve two ounces of beeswax and pour into small ointment or salve jars.

HEALING CRISES

A healing crisis arises as the body slowly regains the strength to retrace past suppressed symptoms in order to eliminate stored toxins. If this occurs, and it need not, it can be recognized by three considerations: first, the pattern of symptoms will be from the most recent to the most distant; second, the symptoms are usually of short duration, ranging from a few hours to days, and are not very severe; third, despite the symptoms, the individual can notice that there is some improvement in one or a number of peripheral symptoms.

A healing crisis, if not too serious, should be interpreted as a positive sign of recovery and healing. Nevertheless, if severe, the taking of any herbs that might be precipitating these symptoms should be suspended for a while or at least diminished until the body is restored to a quieter state. This can be said for the use of any herbs, foods, or drink that could be causing a severe reaction.

HERBS AND PREGNANCY

A woman who is pregnant must be cautious in the use of certain herbs. Sensitivity depends on the individual but herbs that are strong blood movers, including those classified as emmenagogues and many that are warming stimulants and carminatives, should be limited or avoided. Also herbs that have a strong downward energy such as laxatives should not be used unless it is well considered or evaluated by one who is more experienced in such matters.

Examples of some herbs to avoid during pregnancy include: pennyroyal, angelica, rue, and lovage. Herbs to be limited or restricted include ginger, garlic, turmeric, and parsley. If in doubt consult an herb book or seek professional advice from an herbalist.

TRADITIONAL GUIDELINES FOR HERB TREATMENT

Diseases are classified as acute, chronic, excess, deficient, hot, and cold.

A predominance of acute, excess, or heat symptoms is considered hypermetabolic or yang natured and requires cool, surface relieving, detoxifying, or eliminative therapies.

A predominance of chronic, internal, deficient, or cool symptoms is considered hypometabolic or yin natured and requires more internal, strengthening, and warming therapies.

Acute diseases are superficial and require surface relieving treatments such as sweating to resolve them. These include colds, flu, fever, and skin diseases which are also located on the surface of the body.

Chronic diseases are internal and require herbs that affect the internal organic processes. This could include tonics and builders as well as detoxifiers and purgatives.

Excess diseases are diseases that manifest with strong and often severe reactions. Thus there can be extremes of coldness or heat, loud, aggressive temperament, heaviness, strong appetite, strong odor, full pulse, and thick coated tongue. These require elimination therapy.

Deficient diseases arise out of weakness and manifest feebly with accompanying signs of emaciation, fear and shyness, pale urine, loose stool, lack of appetite, thin, small pulse, and a pale uncoated tongue.

Hot diseases are characterized by feelings of heat, fever,

inflammation, infectious viral or bacterial diseases, burning sensations, redness, thirst, constipation, dark urine,
thick yellowish or red-stained discharges, heavy menses,
fast pulse, a thick, yellow-coated tongue with a bright
cherry-red tongue-body.

Cold diseases are characterized by feelings of coldness
and chills, paleness, lack of thirst, clear urine and mucus
discharges, loose stool, slow pulse, a white-coated tongue
with a pale tongue-body.

Herbs that are strengthening and building have sweet,
acrid, or spicy flavors and are more warming yang-natured
tonics.

Herbs that relieve excess have bitter or sour tastes and
are detoxifying, antibiotic, alterative (blood purifying),
purgative, and diuretic.

Herbs that treat and relieve the surface are spicy-tasting
diaphoretics and stimulants which induce perspiration.

Herbs that treat internal conditions include all other
properties.

Herbs that are heating are spicy tasting and have circulating, stimulating, and warming energies. These include
herbal stimulants, warming tonics, carminatives that aid
digestion and emmenagogues that stimulate menses and
blood circulation.

Herbs that are cooling have bitter, sour, or salty flavors
and include alteratives (blood purifiers), purgatives, and
demulcents which are moistening and lubricating.

Most complex diseases manifest as a mixed conformation of hot and cold, excess and deficient, external and internal. Since this is the most common way diseases
manifest, one may need to achieve a harmonized balance
of combining heating and cooling, excess eliminating and
building, external and internal remedies, according to the

individual case. This can be quite complicated and beyond the scope of the lay practitioner. However, using the general remedies and approaches in this book together with a light, easily digestible, balanced diet is a good way to prevent and avoid errors of judgment.

A balanced diet which I recommend is based upon traditional diets from around the world that emphasize the use of cooked whole grains, cereal porridge, a small amount of legumes or beans as a protein complement, steamed vegetables, and the restriction of meat proteins, raw foods such as raw fruits and vegetables, and cold drinks.

I realize that this macrodiet is in opposition to that recommended in many sections by John Lust, but it must be understood that there are many approaches to healing. Each of these arises out of the needs of the individual, his or her life-style, and climate and environment.

Individuals with a hot, external, excess, hypermetabolic, yang condition will respond better to a more eliminative diet of more raw vegetables, fruits, and juices. The use of heavy, rich foods such as dairy, meat, and sugar is counterindicated.

At different periods people have gravitated toward and away from eating heavy proteinaceous foods. Many naturopaths, such as John Lust and others, were working and recommending treatments to individuals who were withdrawing from rich, heavy foods and thus tended to emphasize the use of raw fruits and vegetables and juice therapy.

Today we find that the pendulum is swinging and there are more and more people inclined toward a lighter, vegetarian diet. These will tend to get more yin diseases and require a warming diet, even to the point of recommending heavier and warming proteinaceous foods. In any case they should avoid raw foods, fruits and juices, and limit themselves primarily to cooked foods.

The balanced, macrobiotic type of diet is appropriate for both deficient and external conditions and conformations. So is the one I generally recommend for most of the diseases described in this book.

The best approach to overcome most diseases is to begin a program of eating only kicharee (see recipe on page 60) or to limit oneself to a diet of whole grains with a small amount of legumes for a period of three to ten days. This will do wonders in beginning to establish a newer, more wholesome way of eating that is ultimately the best approach to preventing disease.

3

DIET AND NUTRITION

The reason there is no one perfect food or diet is that what we need is determined by a variety of individual conditions and factors. Some of these include climate, geographical location, ancestry, physical and emotional state, work, and life-style. Thus, what we choose to eat becomes an expression of all aspects of our being.

While, for the most part, people are the same in their basic nutritional needs (protein, carbohydrates, minerals, vitamins, etc.), amounts for each may differ according to environmental as well as constitutional and hereditary factors. What may be a natural and appropriate food for an aboriginal living in a complete state of interdependence with his or her natural surroundings is quite different from the requirements of an American truck driver. Similarly, a pure vegetarian diet that works well for a Hindu or Buddhist monk living in a warm subtropical climate is adjusted by the Tibetan Buddhists to include yak meat because of the severe, cold climate of the Himalayas.

Food serves many functions and must feed all parts of our being; this includes both our physical and emotional selves. Unfulfilled emotional needs often translate into overindulging in sweets. This, for so many, is both a cause and a reflection of the deeper levels of disease.

From another perspective, consider how within our cellular genetic memory there lies the highest evolutionary hopes of all our forebears. From this, we can see one aspect for the underlying basis in many cultures of ancestor worship, which, on a practical level, may imply a profound biological urge to honor and nurture every part of our being. Certainly there are already a few dietary characteristics that have been identified as being racially specific, such as African Negroes' intolerance of cow's milk. It may well be that there are genetic predispositions in all of us that establish a need or intolerance for certain foods.

Natural healing with food and herbs takes one of three paths: to build, to maintain, and to eliminate. Maintaining is for those conditions for which there are no cures; elimination is for diseases associated with excess and toxicity; building is for diseases that arise from deficiency.

For John Lust and so many other natural health exponents living in industrialized Western countries, a diet of raw vegetables, fruits, and fresh squeezed juices, along with the elimination of animal protein and refined foods such as white sugar, seemed to work wonders in bringing about improvement or total cures of many acute and chronic diseases. The reason was that the majority of people in these countries regularly consumed a much higher intake of meat and dairy as well as an abundance of refined foods. Constitutionally, this would produce excess-type diseases with symptoms of aggressiveness, hypertension, and constipation caused by blood and lymphatic congestion. These diseases tend to respond very positively to a lighter, vegetarian diet.

Today, in the West, there has been a trend away from such a way of eating, with increasing numbers of individuals evolving their diet around the complete avoidance or limitation of all forms of animal protein. Some of this is due to the awareness of the dangers of saturated fats, which raise cholesterol levels and contribute to arteriosclerosis, but another significant aspect is the influence of ethical and moral ideas centered around the concept of nonviolence to animals.

Whatever the reason, individuals who have been practicing a more vegetarian style of eating for a number of years, if they develop a sickness, often do not respond well to such extreme eliminative yin diets of raw fruits, vegetables, and juices. In fact, just the opposite: They respond to a high-protein diet with cooked foods and the inclusion of some form of animal protein in the form of meat or dairy.

Thus there is an appropriateness for the use of a raw-food vegetarian diet for those with excess diseases as well as an appropriateness for a predominantly cooked macrobiotic type of diet emphasizing whole grains, cooked vegetables, and occasional organic animal protein for those living in colder climates and whose physical stress requires it. One must determine this according to each individual and their recent dietary history.

It is intriguing to realize how people of poorer, more underdeveloped countries, lacking the food abundance and variety of the United States and European countries, often had the opposite problem of no food or food of poor quality, lacking sufficient protein. Since the documented medical experience and knowledge of countries such as China and India, for instance, extends far back in antiquity, encompassing periods of both feast and famine as well as dramatic climatic and environmental changes, they were able to develop an appreciation for differential diagnosis and individual constitutional differences that might affect health.

The Chinese describe these differences in terms of the bipolar opposites called yin and yang, with deficiency diseases being yin and excess diseases being yang. Thus all foods and herbs that are eliminative or catabolic are classified as yin while those which have stronger building or anabolic properties are classified as yang.

Healing, according to Chinese medical theory, involves treating yin-cold-deficient type diseases with yang-warm-building foods and herbs such as cooked meat, while yang-hot-excess diseases are treated with yin-cool-eliminative foods and herbs such as raw fruits and vegetables. Whole grains such as brown rice or millet along with legumes and beans are considered more balanced, so that these constitute the main or central part of the diet because of their ability to balance both yin and yang conditions.

It is generally more difficult to treat yin or deficient individuals because they are limited in their capacity to digest and assimilate richer foods. Individuals with a stronger yang constitution who are motivated to make some significant dietary and life-style changes often respond dramatically to simple eliminative diets of fresh-squeezed fruit and vegetable juices and a raw-food vegetarian diet that is given for them to follow for a period of a few weeks or even months.

Because of these differences we can see why in Traditional Chinese Medicine there are health foods based on eating vegetarian foods and health foods based on the incorporation of various kinds of animal protein. For one who is yin and weak, meat cooked with certain tonic herbs is considered a tonic. For those who have a more yang condition, lighter vegetable foods, soups, and teas are used.

Food is considered the best tonic, and a superior tonic is the use of herbs cooked with food. Therefore, a typical tonic to increase energy, build up the whole body, and strengthen the immune system is to first cook approximately six ounces each of Oriental ginseng and astragalus *membranicus* root in a quart and a half of boiling water for a half hour and then to add beef, lamb, or chicken to make a soup. For women, to build blood and aid circulation, three to six ounces of dong quai root *(Angelica sinensis)* is similarly cooked with slices of fresh ginger root. Individuals with a weak endocrine system and adrenals are given stews with oysters and certain tonic herbs such as tree fungus and cooked rehmannia *glutinosa*.

The primary prerequisite for health is a healthy state of mind. The other prerequisites are getting increasingly more difficult to secure and include clean air, pure water, whole organic food, and sufficient rest as well as physical exercise. We must try to avoid foods and drinks with preservatives, pesticide residues, artificial coloring, hormones, drugs, refined sugar, white flour, and excess salt. We should limit foods such as meats that are high in saturated fats as well as overcome dependencies on stimulants such as coffee, alcohol, or other drugs that overly stimulate.

For many, just accomplishing these internal ecological changes will be a big achievement for which they will reap the rewards of increased well-being and, in many cases, a cure for many types of degenerative diseases. Even after this is accomplished, fine-tuning our degree of wellness must be achieved by effecting a balance of the yin and yang, negative and positive aspects of foods according to climate, season, and life-style.

Balance will probably never be a popular or commercially viable concept. The downfall of the human experience has always centered around the idea that "more is better." "More" in the sense of diet may mean too much of a certain food or, if following a pattern of restriction, too little. What too much or too little may be is particular to the needs of each individual, so that any dietary regime that is suggested or recommended may serve its intended purpose for a while, but will eventually have to be modified and adjusted for ongoing use. This is why the macrobiotic diet does not simply consist of limiting oneself to a particular kind of food but instead encourages the regular eating of broad varieties of whole, pure foods from the food groups outlined on pages 63–72, following the principles of yin and yang. Those who do not seem to do well on the macrobiotic diet are generally too limited and restricted in their choice of foods.

Since an imbalanced diet generates addictive cravings that make it self-perpetuating, the most efficient progress in detoxification and healing is to begin by following the expansion or contraction fast according to your individual need. The expansion fast encourages the use of more raw fruits, vegetables, and juices to encourage the discharge of yang toxins from excess meat, sugar, dairy, and refined foods. The contraction diet encourages the elimination of excess fluid in and around the cells and thereby discharges more yin toxins in the form of excess coldness and dampness.

EXPANSION

This is an eliminative approach beginning with the four-day cleansing fast. It is especially for those with a more yang-excess constitution or disease. It is cooling and detoxifying to the blood and lymphatic system.

FOUR-DAY CLEANSING FAST

Drink an eight-ounce glass of fruit or vegetable juice or herb tea every two waking hours throughout the first three days. Begin with a glass of prune juice in the morning with approximately half to one teaspoon of cayenne pepper or composition powder (formula number 17). Along with this take one tablespoon of pure virgin olive oil. The olive oil should be taken three times a day along with the cayenne pepper or composition powder and two tablets of triphala. This is all that is taken for the first three days.

On the fourth day continue the cayenne or composition powder and olive oil but begin the process of breaking the fast by taking warm vegetable broth, thin whole-grain porridge, salads, or fruit. Try to continue this diet for several more days if possible, as many as fourteen.

If possible begin the first four days with an enema, using a combination of two ounces of anise seed tea steeped in two quarts of boiling water, covered, a tablespoon each of sea salt, honey, and olive or sesame oil. The enema will greatly aid the eliminative process and is both cleansing and somewhat nutritive to the nervous system.

Anise seed is used because of its mild warming, stimulant, and carminative properties. It will aid in stimulating peristalsis and liver function, while helping to remove trapped pockets of gas in the colon. Salt helps to cleanse the intestines by increasing fluid lubrication. Honey is nutritive and healing. Olive or sesame oil is used to overcome dryness, which is a cause of constipation and eventually colitis in many individuals.*

There are a variety of fruit juices that can be used according to their specific therapeutic properties. To reduce excess fat, use lemon and water; for arthritic tendencies, use cherry juice; for urinary problems, use cranberry juice; for general purposes and to aid the liver, use apple juice.

Among vegetables, the carrot is one of the most healing foods. It is detoxifying to the blood and liver, strengthens the eyes, lubricates the intestines, clears the skin, and aids digestion. Thus, fresh carrot juice is one of the most healing foods for the liver—probably due to its high content of beta carotene and vitamin A.

Celery is also cooling and detoxifying, with mild diuretic properties that help reduce blood pressure and arthritic problems. It can be combined in equal amounts with carrot juice for any of these conditions.

Beets, especially black beets, also have a cool energy and are remarkably high in assimilable iron. Therefore they are best to use for anemia, heart problems, constipation, and liver toxicity, as well as for restlessness and anxiety. Beets can be used in soup or juiced and taken with carrot juice.

Generally a vegetable juice fast is milder in its detoxifying properties than fruit juice so that it can be chosen

---

*Actually, water enemas ultimately tend to aggravate dry conditions in the intestines.

based upon the specific conditions for which each vegetable is useful, or to proceed more gradually. Because vegetables are not so extremely yin as fruits, containing less sugars that will overstimulate the pancreas, they are better suited for occasional cleansing and fasting for vegetarians.

Cayenne pepper and composition powder are used to help overcome any low states associated with detoxification. This is because these serve as natural stimulants which do not rob the body of energy, and yet they are one of the best herbs to use to break up congestion, promote circulation of blood, and relieve lymphatic congestion. Cayenne is also a good household remedy to use externally or internally to stop bleeding.

Olive oil is used to stimulate the secretion of bile by contracting the gallbladder. By so doing, it helps to soften and expel gallstones. It is also a mild laxative which, along with triphala, will encourage the internal cleansing and detoxification process.

CONTRACTION

Contracting and drying is an approach which tones internal organs and other flaccid tissues and cells by eliminating excess interstitial fluid. It is particularly useful for yin conditions where there is flaccidity, weakness, and general loss of tone.

This condition is often associated with lymphatic congestion and general fatigue and is seen on the tongue by slight tooth indentations around the periphery. Anyone who has extraordinary thirst should not try this fast because they are actually suffering from a fluid depletion.

The method is to restrict all drink and fluids except

those that occur naturally in food. This is done only for a limited period of three or four days, maximum.*

FOUR-DAY BROWN RICE DIET

One bowl consisting of two-thirds cooked brown rice and one-third Japanese azuki or black beans is eaten three times a day. If preferred, only the rice can be used without the beans. This can be topped with pan-toasted and ground sesame seeds. Each mouthful should be well chewed.

The combination of rice and beans can be alternated but the azuki beans are particularly good for the kidneys and urinary system while the black beans are good for the reproductive organs and blood, making them especially useful for gynecological problems. Another delicious traditional East Indian therapeutic food can be used which combines brown rice and green mung beans together with a balanced combination of curry-like spices.

KICHAREE: FOOD FOR THE GODS

Presoak one or two cups each of brown rice and green mung beans in twice the amount of water for eight to twelve hours and cook. In a large skillet, heat a tablespoon or two of ghee and lightly sauté one teaspoon each of whole cumin and whole coriander seeds along with one teaspoon each of ground cumin and coriander seeds, a pinch of sea salt, and a tablespoon of turmeric. Be sure the rice and beans are cooked before preparing the spices in

---

*The famous Bircher Bennet spas in Europe used to alternate fast days with days during which only measured portions of red wine were given while fasting because of its drying effects.

the skillet. As the delicious aroma of the ghee and spices begins to arise, stir in the precooked rice and mung beans, mixing them thoroughly with the spices. The kicharee is now ready to serve.

Kicharee is considered the most healing food of India and tradition states that it contains all of the elements necessary to sustain life. It is further claimed that adhering to a strict diet of kicharee for three weeks can treat and possibly cure all diseases. The mung beans in kicharee have the unique property of being a protein-rich legume which also detoxifies the blood, neutralizes acidity and normalizes blood pressure while providing nutritional strength and sustenance.

The kicharee diet can be undertaken to promote the rapid healing of most acute and chronic diseases. It is ideal to use in association with herbal therapy because it will provide nourishment without interfering with the action of the herbs.

Kicharee is an ideal cleansing diet for vegetarians or can be enjoyed as a regular part of one's diet. It can be made more as a soup by adding sufficient amounts of water or, if preferred, as a stew, with the addition of other vegetables such as onions, carrots, and/or mushrooms, topped with a spoonful or two of fresh yogurt.

CONGEE

Congee, or rice porridge, is very similar to kicharee. In fact, kicharee, when made more into a thin porridge, could be called mung bean congee since the type of congee one makes is identified by the accompanying food or herb with which it is prepared.

Eaten as an easily digestible breakfast food by traditional Chinese and Japanese people, congee is also the best food to serve when nothing else can be digested or assimilated. Thus, when cooked with tonic herbs, it is the best food for the very aged and weak.

Basically, congee is made by cooking one part by volume of brown rice to seven to ten parts water for a period of six to twelve hours over a low flame. This can be done overnight or during the course of a day in a double boiler or slow cooker.

Tonic Chinese herbs such as astragalus, ginseng, and dong quai, with or without small amounts of lean meat, can be cooked with the rice to increase its tonic properties.

GHEE

Ghee, or clarified butter, is made by heating raw, unsalted butter to the boiling point and then lowering the heat. The foamy white milk solids will accumulate at the top or bottom of the pan. The sediment is skimmed off with a spoon and the remaining clear liquid is then poured into another container. It can then be stored in a wide jar by the stove for use as a cooking oil.

Be careful not to overheat the butter during its preparation as it can burn and become ruined. The white scrapings and sediment can be saved and used for vegetables, sauces or other dishes, but unlike ghee, it must be kept refrigerated or it will spoil.

Approximately two pounds of butter will yield a pound of ghee. Ghee can be kept for a considerable time (up to six months) without refrigeration and is the most perfect cooking oil. This is because it is least likely to become rancid and at the same time it imparts a delicious aroma and flavor to simple foods.

THE BALANCED DIET

The balanced macrodiet mentioned in the text is as follows:

WHOLE GRAINS:
40% TO 50% OF THE DAILY DIET

Including brown rice, millet, rye, wheat, corn, oats, barley, amaranth, and quinoa. The individual grains have various unique therapeutic properties:

Brown rice is considered the most balanced food, suitable for most climates and conditions. It is good for the stomach, intestines, lungs, and pancreas. According to Chinese medical theory, rice is contraindicated during high fevers because it changes into glucose, which will further aggravate and raise the fever. This may, however, only refer to the use of white rice.

Millet is the only alkaline grain and can be tolerated when individuals have an allergy to other grains. It is good for the stomach, spleen, and pancreas.

Wheat is highly nutritious. Soaked and slightly sprouted, it is excellent to give as a calming sedative. Some, however, cannot tolerate the gluten in either wheat or rye and will develop mild to severe allergic reactions.

Oats are a good grain to use for low energy and fatigue. They are also healing for stomach ulcers. The bran has been recognized as being very effective in preventing and overcoming high cholesterol.

Barley is cooling, detoxifying, and soothing. It is good for helping to cleanse the lymphatic system.

Corn is good for the heart. Therapeutically, it will help to stop bleeding, promote urination, dissolve gallstones, and treat hepatitis. The silk tassels of the corn are made into a tea and taken for urinary problems. Cornseed tea can be used as a treatment for blood in the urine.

Quinoa are seed grains introduced from the South American Andes, where they are a staple. They are higher in protein than other grains and well tolerated by many who are unable to digest the starches of other grains.

LEGUMES AND BEANS:

10% TO 20% OF THE DAILY DIET

Including azuki beans, black beans, green mung beans, lentils, garbanzo beans, soya beans, and soya products such as tofu, tempeh and miso paste, kidney beans and peas. Like other foods, the various beans have their special therapeutic properties and uses as follows:

Azuki beans are good for the urinary tract and especially the kidneys. A tea of the beans can be taken three times a day for bladder and kidney infections. Boil two tablespoons in a cup of water for twenty or thirty minutes.

Black beans are known to be especially good for the blood and reproductive organs. They are good to use with brown rice for anemia and to impart strength when recovering from illness.

Mung beans as described above detoxify and neutralize acids in the blood and lower high blood pressure.

Soya beans and soya bean products are very high in protein, equal to or better than meat. They are difficult to digest and so are made into soya bean cheese called tofu or cultured by the Indonesians to make tempeh.

VEGETABLES:
20% TO 30% OF THE DAILY DIET

Including all seasonally available root vegetables, green leafy vegetables, and a small amount of seaweeds for trace minerals. One should limit vegetables in the nightshade family, which includes tomatoes, potatoes, peppers, and eggplants, as these are thought to contain a substance that interferes with calcium absorption.

Besides the therapeutic properties of the vegetables described above as part of the expansion juice fast, others are also worth mentioning:

Spinach is cooling, anti-inflammatory, diuretic, and demulcent. It is high in iron and can be used for constipation, thirst, and night blindness.

Squash is cooling and anti-inflammatory. It promotes urination, relieves thirst and dryness, treats edema, and is also useful in hot weather.

Parsley is slightly warm, promotes digestion, treats urinary infection, and helps promote the eruption and termination of measles.

Mushrooms have a cold energy, are good for all inflammatory conditions, and in hot weather, they lower blood pressure, are antitumor and promote urination.

Cabbage is cooling, anti-inflammatory, moistening to the intestines, and stops coughs.

FRUITS, NUTS, DAIRY, EGGS, MEAT:
10% TO 20% OF THE DAILY DIET

Fruits should be eaten in moderation and as seasonally available as possible. Fruit juices, containing concentrated fruit sugar, can cause a hypoglycemic reaction and should either be avoided altogether, or served diluted with water.

Nuts are difficult to digest because of their high oil content. Further, the oil of nuts when shelled is susceptible to harmful rancidity. A small amount, however, is a good source of supplemental protein.

Milk can be an important source of protein especially for vegetarians. If used moderately during the course of a balanced diet, there should be no problem. Individuals who have a tendency toward mucus congestion and to form cysts and tumors should avoid milk.

There is a controversy concerning the pros and cons of the pasteurization of milk. If we could be assured of the freshness as well as the proper care and handling of the animals, the use of raw, unpasteurized milk would be best. Milk, however, is a perfect medium for the proliferation of bacteria and various microorganisms; even after pasteurization, which only raises the temperature to 161°F for fifteen seconds, considerable amounts of these microorganisms still remain. Perhaps, part of many individuals' negative reactions to milk lies in the stress to the immune system caused by the introduction of unfavorable microorganisms into the colon.

For these and perhaps other reasons, most traditional people boil milk before using it. Boiling heats it up to 212°F, which is much better. Further, cooking milk in this way helps to break down the large protein molecules that tend to cause mucus congestion and milk allergies. (Cultured milk such as yogurt dos this for us while providing a good source of lactobacillus for the intestines.) For these reasons it is good to boil even pasteurized milk before using it.

One of the pitfalls of the macrobiotic diet is its rigid

avoidance of dairy. This is largely because macrobiotics originates from Japan, where there is hardly enough room to raise milk cows and maintain an active dairy industry. Consequently, there is no significant tradition involving the use of milk in Japan, where fish is the primary source of animal protein.

For many vegetarian adults and children, milk can make the difference between health and deficiency diseases. For this reason, the Hindus consider milk the most perfect food and rely on it as an important part of their diet. For people in the West it is probably a good idea to use low-fat milk (1%) as opposed to whole milk (3.5%).*

There are many wonderful traditional recipes among the Hindus for the use of milk. It can be heated and used with cereal in the morning, and vegetables are sometimes cooked in it. Yogurt is a standard food that is added in tablespoon amounts to balance hot spicy foods. Because it has a cold energy, the Hindu people never take yogurt in the evening or during cold weather. A delicious drink called lassi is made by combining yogurt with lemon water and honey.

Another preparation is called "paneer" and is made by bringing to a boil a half gallon of low-fat milk and slowly adding sufficient lemon juice so that it will curdle and the whey which rises to the top becomes clear. Let it boil a short time longer, then remove it from the stove and allow the whey to further separate from the curds. The whey, which is liquid, can then be poured off into a separate container while the curds are retained. The curds thus

---

*It is interesting to consider how, since the Hindus take animal protein in the form of milk, there is really no ongoing cultural tradition for the complete avoidance of all animal protein from the diet.

produced are one of the best tolerated forms of dairy and can be used as one would use cottage cheese, ricotta, various spreads and toppings, and cooked in vegetable dishes.

Eggs are a good source of protein, and despite the controversy over their supposed high cholesterol content, in the context of a predominantly vegetarian diet, two eggs once or twice a week should not offer any problem.

One of the problems with most commercial eggs is the highly stressful and harmful environment in which the hens are maintained. It has been found that commercial "nest eggs," which come from hens that are allowed to range free, are far superior to commercially produced eggs. They have less cholesterol and higher B_{12} and are considerably more flavorful. Eggs can be eaten soft boiled or made into an omelette. Fried eggs are not so good because of the additional oil content. Eating one or two eggs a day for a month is ideal as a building food for those who are run-down, anemic, or underweight.

Meat is the most efficiently assimilated and concentrated protein source. It is also an important source of iron and all the B vitamins including B_{12}. However, because it is so well utilized, there is the danger that any of the poisons of the animal, including those that are generated from stress and fear, remain in the blood and are consequently absorbed by the individual who ultimately ingests the meat. A further harm stems from the fact that most commercial livestock are hardly raised in optimum conditions. Subjected to extreme overcrowding, many animals that are diseased are slaughtered. Thus they are routinely injected with various chemicals and antibiotics to control the disease symptoms, as well as steroids and growth hormones to increase their weight and market value.

Another consideration is the ethical issues involved in

supporting an industry that is known to be one of the worst ecological offenders. Besides the destruction of precious rain forests in other countries to provide livestock grazing, thousands of acres of precious national forest in North America are destroyed yearly to accommodate the grazing of cattle. The delicate ecology of our national parks and deserts are being subjected to and ruined by the presence of free range cattle. Pollution is a serious problem since the droppings and waste of cattle and livestock are among the sources of water pollution in the country. Finally, the inhumane methods of managing and slaughtering livestock are an insult to one's conscience and sensibilities.

From a practical standpoint meat is one of the most inefficient foods. One can produce ten times the amount of wheat on the same land as is required for grazing cattle. If less meat were produced and in its place were the cultivation of various key food crops, world starvation would be greatly curtailed or eliminated altogether.

There are also many health hazards presented by eating excessive amounts of meat laden with saturated fat. The excessive consumption of red meat and dairy with insufficient exercise is known to be a primary cause of high cholesterol, arteriosclerosis, and heart disease. These foods are also implicated in causing or contributing to other diseases of the kidneys and liver, for instance.

It is no wonder that there is such a strong urge among increasing numbers of people to use less meat in the diet. Still, there is the inescapable fact that while a lot of meat is harmful to a number of people, many may actually require it as a regular part of their diet. For some it may be based on an inherent genetic predisposition that requires animal protein as part of the diet; for others it is based on inherent deficiencies.

Meat is considered a "first class" protein as opposed to vegetable proteins, which are regarded as "second class." This is based on the superior bioassimilability of animal protein over vegetable protein. For those who have deep-level deficiencies, animal protein, whether it be in the form of boiled warm milk with honey, or in fish, eggs, or meat, seems to make a big difference in terms of overall metabolism and health. It may take some experimentation for each individual to determine how much they actually need, based on their individual biological requirements. The percentages I offer here are only approximate.

However, one thing is absolutely clear: Because animal sources of protein are better absorbed and assimilated, only the purest and the finest dairy, eggs, and meat should be consumed. It should be from animals raised free of antibiotics, steroids, or other drugs and the animals should have been raised, maintained, and slaughtered in as humane a manner as possible.

The notion of avoiding the consumption of these important foods based on moral grounds is an individual decision. Considering that life ultimately feeds upon life, it is impossible to eliminate all violence. However, if one is sick or weak, the consideration of passive, self-inflicted violence needs to be compared to whatever violence (hopefully as little as possible) is involved in including animal protein as part of one's diet.

Without meat one is left with a high-carbohydrate diet, since even beans, which are the basic source of protein for vegetarians, are also very high in carbohydrates. For many, perhaps the majority, this causes a tendency toward abnormal weight gain, based on the propensity of insulin to convert excess, nonutilized carbohydrate to its storage form, as fat. Therefore eating more protein, especially low-fat animal protein, increases body metabolism and allows one to utilize and burn up stores of fat.

Many who have abused their bodies through the practice of eating a protein, iron, and B$_{12}$ deficient diet for years seem unable to recoup their health without the inclusion of some red meat at least two or three times a week in their diet. Many chronic deficiency diseases suffered by long-term vegetarians such as candidiasis, chronic fatigue syndrome, anemia, weak digestion, depression, and moodiness, among others, can be traced to an improper vegetarian diet or a diet severely lacking in protein, B$_{12}$, iron, and other essential minerals that are found in meat.

A Chinese Taoist practice to detoxify meat is to presoak it in cold water for a few hours to dissolve and eliminate as much of the blood as possible, since it contains the greatest concentration of the animal's toxins. Another method is to prepare and eat meat with ginger, which enhances its digestibility and assimilation.

Now a brief presentation of the therapeutic properties of different forms of animal protein:

Lamb is good for improving circulation and overcoming coldness.

Beef is good for hypoglycemia, underweight and weakness.

Organ meats tend to strengthen a corresponding weak organ within our own bodies. For this reason, traditional Native American hunters would first offer the heart and liver of the animal to be eaten by one who is weak or recovering from sickness.

Chicken is warming and is useful for promoting circulation. Eliminating the skin of chickens and turkeys is beneficial to those who are on a low-fat diet.

Like fowl, fish is eaten because of its value for a low-fat

diet. Unlike other meat proteins, most saltwater fish generally have a metabolically cool energy, making them not so useful as red meat for raising overall body metabolism.

Shrimp, however, do have a warm yang energy and are good for general weakness and deficiency. They are also good for male impotence because of their ability to stimulate body metabolism.

Oysters are used regularly by Chinese women (about two or more daily) because they seem to increase estrogen. Thus they are particularly useful for infertility and for treating menopausal disorders.

SUMMARY

From the preceding text we see again how diet and health are a question of balance rather than a simple issue of what is good or bad for us. All foods possess a positive (yang) or negative (yin) energetic balance apart from any of their individual biochemical nutrients. This balance derives from and is relative to all aspects of our inner and outer environment. Thus, not only is eating high-quality food essential, but so is eating it in proportion to the various categories of grains, legumes, beans, vegetables, fruit, meat, and dairy to harmonize with our individual needs according to climate, life-style, and all other factors.*

Just because certain foods such as dairy, eggs, and meat,

---

*It is interesting to consider how, even before science discovered the importance of the human immune system, the philosophical wisdom of the Chinese wisely states that in an impure world it is not good to be too pure and, therefore, we should allow a small amount of toxins into our systems each day to maintain balance with our surroundings.

which were of poor quality and eaten in excess, proved harmful to so many does not mean that, by improving their quality and eating them in more moderation, they cannot be unique and important sources of B_{12}, protein, iron, and other valuable nutrients and minerals. Further, in the context of a diet consisting of 80 to 90 percent vegetable-derived foods, high-quality, humanely raised animal-derived foods in the form of dairy, eggs, and meat can be of important health benefit to some. While over-consumption of animal foods high in saturated fat can be harmful, a diet deficient in easily assimilable first-class protein found in animal protein foods can over time cause profound nutritional deficiencies that eventually are a cause for many serious chronic deficiency diseases.

4

ACUPUNCTURE AND
RELATED THERAPIES

Acupuncture is one aspect of Traditional Chinese Medicine (TCM) which includes herbal medicine, food therapy, and a form of psychotherapy. While acupuncture has received the widest recognition in the West, to the Chinese, the use of herbs is often of much greater value. Nevertheless, acupuncture as a systematic approach seems to be a unique contribution of the Chinese that dates back some three thousand to five thousand years, depending upon which authority is followed.

Acupuncture is an ancient system of healing based upon the stimulation, with the insertion of fine needles, of specific points along the entire body. The term *acupuncture* is comparatively modern. The original term was "ching lo" therapy or meridian therapy, which describes the process of stimulating and thereby opening the fourteen meridians or pathways on which the over 365 systematized points of acupuncture are charted. These meridians in many instances seem to correspond to various inter-connecting nerve channels and are characteristically named by one of the twelve major internal organs such as the stomach meridian, spleen meridian, kidney meridian, etc.

The concept of "ching lo" or meridian therapy admits of a much broader range of stimulation than of only the use of needles. Traditionally the Chinese have used many methods including a massage technique called acupressure, the use of heat in the form of moxibustion and the placement of small bamboo or glass cups by a vacuum or suction method. Today, acupuncture continues to evolve with the use of small magnets or painless light lasers to acupuncture points.

Despite its complex theoretical base and its outstanding professional clinicians, acupuncture, like herbalism, evolved out of the practice of village folk healers who, perhaps through trial and error, learned of the therapeutic effect of stimulating certain points in the body. The knowledge of these special points was passed down through generations as "family secrets." At various times, historically, these secrets have been called forth, compiled and organized into the system we know today.

Certain related modalities associated with the practice of acupuncture can be easily assimilated into a self-healing program. This may be useful because there are many areas where one may not have easy access to an acupuncturist or where the cost of treatment is prohibitive. The following simple modalities can be easily learned and for certain conditions prove to be of great benefit.

MOXIBUSTION

Moxibustion is a method of applying heat with mugwort herb *(Artemisia vulgarus)* on or near a chosen point on the surface of the body. There are two basic methods. Direct moxibustion is where a small cone of the herb about the size of a grain of rice is placed directly over the point, ignited with an incense stick and left to briefly burn until it goes out. This is very powerful for recalcitrant problems but may leave a small blister.

The second method, which is more appropriate for self-healing, is to hold a pre-ignited moxa roll near the skin until it gets hot, backing away for a few moments, and repeating several times until there is a mild rebefacient or reddening of the skin surface. This does not leave a blister if done properly.

Many people enjoy the sensation of applying heat to injured areas of the body because in many instances it seems to provide immediate relief from discomfort. Moxa seems to work primarily through the action of the heat, which dilates the vessels and capillaries, allowing for better circulation of blood through the area and, consequently, the normalizing of cellular metabolism. A secondary action is provided by the actual herb itself, which has antispasmodic pain-relieving properties.

Moxa is ideal for conditions associated with coldness and poor circulation. It works phenomenally well for arthritis and rheumatic problems, when applied over sore and aching joints and muscles, and to relieve whiplash, certain bruises and injuries, lower back pain, abdominal pains and menstrual pains.

CUPPING

Cupping, a mode of therapy widely used by the Chinese, is actually found as a common folk treatment in traditional cultures throughout the world, ranging from Mediterranean countries to Central and South America.

Cupping consists of creating a temporary vacuum in a small cup or bamboo receptacle and then quickly applying it to the surface of the skin. The vacuum is created by holding the cup upside down close to the surface upon which it is to be applied, passing a flame under the cup and quickly placing it over the area of pain.

Certain cups work better than others. Glasses or cups that hold about a half cup of liquid and have a slightly rounded shape work best. The sawed-off joints of bamboo are light and easily utilized, but the rough open lip of the bamboo must be smoothed and sanded so as not to injure the skin when suction is applied.

Cupping is applied usually to the back, neck, arms, and legs, and directly over areas of pain. Cups relieve pain by drawing the congested blood and fluid, usually lacking in nutrients and full of painful lactic acid waste, to the surface of the skin for dispersal and elimination, thus allowing for the free circulation of freshly oxygenated blood to the deeper tissues and cells underneath.

DERMAL HAMMER

A dermal hammer is a small hammerlike device, usually made of lightweight metal or plastic, which has at one end a simulated hammer about a half inch in diameter with many fine protruding needles. It is used by gently tapping over the affected points or areas of the body.

The use of a dermal hammer is a mild surface treatment particularly suited to the treatment of skin diseases such as psoriasis, eczema, rashes, wrinkles, and other skin problems. It also can be used on the scalp to stimulate hair growth and occasionally works quite well. It relieves localized aches and pains on the neck, limbs, and back and, finally, because it is so gentle and painless, it is used for treating small children. Acupuncturists use it specifically to relieve pains such as carpal tunnel syndrome or chronic pains of the wrist and forearms.

The method of treatment is to tap gently around or directly over the affected area. A stronger treatment consists of tapping until there is a superficial reddening, even to the appearance of tiny drops of serous fluid. A gentler treatment gives only the tiniest blush to the surface of the skin. Because of its mildness, the treatment will probably need to be repeated at least once daily for one to several weeks and in the case of baldness, once daily for several weeks up to three to six months. One should sterilize the dermal hammer between uses by pressure cooking for twenty to thirty minutes.

Moxa, cups and dermal hammers are available from oriental medical suppliers.*

---

*One source for moxibustion sticks, therapeutic cups and dermal hammers is Oriental Medical Supply, 1950 Washington St., Braintree, WA 02184; Tel: (800) 329–1839.

5

A BRIEF INTRODUCTION TO HOMEOPATHY

Homeopathic medicine was discovered during the late 1700s by Dr. Samuel Hahnemann, a German doctor who was frustrated by the medical practices of his day. He observed that the popular use of cinchona bark (the source of quinine) for the treatment of intermittent and remittent fevers actually brought on these fevers as well. This observation was followed by a number of experiments with various other remedies on himself, family, and other subjects, which led to the founding principle of homeopathy: "Like Cures Like."

Therefore, to determine the suitability of a given remedy for a variety of conditions and symptoms, Hahnemann's followers to this day undergo a series of "provings" during which a number of people agree to take increasing doses of a given remedy and carefully note the reactions, physiological as well as psychological, that are experienced. These then become the basis for the descriptive indications for the remedy as is published in homeopathic materia medica books.

Obviously in many cases poisonous or toxic reactions are known from the reaction of individuals who for whatever reason ingest them, and these may not be as a result of "provings" but are extracted from toxicological data and, for the homeopath, serve the same purpose. Consequently, the various reactions and symptoms individuals have experienced as a result of ingesting, for whatever reason, poisons such as strychnine or arsenic or allowing themselves to be bitten by a venomous insect, snake, or animal become part of the description for the use of the homeopathic remedy made from these substances.

POTENTIZATION

Hahnemann did not believe in testing poisonous substances on animals, perhaps for ethical reasons, but even more relevant it was because he did not believe that the effect of a substance on an animal was necessarily the same as it would be on a human. As a result he initiated the principle of the minimum dose. In fact he found that the more diluted a substance was, the more profound its effects not only on the body but on the mind as well.

Since then, homeopathic medicines are potentized by carefully diluting one part of the original substance, or "mother tincture" as it is called, in either ten or one hundred parts neutral solution. If it is diluted in ten parts it is marked as 1X, 6X, 12X, 30X, more or less indicating the number of times it has gone through the dilution process. If it is diluted in one hundred parts of neutral solution it is correspondingly marked 1C, 15C, 30C, etc., with "C" standing for centesimal potencies. In between each dilution the mixture is percussed to allow for further saturation and potentization.

The process actually involves, for instance, mixing one part of a mother tincture of an herb, mineral, animal part, pathogen, etc., with either nine or ninety-nine equal parts water or alcohol or, for a dry remedy, powdered lactose (milk sugar). This would produce the first potency, either an "X" (decimal) or "C" (centesimal) strength. To produce the second, one would repeat the process taking one part of the first dilution and mixing it with nine or ninety-nine parts of the neutral solution or lactose. Percussing or shaking the mixture between each dilution is vitally important and this is done by striking the bottle against a firm surface between each dilution. For dry powders, the remedy must be carefully mixed and ground in a mortar and pestle or the equivalent.

As stated, the higher the potency, the more profound the reaction. This has brought the founding principles of homeopathy at odds against the prevailing understanding of science, since beyond 12C one is unable to find a molecule of the original substance. Dilutions from 200C up to several million are used and in many cases seem to produce dramatic positive results.

Historically, homeopathy had the best record for dealing with deadly streptococcal infections (strep throat) and later with various epidemics. At the beginning of the twentieth century 20 percent of the physicians in the United States practiced homeopathy, and at one critical historical junction, homeopathy seriously rivaled standard allopathic practice. Eventually, with the rise of pharmaceutical interests that influenced medical education, homeopathy was deemed unscientific, and medical schools stopped offering instruction in its use. Homeopathy is currently widely practiced throughout many parts of the world, especially places where pharmaceutical or even herbal medicines are too expensive. Obviously it requires very little raw material to manufacture homeopathic medicines, so that in countries such as India, for instance, homeopathy is widely accepted and practiced. Fortunately, in Western countries, homeopathy, along with other alternative medical practices, has been experiencing a popular revival.

One of the problems with homeopathy in relation to current practice is that like other traditional medical systems, such as Traditional Chinese Medicine, it is not oriented toward the treatment of named diseases as much as it is of the various symptoms that may comprise a specific disease. To find the correct homeopathic remedy for symptoms of the common cold or headache, for example, can depend on a number of symptoms; for instance, if it is induced by a sudden shock to the system, whether it is aggravated by hot or cold, whether there is mucus or not, whether the symptoms are predominantly right- or left-sided, whether they are accompanied by other symptoms, from strange skin reactions to various emotional reactions. The best remedy is that which corresponds to most of the important presenting symptomology of the patient. To find the right remedy is especially vital to treating more complex problems.

Throughout this book, I have tried to mention a few homeopathic remedies that are most likely to be indicated for a specific condition; in fact, they may not be the most efficacious for a particular patient with a different symptomatology. I would suggest that if one does not achieve expected results within a reasonable period and homeopathy becomes the treatment of choice, one should seek the services of a qualified homeopathic practitioner who is able to use the higher-potency homeopathic remedies not commonly available to the layperson.

Today one can often find homeopathic medicines sold in natural food and drugstores throughout the country, and many of these are combined remedies. In many cases these are effective, especially, of course, for minor acute symptoms.

In conclusion, I think that homeopathy has the potential for achieving the most profound changes, physiologically and emotionally. They also require faith, patience, and the skill of a homeopathic practitioner. With the higher potencies being impossible to measure or analyze by any known methods of scientific evaluation and the results in the treatment of long-term, chronic, or constitutional imbalances often occurring over a period of months or years, homeopathy is vulnerable to exploitation by individuals knowingly or not who use a variety of questionable or dubious methods for prescribing. This is further complicated by the fact that in some instances the remedies prescribed in this way seem to have a positive effect on some patients regardless of the method of prescribing.

Sound confusing? It is, but I have personally experienced and seen a number of positive cases that were unresponsive to all other methods of treatment respond favorably to homeopathic treatment.

6

TWENTY POPULAR HERBS

ST. JOHNSWORT (HYPERICUM PERFORATUM)

Clinical trials conducted by German researchers found this herb effective for mild clinical depression. Double-blind, placebo-controlled studies published in reputable journals, including the *British Medical Journal* (December 11, 1999), show that standardized extracts of St. Johnswort are significantly better than dummy pills, as good as imipramine, and substantially less likely to cause side effects. The Latin name is derived from the Greek meaning "to counteract the evil eye" based on its traditional use, where it was once hung over the door to ward off evil influences. Extracts of the herb also have been found to be an effective antiviral agent against viruses causing colds, influenza, herpes simplex, hepatitis and AIDS. Other traditional uses were primarily for affections of the nervous system, including menopausal neurosis, hysteria, spinal injuries, neuralgia, sciatica, and muscular rheumatism. As an astringent and diuretic it is used to treat a wide variety of conditions, including inflammations of the genitourinary tract, diarrhea, dysentery, parasitic infections, and bed-wetting. It is also useful as both an oil and ointment applied topically to ulcers, sores, swellings, bruises, and some cancers. *Hypericum* is considered a safe and effective treatment and an alternative to standard pharmaceutical antidepressants. In animals who graze on *Hypericum,* higher sensitivity to the sun has been shown. Probably some of the therapeutic effect of *Hypericum* is in its ability to interact with direct sunlight. However, excessive indulgence is to be avoided. Negative herb-drug interactions are unlikely. While the combined use of *Hypericum* with orthodox medications has even shown an increased favorable response, it is advisable to exert some cautious watchfulness with the prolonged usage of St. Johnswort with serotonin reuptake inhibitors (SSRI) and monoamine oxidase inhibitors (MAOI).

Use St. Johnswort:

- for inflammation
- for nerve injuries and pains
- as an anti-inflammatory for viral and bacteria-based diseases
- externally for bruises, injuries, wound healing
- for mild depression with the standardized extract, with 1.0 to 2.7 mg of total hypericin per day

Effective minimum dose: 3 to 6 grams of the dried herb in tea or the equivalent as an alcoholic extract (about a teaspoon two or three times daily of the 1:5 liquid alcoholic extract).

ECHINACEA *(ECHINACEA PURPUREA* ET SPECIES)

This plant (also known as purple coneflower) is native to North America, but most of the research on it has been conducted in Germany. There are various species, and all seem to be therapeutically effective, but the most common species in trade is *Echinacea purpurea*. Traditionally the root is preferred, but nearly equal therapeutic effects are claimed for the use of the aerial portions (leaves and flowers) as well. Echinacea is regarded as a nonspecific immunostimulant, and as such is used for the treatment and prevention of colds, flus, and allergies. Traditionally it is effective for a wide variety of infections whose origins are bacterial, viral, or protozoal. It can be used for gangrenous and purulent conditions anywhere in or on the body. For these conditions its effects are enhanced when used topically as well as internally. The effective dose is approximately 3 to 6 grams of the dried root or aerial portions divided into two or three doses per day. For acute conditions it should be taken more frequently, four to six times per day, and should be tapered off as symptoms subside. Of the 1:5 extract, take half to one teaspoon as a single dose.

Use echinacea for:

- internally for inflammations and infections
- externally for infections and inflammations
- prevention and treatment of colds and flus

ST. MARY'S THISTLE *(SILYBUM MARIANUM)*

It is also commonly called milk thistle. The primary part used is the dried seeds. However, the whole herb made into a tea functions well to promote normal liver function and enhance the secretion of bile. Its major use is as a liver protective agent for all liver diseases, including all forms of hepatitis. It is also an effective antioxidant. Either alone or together with dandelion root it is an effective treatment for a wide variety of liver complaints, including all forms of hepatitis and cirrhosis. Even after a month of use it will bring down abnormally high liver enzymes. It is also useful for the prevention and treatment of gallstones, diabetes, and cancer.

The effective therapeutic dose of the powdered seeds is 4 to 9 grams divided into two or three doses per day.

Use milk thistle for:

- all liver and gallbladder diseases
- enlarged liver and spleen
- hepatitis (all kinds) and liver psoriasis
- protectant from toxic poisons affecting the liver
- as an antioxidant

SAW PALMETTO (SERENOA REPENS)

Saw palmetto berry tea was used by Native Americans to treat genitourinary problems, and physicians actually prescribed an extract of the berries to treat prostate problems until nearly 1950. Double-blind studies have confirmed that saw palmetto berry extract can relieve symptoms of prostate enlargement (such as frequent urination or restricted flow) as effectively as some prescription prostate medicines with no adverse side effects. Traditionally saw palmetto berries were used for chronic respiratory conditions associated with mucus. It was also used to reduce the irritation associated with cystitis. Saw palmetto is also reputed to be an effective endocrine agent for both men and women, having mild aphrodisiac effects and even claimed to promote the enlargement of underdeveloped breasts in women. The effective dose ranges from 4 to 9 grams of the dried berries divided into two or three doses per day. The taste is a strong disincentive for its use as a tea. Therefore, it can be taken in a 1:2 extract (the liposterolic compounds are most effectively extracted with ethanol). It also is taken in pill or tablet form. It combines well with other herbs for benign prostatic hypertrophy such as pumpkin seeds, pygeum root, and nettle root.

Use saw palmetto for:

- enlarged prostate (benign prostatic hypertrophy)
- accompanying prostate symptoms, including frequent urination
- underdeveloped glands in either men or women
- cystitis
- chronic respiratory conditions

GINKGO

Ginkgo biloba has been used in China for thousands of years for a variety of purposes. In the 1960s German scientists were examining a number of plants for their ability to enhance circulation. The leaves of the 150-million-year-old revered ginkgo tree was found to be the most active. Soon after, a highly concentrated 50 to 1 standardized extract was prepared and found effective in enhancing memory and cognitive function in the elderly and slowing the onset of Alzheimer's disease. Its current popularity is due to its reputation for aiding memory. Clinical trials have proven that this herbal extract can increase circulation throughout the body as well as the brain and thereby slow mental decline due to Alzheimer's disease, although it is not a cure. Other disorders associated with restricted peripheral blood flow, such as Raynaud's syndrome, diabetic vascular disease, macular degeneration, asthma, allergic reactions, ischemia, thrombosis, and sexual dysfunction also have been found to respond to the use of ginkgo extract. Ginkgo leaf extract also has been found to serve as an effective antioxidant for the prevention and treatment of a variety of chronic degenerative conditions. Caution needs to be used for patients who are already taking anticoagulant medications including warfarin, coumadin, and aspirin. The recommended dose, based upon research, is 120 mg of the 50:1 standardized extract.

Use ginkgo:

- to improve short-term memory
- to assist and benefit circulation
- to warm cold extremities
- for macular degeneration
- for asthma
- to help dissolve and prevent blood clots
- for impotence

GARLIC (ALLIUM SATIVUM)

This root is extremely popular as a culinary flavoring, but it also has a long tradition of use as a medicine. It is known to help lower cholesterol and regulate blood pressure, and its anticlotting properties make it useful for preventing and treating blood clots. It also has antifungal and antibacterial properties. Garlic is effective particularly for upper respiratory conditions, colds, flus, bronchitis, and allergies. It is also excellent for the prevention and treatment of worms and parasites of all kinds. Garlic oil, made by macerating finely chopped garlic in olive oil, can be applied topically for itches, tineas, and fungal infections. An excellent way to take garlic internally is either by taking a teaspoon frequently throughout the day or by simply dipping bread in it and eating it freely. One or two drops of garlic and olive oil inserted into the ears is an excellent treatment for childhood ear infections. Because garlic has antibacterial properties it can be used internally or topically for all kinds of infections, either bacterial or viral. Comparative studies in China indicate that people who consume large amounts of garlic on a regular basis are less prone to stomach cancer. American folk wisdom holds that plenty of garlic at the first sign of a cold will speed recovery. One may need to be careful if taking high doses of garlic daily along with pharmaceutical anticoagulant agents. Since there are few or no contraindications, garlic can and should be taken in frequent doses throughout each day.

Use garlic:

- for infections and inflammations
- externally for injuries, bruises, fungal infections
- internally for upper respiratory diseases
- for parasites, either internally or externally
- for cardiovascular diseases

GINSENG

There are several types of ginseng. The primary ones include *Panax* ginseng from Asia, which is used as a tonic to raise body metabolism and increase energy and vitality; American ginseng *(Panax quinquefolium),* which is less stimulating and nourishes blood and body fluids; Siberian ginseng *(Eleutherococus senticosus),* which is used to counteract stress and increase stamina and endurance. The best quality is from seven-year-old roots and older, but four-year-old roots may also be used. *Panax* ginseng is given to those over fifty years of age to prolong longevity and counteract stress. Ginseng is believed to increase the utilization of nutrients and oxygen in the cells. It also may lower blood sugar, so diabetics should monitor their blood sugar carefully while taking it. Ginseng also has anticoagulant properties, and people who are taking pharmaceutical drugs for this should be sure to tell their doctor, especially if they may need to undergo an operation. Dose ranges from 1 to 10 g per day and may be as high as 30 g.

Use *Panax* ginseng for:

• low energy
• poor metabolism and digestion
• longevity

Use American ginseng *(Panax quinquefolium)* for:

• low energy
• dryness of the mouth and respiratory passages
• upper respiratory weakness

Use Siberian ginseng:

• for stamina and endurance
• to counteract stress

KAVA *(PIPER METHYSTICUM)*

The root of the kava kava tree has been used as a medicine and ritualistically by island natives throughout the Pacific region (with the exception of New Zealand, New Caledonia, and the Solomon Islands) for over a thousand years. It has the effect of relieving anxiety and relaxing the body without diminishing mental acuity. It is not dissimilar to procaine or zylocaine, and similarly is a mild pain reliever; when taken by mouth it will exert a mild temporary numbing sensation. Kava has anti-inflammatory properties, and in Fiji it is used to treat genitourinary complaints and filiariasis, and as a treatment for colds, coughs, and sore throats. It is effective for venereal diseases, especially gonorrhea. Its most common and immediately experiential use is to relieve anxiety and promote sedation. Excessive and overly frequent use has resulted in temporary skin irritation and itching in rare instances. Dopamine antagonism also has been reported in some instances. Today it has become very popular as a mild sedative and sleeping pill. One caution: Do not combine kava with alcohol or other sedatives, tranquilizers, or sleeping pills. In general it should not be taken during pregnancy or by nursing mothers. Dose: 2 to 3 g of the dried root in one or two daily doses. Of the liquid 1:2 extract, about half to one teaspoon once or twice daily. The standardized extract should be 100 to 200 mg of kava lactones daily.

Use kava:

- for anxiety and nervousness
- for insomnia
- for genitourinary tract infections
- for coughs, colds and sore throat
- internally and topically to relieve pain
- for toothache

DONG QUAI (OR DANG GUI) *(ANGELICA SINENSIS, A. POLYMORPHA;* JAPANESE VERSION IS *A. ACUTILOBA)*

Dong quai is the second most popular Chinese herb in the West, next to ginseng. The root of this *Umbelliferae* herb has been used for centuries by Chinese healers for diseases of the female reproductive tract, as well as for menstrual cramps, irregular periods, and problems with menopause. As ginseng is used as an energy tonic, dong quai is used primarily by women as a blood tonic. It is an anti-inflammatory, anti-anemic, antiplatelet, gynecological tonic and a mild laxative and anti-arrhythmic, and it will prevent and treat peripheral vascular disease, angina, and stroke. Women with fibroids or heavy menstrual bleeding should probably not use dong quai. It should be used with caution or not at all by individuals who are taking warfarin or other anticoagulant, antiplatelet medication. It is contraindicated especially during the first trimester of pregnancy unless prescribed by a qualified herbalist. Dose is 3 to 15 g per day of the dried root decoction in water.

Use dong quai:

- for dysmenorrhea and other menstrual irregularities
- for anemia and poor or impaired blood circulation
- for cardiovascular disease, including arrhythmias and angina
- as a mild laxative
- for menopause

GOLDENSEAL *(HYDRASTIS CANADENSIS)*

This North American native is popular in combination with echinacea to help fight off respiratory infections. It does contain compounds such as berberine that have some antibacterial properties, but there is very little evidence that it is effective in preventing colds. Presently, due to overharvesting and loss of native habitat, it is severely endangered, to the point that no one should sell or purchase wild harvested goldenseal. In fact, for all practical purposes the organically cultivated goldenseal is nearly of equal value. Goldenseal has been widely used. One useful application is as a simple bitter tonic compound combined with other herbs such as anise seed, licorice, cardamom, and angelica root, macerated in vodka or gin, and taken in spoonful doses twenty or thirty minutes before meals to stimulate appetite and aid digestion. It is also effective as an eyewash for conjunctivitis and for constipation, ulcers, gastritis, and menstrual irregularities. One of its most effective uses is as a treatment for amoebic or bacterial dysentery. However, many of the uses can be accommodated by cheaper herbs such as Oregon grape root or East Coast barberry root, both of which also contain berberine as one of their principal chemical constituents. The dose of the powder, either in capsules or tablets, ranges from 250 to 540 mg, taken two or three times daily. Taking goldenseal long-term, more than two weeks to a month, in higher dosages is generally not recommended, since it can cause gastrointestinal atony. This may not be true if it is taken in a formula with other herbs and in less quantity. It also can be taken as a tincture or tea, but be warned: Goldenseal sets a standard for bitterness that is quite unforgettable. Persistent popular myth credits goldenseal with being able to mask illicit drugs in urine, but this appears to be fiction. As a single herb, in more significant dosages, goldenseal may be contraindicated for high blood pressure, heart failure, irregular heartbeats, and pregnancy. It should be restricted or used with caution when taking anticoagulant drugs such as coumadin, benzodiazepines, high blood pressure medicine, beta blockers such as Inderal, calcium channel blockers such as Calan and Procardia and Lanoxin.

Use goldenseal:

- for inflammations
- as a bitter tonic for loss of appetite
- as an eyewash for conjunctivitis
- for bacterial or amoebic dysentery
- for constipation
- for cancer
- for menstrual pain
- for ulcers and mouth sores

SENNA *(CASSIA* SPECIES*)*

Herbal laxatives are historically as they remain today, the most widely accepted use for herbs. Their use dates back at least to ancient Egypt, where senna was recognized as a powerful laxative. It is available in such over-the-counter laxatives as Ex-Lax and Senokot. Many diseases are aggravated or caused by chronic constipation. Even a daily bowel movement may be insufficient. Probably most people would benefit from taking a safe herbal laxative one day a week on average. Whenever taking an herbal laxative it should be combined with a smaller amount of a carminative such as ginger to prevent abdominal cramps. In addition to constipation, senna can be considered for a variety of other conditions, including fevers, intestinal parasites, skin eruptions, psoriasis and tumors, and topically as a wash or fomentation for burns. Generally, when taking one of the over-the-counter senna-based products, follow the instructions for dosing. We do not recommend the regular use of strong laxatives, including senna, as this can result in loss of important minerals such as potassium. Excessive use can cause diarrhea, intestinal cramps, rash, and severe weight loss.

Use senna for:

- constipation
- intestinal parasites

BLACK COHOSH (*CIMICIFUGA RACEMOSA*)

Black cohosh is popularly used for menopause symptoms. Traditional usage includes menstrual irregularities, diarrhea, fluid retention, and inflammation. It is also effective for rheumatic and arthritic conditions. In general it is contraindicated during pregnancy, especially during the first and second trimesters. It also should be used cautiously with drugs intended to lower blood pressure. Recommended dosage in capsules or tablets ranges from 50 to 500 mg.

Use black cohosh for:

- menstrual irregularities such as hot flashes
- menopause irregularities
- arthritis and rheumatic conditions

VALERIAN (*V. OFFICINALIS*)

Valerian is popularly used as a sedative, for insomnia and excitability. The dose ranges from 250 to 800 mg. Valerian should be avoided when taking alcohol, drugs that depress the nervous system or Antabuse. High doses of valerian, 2.5 g or more, at one time have been known to affect the liver adversely. Generally it is safe to use in recommended doses, and in any case is far safer than any of the pharmaceutical sedatives, which, unlike valerian, tend to be addictive over time.

Use valerian root for:

- insomnia
- nervousness

ALOE *(A. BARBADENSIS)*

Aloe is justly one of the most popular herbs for topically soothing and promoting the healing of burns, wounds, skin irritation, and itching. In addition, the commercially available gel is taken internally for promoting general health and in the treatment of stomach ulcers, diabetes, and colitis, to name only a few conditions. Recent research has found that aloe can alter the body's DNA, substantiating the claim that it may be good for the treatment of cancer. In India, liquid aloe preparations are used to help women maintain their attractiveness, suggesting that it may have female hormonal-enhancing properties. Follow the recommended dosage on the commercial products. In prescribed dosages, aloe is one of the safest of all herbs. However, some possible contraindications might be using aloe with digoxin (Lanoxin), drugs such as Bumes, Demadex, Edecrin, Lasix, and Sodium Edecrin that are known to cause potassium loss. Aloe should not be taken regularly if one is taking heart medication or steroids.

Use aloe:

- topically for burns, wounds, itching, skin irritation
- internally for ulcers, diabetes, colitis, cancer

ASTRAGALUS ROOT (A. MEMBRANACEUS)

Astragalus root is a traditional Chinese herb that improves energy and vitality with a very special benefit for the immune system. If one is prone to frequent colds and flus, astragalus will correct the problem better than any other herb. Constituents in astragalus (astragalan) have been found to have antiviral and anticancer properties. It is a specific herb used to offset the negative effects of chemo and radiation therapies. One of the ways it stimulates the immune system is by stimulating interferon, making it useful for all immune-deficiency diseases. Taken internally, astragalus alone, or together with reishi mushrooms, will increase one's ability to heal. Astragalus root seems to exert a beneficial effect on the cardiovascular system and in patients with angina and congestive heart failure. The unique properties of astragalus are that it increases vitality, improves digestion while at the same time having antipathogenic properties against bacteria and viruses. Astragalus also is used in ointments to induce wound healing and, finally, its seems to have aphrodisiac properties. Astragalus is quite safe and not unpleasant to the taste. It is a good idea to do as Chinese families do: have a pound on hand and throw a few slices into soups and when cooking rice. While there are no adverse effects in normal use, in general it should be used with caution when taking anticoagulant drugs such as coumadin, and with phenobarbital and beta blockers. It may also interact with decongestants given for colds, though from considerable experience this has not been a problem. Dose: for general use and for colds and flus, take 9 to 15 g in tea.

Use astragalus root for:

- immune deficiencies
- healing of wounds and injuries
- cancer and AIDS
- low energy
- weak digestion

VITEX *(VITEX AGNUS CASTUS;* ALSO CHASTEBERRY)

Vitex is the fruit of a large European shrub. It is primarily used for menstrual irregularities. Research has shown that it specifically regulates prolactin secretion from the pituitary gland and progesterone. The dose is from 20 to 40 mg two or three times daily or thirty to sixty drops of the 5:1 tincture twice daily. In general, it is very safe, with few reported side effects. It should be used with caution when undergoing hormone replacement therapies with drugs such as Premarin, Prempro, Premphase, Provera, etc. Animal experiments suggest that it may effect dopamine in the brain. Therefore, there may be possible interactions with compounds such as Haldol, L–Dopa, Parlodel, and Wellbutrin or Zyban.

Use vitex for:

- menstrual irregularities
- fibroids
- cysts of the ovaries and breasts
- menopausal irregularities

CHAMOMILE FLOWERS *(MATRICARIA RECUTITA)*

Chamomile flowers are, along with mint, one of the most popular herbal beverages in the western world. It is known as a calmative, and research has found that ingestion of chamomile acts as a wonderful mild sedative and antispasmodic. It is also known as "Band-Aid for the stomach," attesting to its positive effects for many digestive disorders. Finally, it can be used as an anti-inflammatory for skin diseases. Chamomile tea is effective for relieving menstrual cramps, especially if combined with ginger. There are a few varieties, but the one most commonly used is German or Hungarian chamomile. Dose: one teaspoon to a tablespoon steeped in a cup of water is the best way to take chamomile.

Use chamomile flowers for:

- gastrointestinal problems
- nervousness
- insomnia
- cramps and mild aches and pains
- colds and flus
- some skin irregularities

HAWTHORN (CRATAEGUS SPECIES)

Hawthorn is recognized in Germany for the treatment of mild heart failure. Traditionally the berries were used but, more recently, the leaf and the flowers have been shown to possess even greater heart benefit potency. In Chinese medicine, hawthorn berries are used to assist in the digestion of protein and fat, substantiating its anticholesterol properties. Hawthorn also has mild sedative properties and can lower blood pressure, relieve angina, and treat irregular heartbeat. Hawthorn is generally very safe, but in general one might be a little cautious if combining it with drugs that lower blood pressure and heart drugs called cardiac glycosides, such as digoxin and Lanoxin. Dose is approximately 510 mg of the berries in a capsule.

Use hawthorn berries, leaves and flowers for:

- heart irregularities
- high blood pressure
- elevated cholesterol
- digestive upset, especially from eating meat, fats, and oils
- nervousness and insomnia

CAYENNE PEPPER (CAPSICUM FRUTESCENS)

Cayenne pepper is a plant that originated in the New World but has been adopted as a common spice throughout the world. There are several subspecies that are mostly delineated in terms of their spiciness, ranging in a "hotness" scale from paprika (which is not hot) to 3,000 to 5,000 British Thermal Units (BTUs) for jalapeño to 50,000 BTUs for cayenne pepper, with the hottest habeneros at 200,000 to 300,000 BTUs. The species *C. annuum* is classified as cayenne and is often known as African bird pepper, and it is used both for spice and herbal medicine.

This is one of the most popular of all herbal remedies, along with other well-known herbs such as garlic and echinacea. In Africa it is eaten daily to both treat and prevent common colds and influenza. In North America, it is the main pillar of the popular nineteenth-century Thompsonian herbal medicine based on the work of maverick herbalist Samuel Thompson. There are many heirs to the Thompson legacy on both sides of the Atlantic. In the UK, the main proponent of Thompsonian herbalism and, of course, the heavy reliance on the use of cayenne for just about every evil to which the flesh is heir, was Dr. Coffin, who in the twentieth-century continued in the practice of the North American Eclectic and Physio-medicalist herbalists and such well-known exponents of Thomsonian herbalism (and of course the use of cayenne) as Dr. Raymond Christopher. In our own time Richard Schultes, a disciple of Dr. Christopher, is known as "Dr. Cayenne" because of his heavy reliance on this great common herb. While cayenne is rich in nutrients, especially vitamin C and carotenes, it is the capsaicin that accounts for its hotness and probably its primary therapeutic properties as a stimulant, anti-inflammatory and, most important, analgesic. It can be used topically in ointments and in creams for sprains, aches, and rheumatic complaints. It is also a treatment for shingles. Internally, paradoxically, it has been found to be effective for gastrointestinal ulcers, especially when taken fresh. It is also used to fight off the common cold and flu, to stimulate digestion, and even to relieve migraine headaches. Over-the-counter creams containing 0.025 percent capsaicin is prescribed for postherpetic neuralgia, diabetic neuropathy, and trigeminal neuralgia. A higher potency product is called Zostrix-HP. Recent research has found it a nasal spray effective for cluster headaches. Research at John Hopkins Hospital has found a nasal spray to be effective for asthma and the treatment of chronic runny nose. Cayenne is also an effective antihemorrhagic and, taken internally and/or applied externally, is very effective in stopping acute bleeding. Cayenne also will help to lower cholesterol and slow blood clotting. To attest to its safety, while it burns, cayenne is safe to use in equal parts with raspberry leaf, goldenseal, and eyebright for eye problems including cataracts and glaucoma (steep one teaspoon in a cup of hot water until cool, strain through a cloth, and use this tea to rinse the eyes twice a day).

Despite its safety and relative versatility as a therapeutic agent, in general if one doesn't want to experience temporary discomfort, cayenne should not be used on broken skin or in the eyes. Water is feebly effective for removing cayenne residue from the skin, so care must be exercised when handling cayenne that one not rub the eyes. For internal use a dose range from 30 to 120 mg can be taken three or more times daily. It is generally not used for people with irritable bowel syndrome or inflammation.

GINGER ROOT (ZINGIBER OFFICINALIS)

The primary active constituents are gingerols, shogaols, gingerdiones, and zingerone, which are responsible for its unique spicy flavor and aroma. It is excellent for counteracting nausea from many causes, such as for motion sickness and morning sickness of pregnant women. For seasickness, one study where the participants took 500 mg every four hours was as effective and better in many cases as the over-the-counter drug Dramamine. For motion sickness, one should begin taking ginger at least a half hour before departing and then repeat every two to four hours. In general, ginger taken with food will assist digestion and assimilation and increase appetite and saliva. It is also effective in preventing gas from beans and other gas-causing foods. It is a wonderful spice to add to heavy foods and desserts such as cake and ice cream or anytime it seems appropriate to increase the movement and assimilation of food through the GI tract. Ginger is also excellent at relieving pain from many causes, but especially spasmodic and "crampy" types of pains. For gastrointestinal cramps and menstrual cramps a strong tea of chamomile and ginger is very effective. Ginger tea taken alone or with honey is effective for treating mucus, coughs, and colds. Ginger is also known to lower cholesterol and keep the blood platelets from clumping. Ginger will increase significantly the absorption of nutrients, drugs, and anything with which it is taken. This is both a benefit and a cautious consideration when, for instance, taking barbiturates. Paradoxically, ginger promotes blood circulation, and despite its benefit when used moderately for morning sickness, in general it should be used with caution during pregnancy. It also is known to increase bile and acid secretion so that those with gallstones or gallbladder disease should also use it with caution. Because of its anticlotting properties, it should be used with caution with drugs such as coumadin, aspirin, Plavix, or Ticlid. Ginger is one of the safest of all herbs, with the dose ranging from 250 to 940 mg.

TURMERIC ROOT (CURCUMA LONGA)

Turmeric root is a condiment used especially in Indian cooking, but in other cultures as well. It is known to have effective anti-flammatory and pain-relieving properties. Like cayenne, turmeric seems to interfere with the transmission of pain reflex to the brain. It is very effective for a wide range of problems, including arthritic and rheumatic problems, digestive weakness, inflammations, and topically together with aloe and cayenne for the relief of various kinds of pains, including shingles. Turmeric is excellent alone or with other herbs for liver and gallbladder problems. However, it probably should not be used alone for gastritis, stomach ulcers, gallstones, or bile duct obstruction.

Use turmeric root for:

- inflammations
- arthritic and rheumatic conditions
- digestive problems

PARSLEY (PETROSELINUM SATIVUM)

Parsley is at the same time one of the most popular and most neglected herbs. Of course it is popular as a colorful garnish on food, and because of its slight bitter taste it is customarily thrown away by most gourmands. Too bad for them, for in many fat-laden dishes it may be the healthiest article on the plate. Medicinally, parsley has a history nearly as extensive as garlic. Its rich green color betokens its high chlorophyll content, which accounts for much of its therapeutic value. It is an antirheumatic, antiseptic, carminative, diuretic, expectorant, stone dissolver, nervine, stimulant, parasiticide, aperient (gentle laxative), antispasmodic, and tonic. It is one of the best remedies for urinary tract infections. The list could go on, but the greatest value of parsley has got to be its widespread fresh availability in produce markets throughout the country.

So why is it not used more frequently? The reason I think is a kind of snobbery, even unconsciously, among many alternative practitioners based in the fact that because it is so ubiquitous it is somehow beneath one's consideration. Whatever the reason, steeping a bunch of parsley leaves in two cups of water is one of the best kidney and urinary cleansing treatments. It inhibits the reabsorption of salt by the body tissues, which assists in its gentle diuretic action. It is three times higher in vitamin C than citrus juices, has a higher iron content than other leafy greens, and is also rich in potassium and other essential minerals. Parsley root is effective for chronic conditions of the urinary tract and the liver. The whole plant can be used for delayed menstruation (it probably should be avoided during pregnancy). It will help to dry mother's milk, making it useful when weaning a child. It prevents cancer, lowers blood pressure and is useful for asthma and other respiratory disease, and the list could go on. Its most common use, based on its high chlorophyll content, is to eliminate bad breath, smelly feet, and bad body odors. The full medicinal daily dose is the standard ounce in a pint of boiling water steeped for ten to twenty minutes.

Use parsley:

- for urinary tract infections
- for bad breath
- for body odors
- for nervine and calmative
- for digestive problems
- for respiratory tract imbalances

PART TWO

NATURAL

REMEDIES FOR

COMMON

AILMENTS

ABSCESSES

OTHER NAMES: Boil, carbuncle, cold abscess, dry abscess, felon, furuncle, whitlow.

DESCRIPTION: The term *abscess* is a general one used for a localized inflammation and accumulation of yellow, white, or green pus. Basically, an abscess is the body's way of isolating, fighting, and finally expelling an infection. Abscesses can form anywhere in or on the body, including on internal organs, but they are usually found just below the skin.

SYMPTOMS: An abscess usually produces localized tenderness, pain, heat, redness, and swelling; slight fever, headache, loss of appetite, and a general feeling of discomfort may also be present. A cold abscess is chronic, not simply coming to a head but giving off a discharge. A dry abscess disappears without pointing or breaking through the skin; it seems to be reabsorbed into the body's lymphatic system for elimination through other channels.

CAUSES: Abscesses may be brought on by the body's lowered resistance to infection, which may result from faulty metabolism and accumulated toxins, poor dietary or hygienic habits, lack of sleep, stress, polluted air, or suppressive medical treatments. The infection may enter through a wound or an abrasion of the skin, or even through a sweat gland or hair follicle.

TREATMENT: Powdered fenugreek or flaxseed poultices as external application are the best remedy to dissolve abscesses. They work slowly and painlessly but lastingly and thoroughly to eliminate the last bit of disease-produced matter. An onion baked until soft can be applied as hot as possible to help draw it to a head.

A so-called whitlow is a boil on the tip of a finger. One remedy is to bore a hole into a lemon and stick the affected finger into it. Similarly, a slice of lemon or lemon juice is effective when topically applied with a gauze bandage (see "Poultices" in Part Three). The effects are those of cooling, softening, dissolving, and extracting. Repeat two or three times a day until the abscess opens and drains. Rinse the wound with chamomile or calendula lotion or cold tea. Apply aloe gel over the wound.

Internally, a combination of the powders or echinacea root, goldenseal, garlic, and chaparral can be taken two or three times a day. Burdock and yellow dock root tea is also very effective to drink. Homeopathic hepar sulph 6th to 30th potency is specific for the healing of any infected, suppurating sores, boils, or abscesses. The cell salts calcium sulph or silicea are both effective for this condition and should be taken in 3rd to 12th potency every hour until symptoms begin to subside, tapering off gradually.

For acute abscesses, Planetary formula Echinacea and formula number 48 (Echinacea, Goldenseal and Olive Leaf Formula) are appropriate and should be taken four times a day for a week or two as needed.

Abscesses that are recurring and chronic can be caused by a deficiency, in which case one may need to use tonic herbs such as astragalus root or the Planetary formula number 84 (Women's Dong Quai Tonifier), which despite its name is a tonic suitable for both men and women.

ACNE

DESCRIPTION: Acne is a disease of the skin. It is quite often though not always associated with adolescence.

CAUSES: Usually it is caused by some form of kidney, liver, or bowel congestion, and digestive problems. Acne can also be caused by a hormone imbalance during puberty during which an increase in testosterone in boys causes a thickness of the skin and an increased secretion of melanin which deepens pigment. It also increases the rate of secretion by the sebaceous glands of the face resulting in acne. Thus herbs that aid general elimination and detoxification through the liver and intestines and increase perspiration through the skin are very useful in the treatment of acne.

TREATMENT: Acne usually responds very well to diet and herbal treatment. One should avoid fried foods, heavily spiced or salted foods, sugar, white flour and pastries, acid foods and drinks. The diet should be the balanced macrodiet of whole grains, legumes, beans, steamed vegetables, a little organic fish or poultry, and nonacidic seasonal fruits in moderation.

External treatment used by traditional Japanese healers is to apply therapeutic cupping and/or moxibustion over the navel.

Planetary formulas that are effective for acne are formulas number 99 (Yellow Dock Skin Cleanser), number

66 (Red Clover Cleanser), and number 89 (Triphala). These can be taken separately or together.

Nutritional supplements that are effective for treating acne are the following:

- mycelized vitamin A: Apply a dropperful topically at bedtime each day until the condition is improved. When improvement is noticed, apply it once every other day. Be aware when doing this of possible increased sun sensitivity.
- A good multivitamin formula that contains therapeutic levels of zinc, vitamin E, vitamin C, selenium, folic acid, B_6, chromium, and other nutrients.
- Acidophilus and bifidus alternated each day in half-teaspoon doses three times daily.

A Chinese patent that one can use for acne and other skin diseases, including psoriasis, eczema, urticaria, and boils, is Ledebouriella Sagely Unblocks Tea Pills (Fang Feng Tong Sheng Wan).

Another alternative is to make a tea consisting of equal parts of the following: sassafras root bark, sarsaparilla root, burdock root, yellow dock, dandelion root, and red clover. Simmer one ounce in a pint of boiling water for fifteen minutes and take three cups daily.

ADDICTIONS

DESCRIPTION AND SYMPTOMS: People can develop addictions to many things. An addiction is any substance or experience that is repeatedly craved which harms us. Thus, there is a strong mental and emotional aspect to all addictions and for some this takes precedence over the biological aspect. Most specifically we will address the issues of sugar, alcohol, coffee, tobacco, and drug addictions, which are the most common forms.

TREATMENT: What is it about sugar that creates such a strong addictive craving in some people? Sugar is the underlying basis for most addictions. First, sugar is the essence of food energy in the body. In humans, mother's milk is very sweet and contains more sugar than cow's or goat's milk.

Many individuals whose work involves a considerable amount of mental activity seem to crave more sweet foods. One reason is that the process of thinking consumes a lot of energy. The more mental one is, the more the need for sugar. Many individuals satisfy this need for the use of sugar by increasing their consumption of fresh or dried fruits.

In traditional herbalism, all wholesome foods including carbohydrate and protein foods are considered sweet in flavor. We can interpret that a lack in either good-quality complex carbohydrates or protein will create a nutritional debt so that one craves more intense and concentrated sweets in the form of sugar.

Most commercial foods contain sugar. The manufacturers know that this makes their foods more appealing and the possible addictive aspect will certainly not hurt business. There are many types of sugars but white sugar is by far the most harmful in that it lacks all the subsidiary rich minerals and nutrients that are normally associated with whole sugar cane.

Whole sugar cane is a very wholesome and nutritious food. However, when it is processed, the high amounts of iron, calcium, and other nutrients and minerals normally found in the pure unprocessed sugar cane juice are removed. In order for the body to utilize white sugar, it must use up some of its innate stores of these essential nutrients. Thus there is a nutritional debt that is created that causes a severe craving for stronger sweet foods that contain sugar.

To overcome the problem, one will have to be patient and begin by using only pure, whole sugar such as succanat, honey, maple syrup, and dried fruits for sweetening. Eventually these will also be limited. But the most important thing is that one establish a diet based upon 50% to 70% whole grains, 20% to 30% beans, legumes, and perhaps a little organic animal protein, and 10% to 20% steamed vegetables. If there is a sweet craving, take some baked or stewed fruits, a baked apple, applesauce, or stewed figs. One should eliminate all refined sugar since consuming even the smallest amount will set up an immediate craving for more.

The emotional basis underlying the need for sugar is a need for inner satisfaction and love that is not being found in daily life. Attempting to understand that there may be such inner needs and then finding more affirming ways to meet them through supportive and positive contact with others is the approach to overcoming the emotional addiction to sugar.

Alcohol addiction can be another form of sugar addiction. Perhaps this is one reason that individuals who go through an alcohol withdrawal program substitute their craving for alcohol, at least in the beginning, with a craving for sugar.

The treatment for recovering from alcohol addiction is, of course, to abstain from alcohol and then to try to create a more wholesome life-style and diet. Herbal treatment is a combination of the following: 1 ounce Labrador tea (leaves), 1 ounce angelica root, 1 ounce scullcap herb. Simmer in three cups of boiling water for ten minutes and strain. If it is available, add five drops of tincture of oak bark to each cup of hot tea (the alcohol will evaporate out) and take one cup before each meal. When Labrador tea is unavailable, simply use angelica, skullcap, and oak bark tincture. Skullcap tea is very effective in overcoming any of the side effects of alcohol withdrawal such as delirium tremens. In addition to the use of these herbs, consider including formula number 12 for the liver.

On the emotional level, alcoholics have a problem facing up to important issues in their lives. Thus, they drown their feelings in alcohol.

Coffee is often not thought of as an addiction but it actually fits the criterion of the definition quite nicely: a substance that is craved that is known to be harmful. Coffee is a pure adrenal stimulant. It robs our body's innate stores of energy but gives nothing in return. The result is that overconsumption of coffee creates physiological imbalances that lead to urinary and neurological disorders, hypertension, skin problems, prostate problems, headaches, and cravings for sweets and sugars because of the body's desperate need to replace the energy that has been lost from the caffeine stimulation of the coffee.

Do not be deceived that it is only the caffeine in coffee that is harmful. Coffee is very acidic and just as much as the caffeine, the acid nature of coffee can equally cause biological imbalances.

The cure for coffee addiction is to stop using it. Frequently one of the complaints of coffee withdrawal is a severe headache and a lack of mental clarity. A combination of the powders of gotu kola, calamus root, skullcap herb, and rosemary taken in 00-size capsules about four times a day will help clear and relieve the headache.

For one who is not already addicted, an occasional cup of coffee to help remain alert while driving a long distance is not a big problem. However, for essential health reasons, coffee should not be consumed on a regular daily basis. As an alternative, try substituting roasted dandelion root tea, which has the additional positive benefit of being good for the liver and stomach. Another possibility is to use one of the many roasted grain beverages that are currently available.

Addiction to tobacco is one of the most difficult to overcome. It has been scientifically established that tobacco is a definite and primary cause of lung cancer and, like alcohol, it also causes birth defects. Certainly anything that affects our lungs and breathing ultimately affects the very source of our vitality.

Tobacco addiction represents the ever-present need for positive energy. The effect of tobacco is a momentary feeling of satisfaction and clarity; that is why the Native Americans used it in their prayer pipes. However, since its effects wear off quite fast, we need another tobacco fix to reinstate our sense of well-being.

The need for tobacco represents many unfulfilled emotional needs including anxiety, boredom, depression, and loneliness. This is one of the reasons that tobacco addiction is so difficult to overcome. While the actual physical craving can be overpowering to some, the emotional investment involved with smoking has to be supplanted with other, more positive endeavors.

One should consider taking up some other physical activity—sports, exercise, yoga, or something that requires a full breathing capacity and is therefore incongruous with smoking. Ear acupuncture can be very effective. Again, for those who have no ready access to an acupuncturist, try using the mustard seed and bandage method over the area associated with the spirit gate, lung, and addictive areas of the ear. Whenever there is a need to smoke, simply massage the tape with the mustard seed to help overcome the craving.

Herbs to help quit smoking should include formula number 1 for the lungs. This should be taken three times daily. Formula number 1 is not only good to help quit smoking but it is also good to help protect and cleanse the lungs of smokers who are not yet ready to quit.

In addition, take a combination of 500 mg of Chinese or Korean ginseng and 50 mg of calamus root every two hours the first three or four days of withdrawal and then gradually taper down. Ginseng is an herb that increases positive energy (its use should not be abused, however), while calamus root is used in India to enhance mental clarity. After a week or two, the actual physical craving for tobacco may be overcome but dealing with emotional cravings and how to handle all the extra time one has without having to smoke becomes a more obvious problem.

Drug addition includes using illegal drugs such as cocaine, heroin, marijuana, and others, as well as legal drugs and sedatives that individuals are able to obtain from medical doctors for the purposes of relieving pain, insomnia, or nervousness.

First, it is very important for the individual to face up to the possible damage and disastrous consequences of any of these addictions.

Second, it is necessary to establish a generally more wholesome life-style so that the need for drugs is considerably less.

After adopting these attitudes, one will find a number of therapies effective for overcoming addiction. Diet, herbs, and acupuncture are all effective in helping lessen the symptoms of withdrawal and the cravings associated with all addictions. However, one may do better if at all possible to seek professional assistance.

A good detoxification tea that will also alleviate and shorten the symptoms of withdrawal is as follows: Combine equal parts burdock root, red clover, dandelion root, skullcap with a quarter part licorice (optional), and 3 slices of fresh ginger. Simmer an ounce of all the herbs in 3 cups of water, except the ginger, for 20 minutes. Add the ginger slices at the end to cool. Take a cup three times daily. This is an excellent herbal detoxification formula. Recommended Planetary formulas include the blood-purifying formula number 66 (Red Clover Cleanser) and the nervine formula number 84 (Stress Free).

AGING

DESCRIPTION: Because aging is not a disease, what we must consider here are two things: the kinds of conditions one is likely to develop as one ages, and premature aging.

CONDITIONS ONE IS LIKELY TO DEVELOP AS A RESULT OF AGING: Many of the conditions that were a minor nuisance when we were younger tend to be exacerbated with age. In general, one's essential body fluids tend to dry up and diminish with age; this includes reproductive fluids, skin moisture, secretions of the endocrine system (hormones), as well as basic secretions such as lubrication of the joints. The result of this can be a number of complaints ranging from sexual dysfunction and arthritic conditions to skin wrinkling and itchiness. Hormonal dysfunctions characteristically affect men and women differently, depending on what hormones are involved.

Men and Aging

For men, the diminishing of testosterone levels brings with it a corresponding reduction (though not necessarily elimination) of their sex drive. At the same time as the prostate tends to enlarge, the onset of BPH (benign prostatic hypertrophy) can occur, causing a variety of urinary problems; i.e., too frequent, not enough, and in advanced cases, pain, etc.

Appropriate exercise and rest is important for managing male hormone shifts and possible prostate enlargement. The prostate gland is located directly behind the scrotum and can be felt through the anus. Direct massaging of this area is helpful. Further, performing regular Kegel type exercise each day, where one repeatedly contracts the spincter muscles of the anus, similar to the motion of trying to stop and start urination midstream, repeated several times in succession throughout the day, is a very effective treatment for maintaining prostate health.

In addition, there are a number of herbs and foods that are particularly helpful for male prostrate problems. The known action of foods and herbs that relieve BPH is to prevent the formation of testosterone in dihydrotestosterone in the prostrate gland. One of the simplest treatments to help maintain prostate health is to eat a few tablespoons of pumpkin seeds (Cucurbita pepo) each day. Taking supplemental zinc is also very helpful for reducing the size of the prostate gland.

A number of herbs have been found to be as effective as pharmaceutical drugs and offer a more natural alternative. Among these are saw palmetto berries *(Serenoa repens)*, pygeum *(Pygeum africanum)*, and the root of the stinging nettles *(Urtica dioica)*.

Planetary formula number 72 (Saw Palmetto Classic) contains all the herbs described above, along with others in a synergistically balanced formulation to alleviate symptoms of BPH in men.

Wulingshen (Xylaria Fungus)

My recent favorite is a Chinese herb that has been called Wulingshen and is also sometimes known as Wuling ginseng. This herb is not even remotely related to ginseng but is a fungus that grows in a discarded white ant terminary. It is popularly regarded as a ginseng for the hormonal system because of its broad adaptogenic or immune tonic benefits, increasing vitality while at the same time inducing a calm, restful state and broadly treating a number of symptoms associated with hormonal imbalances.

While useful for all ages, this herb is like a panacea for all aging imbalances.

Immune system and anticancer activity: It increases the immune system by increasing white blood cells. At the same time it increases the cytotoxic action of macrophages in destroying tumor cells by stimulating the production of lymphokine interleukin.

Anti-anemia function: It is effective in increasing red blood cells and thus counteracts anemia.

Sedative, sleep-enhancing, and memory-enhancing properties: It is a mild sedative and promotes patterns of sound, restful sleep. In conjunction with this it has a unique brain protective action, enhancing memory and alleviating depression.

Antifatigue: Like ginseng it increases energy and counteracts stress, as demonstrated in a number of animal studies.

Antisenility action: Studies on the fruit fly have shown that it significantly increased the lifespan of the female fruit fly.

Urine output and frequency: It increased the urinary output of rats some 140 percent, and in humans this means better urinary output and ultimately less frequent urges. It also enhanced urea-nitrogen filtration, thus aiding overall detoxification.

Wulingshen has been proven in a number of studies conducted by the manufacturer in China to be effective for a wide range of hormone-related problems in both men and women. Studies on men involving BPH have found it to be over 90 percent effective in reducing prostate size and regulating urine flow. Similarly, for women, it has been found to be highly effective for regulating menstruation through all ages as well as the symptoms leading up to and occurring during menopause.

At the time of this writing, this herb is available solely from China and is also available directly from Planetherbs (www.planetherbs.com).

Women and Aging

For women, the entire phase of perimenopause, menopause, and postmenopause have their own considerations and problems. With women, after puberty and the onset of menstruation (which can occur anywhere from the ages of twelve to fourteen for most girls), the next important change is when menstruation ceases. Again, this is variable and can range from mid-forties to age sixty in some.

There is a wide variation as to how women experience the change. For some it is hardly noticed, while others experience a wide range of uncomfortable symptoms as their hormones decrease.

The precise definition of menopause is the period beginning one year after the monthly cycle has stopped. However, the period leading up to menopause (perimenopause) can go on for years before there is a noticeable stopping of menstruation. There are a wide variety of symptoms that occur throughout this period, ranging from hot flashes, difficulty sleeping, poor memory, mood changes, headaches, vaginal dryness, and night sweats. These symptoms can go on for weeks or years depending on individual differences.

To alleviate symptoms, doctors can offer hormone replacement therapy (HRT) as a temporary solution. This usually involves taking supplemental estrogen and/or progesterone. Estrogen replacement is controversial and has been associated with an increased risk of breast cancer, so alternatives in the form of estrogenic food and herbs are a welcome alternative to what for some women is a difficult dilemma.

The first recommendation that is good for both sexes is to maintain a good, regular exercise program. Isoflavones can be an important key to the regulation of hormones. These are compounds found in some herbs and foods that are able to occupy the hormone receptor sites in the body and either block hormone absorption if it is too much or enable it by converting to the needed hormone when it is too little.

Vitamin E at the dose of 800 IUs daily, bioflavonoids, and Vitamin C have been recognized by a number of women over decades to be effective in relieving hot flashes and other menopausal symptoms. These positive experiences have been confirmed by a number of studies.

Of course Vitamin E, the anti-aging vitamin, is specifically good for coronary health as well.

A number of herbs have been found to be effective for the years leading up to and during menopause. Black cohosh *(Cimicifuga racemosa)* was used by Native American women, immigrant European women, and in the famous Lydia E. Pinkham's Vegetable Compound for "women's problems."

Recent studies in Germany have confirmed the estrogenic activity of black cohosh. It has been found to reduce the symptoms of hot flashes and uncomfortable vaginal dryness associated with decreased estrogen.

Chastetree berry, or vitex *(Vitex agnus-castus),* is a well-known European herb that is used for normalizing female sex hormones. It has particular benefits in helping normalize both progesterone and estrogen levels and alleviating all menstrual irregularities including depression associated with premenstrual syndrome and the menopausal years.

Red clover *(Trifolium pratense)* is related to the pea and bean family, and like its relative, the soybean, is high in potent isoflavones and will naturally increase estrogen. At the same time, red clover is one of a number of herbs that has been found to have anticancer properties. Both the flowers and the attached leaves are used. Simmer an ounce of red clover in a pint of water and take one or two cups daily. Red clover also possesses effective blood-thinning components so that those who are already taking blood thinners, or are at risk for bleeding, should not use it. In general, it is a good idea to use a single herb like red clover for no more than two weeks at a time, then pause for a week or so before resuming.

Dong quai *(Angelica sinensis)* is commonly used in traditional Chinese medicine as a blood tonic for women and to help regulate menstruation. It works by promoting circulation through the uterine cavity and thus enhancing all related functions.

Planetary Herb formula number 56 (MenoChange [Cimicifuga-Vitex] Compound) is particularly useful for menopause support. It contains black cohosh, vitex, dong quai, and wild yam and is a carefully balanced formula with a variety of other herbs to alleviate uncomfortable symptoms including hot flashes associated with menopause. (See the section on gynecology).

While decreasing hormones is one of the most noticeable causes of aging in both men and women, there are other symptoms and tendencies as well. In both sexes, but more so in women, thyroid function slows with age, and the associated slower metabolism of food often results in weight gain. There is a greater risk of cardiovascular disease and osteoporosis. Another common complaint associated with aging is arthritic and rheumatic problems. Check under the corresponding topics for natural remedies for these problems.

Premature Aging

Premature aging generally refers to symptoms of aging such as wrinkling and drying skin, brittle bones, gray hair, and loss of sexual desire one gets in their thirties or early forties. There is certainly a strong genetic influence here, but life-style can make a tremendous difference in when and how one ages.

It cannot be overstressed how any longevity program must be based on a balanced program of moderate exercise, wholesome diet, clean air, restful sleep, and lessening stress.

Importance of Exercise

While an excess of aerobic or strenuous exercise will actually compromise longevity, a moderate program of twenty to forty-five minutes once daily or at least three times a week is highly beneficial. The most beneficial forms of exercise are those that combine mind and body together and involve maintaining flexibility. These include Asian practices such as yoga, tai chi, and qi gong. These combine physical postures with mental focus directing one's energy to specific areas of the body. By so doing one achieves the maximum amount of circulation with the minimum loss of vital energy. There are literally thousands of different postures so that anyone with virtually any physical handicap can, with guidance, develop a practice that will optimize their circulation and vitality.

Free Radicals

Free radicals are implicated in aging and all chronic degenerative diseases. A free radical occurs when one of the paired electrons circling the nucleus of an atom is thrown off. This leaves the atom in an unstable condition, and the free radical electron continues to seek other electrons from nearby molecules at the rate of billions per second, causing further free radical damage and molecular instability. Thus a chain reaction of cell-damaging free radicals occurs, adversely affecting various cells and parts of the body.

While free radicals are the quintessential toxins of the body, they are nevertheless formed as a natural by-product of normal bodily metabolism of air and food. They are also formed as a result of physiological and emotional stress. Some of the causes of free radicals are environmental toxins including air pollution, cigarette smoke, inhaled fumes, automobile exhaust, smog, radiation, overexposure to sunlight, X rays, environmental chemicals, petrochemicals, asbestos, alcohol, cured meats, chemotherapy, pharmaceutical drugs, and chemotherapy, and the list could go on and on.

Nor are free radicals all bad. For instance, one of the ways our immune system attacks and kills bacteria, viruses, and other toxic substances is for our white blood cells to seek out and attack these particles with an oxidative burst.

While oxygen is necessary to sustain life, to a certain extent, oxygen from the air we breathe will cause free radicals to form. Just as exposure to oxygen will eventually cause iron to rust, fats to turn rancid, rubber to lose its elasticity, and paper to turn brown, all cells of all plants and animals, according to Dr. William Pryer, a researcher at Louisiana State University, "show a continuous level of oxidative damage" (Anderson, et al. 1996).

So what are some of the ways free-radical damage is implicated in the process of aging? First, free radicals tend to target molecules such as proteins. This includes collagen and elastin, which keep our skin soft and pliable and free of wrinkles. Because proteins are part of the immune system, free radicals lower our resistance to disease. Proteins are also part of the hormones of the body, so free radicals will adversely affect them as well. Free radicals also attack fatty acids or lipids and contribute to cardiovascular disease. The absorption of nutrients at the cellular level is compromised because free radicals damage lysosomes, which are enzymes necessary for the assimilation of cellular nutrients. The result is low energy.

Finally, the brain is affected because by consuming 20 percent of the oxygen in a resting state and more during exercise, it is exposed to ten times the amount of free radicals compared to any other part of the body. Thus, with age, we have symptoms of diminished mental capacity, memory loss, and dementia.

The extent and severity of free-radical damage depends on one's genetic makeup, current health status, nutrition, and stress level. The body has its own innate ability to counteract free radicals through the production of glutathione, which is one of the most powerful antioxidants. In addition, fresh fruits and vegetables are high in a variety of free-radical–fighting antioxidants.

There are also a number of vitamins, minerals, herbs, and food supplements that are known to serve as powerful antioxidants. Among these are vitamins A, C, E, and the mineral selenium. In addition, the flavonoids found in vegetables, berries, citrus fruits, and herbs such as amla fruit *(Emblica officinalis)* from India all possess powerful free-radical–fighting antioxidants. Many herbs are high in flavonoids, including ginkgo biloba, astragalus, hawthorn, green tea, and turmeric, to name a few. Other powerful antioxidants include pycnogenol from grape seed and pine bark, coenzyme Q10, lipoic acid, and N-acetyl cysteine (NAC).

It has been found that a deficiency of the mineral selenium is directly implicated in statistically significant higher incidences of cancer. One study is that of Dr. R. J. Shamberger of the Cleveland Clinic, who found in 1969 that the lowest incidence of cancer in the United States occurs in Rapid City, South Dakota, which in turn has the highest amount of selenium in the soil. In Lima, Ohio, residents have twice the normal cancer rates, compared with those in Rapid City, with blood selenium at approximately 60%. A similar relationship between selenium and cardiovascular disease was also evident in this study. In Venezuela, where the amount of selenium in the soil is high, the death rate from large intestine cancer was only 3.06% while in the United States the rate is 13.69%. As part of their traditional diet, the Japanese are known to consume a high amount of selenium. Lung cancer in Japan is at 72.65 per 100,000 compared to 136.86 per 100,000 in the United States.

Obviously, to offset the negative effects of aging, one should be taking a generous amount of fruits and vegetables, a good multivitamin with additional vitamins E and C (up to 2,000 mg daily), and an all-purpose antioxidant formula containing lipoic acid, pycnogenol, and N-acetylcysteine.

Tonic Herbs and Herbal Formulas

Asian tonic herbs have been known for thousands of years to play an important role in promoting longevity. Following are a number of them that are highly efficacious.

Ginseng (*Panax* species) is the most esteemed herb for promoting longevity. There are two main types; Chinese ginseng (*Panax* ginseng) and American ginseng *(Panax quinquefolium)*. The difference between the two is that the American ginseng is more bitter and therefore more cooling and anti-inflammatory than the Asian species. American ginseng nurtures the blood and fluids more, while the Asian species increases vital energy. Both work by enhancing intracellular energy by increasing mitochondria replication. Ginseng is recommended whenever there is low energy, weak digestion or metabolism, and low libido in anyone of any age. However, since these are sure to be an increasing issue with age, it can be taken in a small amount daily after a man has turned fifty. The Korean red ginseng is warmer and more invigorating. It is specially steamed to enhance its properties and to prevent insect infestation. American ginseng is recommended if one is prone to high stress and nervousness, and for women. Either can be used for any condition caused by internal weakness and deficiency. Dosage on a daily basis can be anywhere from 6 g once daily as a maintenance dose or more if there is a specific indication. Siberian ginseng (*Eleutherococus senticosus*), while in the ginseng family, is distinctly different and not as strong. It is used to increase stamina and vitality, but it is not as regenerating as Chinese or American ginseng. *Codonopsis pilosula* (Dang shen) is not a *Panax* at all but is recognized as having the same properties as the more expensive ginseng but about half the strength. It is commonly substituted for *Panax* species in formulas if the practitioner deems that the more expensive variety may not be needed.

As with herbs generally, taking an herb like ginseng has a broader effect than if one were to take it by itself. Planetary formulas numbers 38 (Ginseng Classic) and 39 (Ginseng Elixir) are based on ancient traditional formulations. Formula number 40 (Ginseng Revitalizer) combines five different types of ginseng with other tonic herbs, including astragalus root, poria mushroom, atractylodes, and dong quai to enhance its action.

SPECIAL TRADITIONAL CHINESE GINSENG THERAPY: My first Chinese herb teacher made it his lucrative specialty to administer the finest-quality ginseng according to the following protocol. He had people in high places coming to him from all parts of California for this treatment. They claimed the most incredible vitalizing and rejuvenating effects. Michael and his wife were visiting a

Chinese pharmacy in San Francisco and we began to speak of this protocol, which began with a special detoxifying diet and herbal formula before taking ginseng. Suddenly we had five older Chinese people all around us confirming that indeed this was the most efficacious way of deriving the most benefit from ginseng.

My teacher used this as an approach for a wide number of degenerative conditions associated with aging. One younger person in his mid-forties claimed that after following this protocol he had so much energy that he was able to drive clear across the country nonstop in three days.

The principle is to first clean excess dampness and stagnation from the body and tonify the vital "yin" fluids with herbs before taking a single high dose of top-quality ginseng. By top-quality we are talking about a range of single ginseng roots that must be purchased from a reliable supplier and may range in cost from several hundreds to several thousands of dollars. Therefore, of necessity, this therapy was reserved for the wealthiest.

The protocol consists of a weeklong detoxification diet, avoiding all fried foods and excess fat, and taking a formula called Liu Wei Di Huang or Rehmannia Six prior to taking a high dose of the best quality ginseng. The formula is available in a slightly modified form as Formula number 67 (Rehmannia Endurance). On the seventh day an entire root of the finest quality Chinese ginseng was carefully decocted in a special covered Chinese ceramic ginseng pot using about two cups of water. The covered ceramic ginseng container is placed in a pot of water and allowed to simmer on a low flame for up to two hours. It is carefully strained, and the resulting tea is taken in one or two doses the same day.

If such a high-quality ginseng root is unavailable, one can use the entire ninety tablets of Planetary formula ginseng dissolved in two cups of boiling water and lightly simmered or kept warm over two hours.

I recommend consuming the dregs after drinking the ginseng if at all possible.

Astragalus root *(huang qi)* is a famous Chinese herb highly esteemed throughout the world as one of the most powerful herbs for the immune system. While it can be used by people of all ages, it is very useful with advancing years as the immune system tends to diminish, making one more prone to infectious diseases. Chinese people frequently cook about 9 g of sweetish-tasting root to make soup stock in which other vegetables, meat, or rice is cooked. This method of using tonic herbs such as ginseng, codonopsis, astragalus, lycii berries, and others in soup taken with food is one of the best ways to take these important herbs. The most famous traditional astragalus formula available is Jade Screen Combination, Planetary's formula number 24. It is phenomenally effective at protecting the body from infectious diseases, especially those of the upper respiratory tract.

Lycii berries *(gay gee)* are sometimes called "red raisins" by Chinese people, who will stock them in the cupboard to add to soups and other special dishes both for their flavor and for their tremendous health benefits. They are extremely high in betacarotene, making them both powerful antioxidants and good for the eyes and blood generally. They are delicious cooked with cereal in the morning. They also act as an aphrodisiac.

Reishi mushroom *(Ganodermum lucidum)* is, along with astragalus, one of the most powerful herbs known for helping the immune system. Because it is very hard and mildly bitter, it doesn't lend itself readily to being cooked with our favorite dishes. However, about 15 g each of reishi mushroom and astragalus cooked in a quart and a half of water, slowly down to a half quart, makes a not unpleasant tea for the immune system. It is excellent for the treatment of cancer and other serious diseases. One of the most effective immune-building formulas is Planetary formula number 43 (Reishi Mushroom Supreme), which combines reishi mushroom, astragalus, and other herbs known to strengthen and support the immune system.

Hou shou wou (Polygonum multiflorum) is a well-known herb that tonifies blood and will counteract anemic tendencies for anyone, but it is especially useful for the aged. It has a long-standing reputation as a longevity herb and has been reputed to restore normal hair color for those who are prematurely gray. The daily dose, which can be divided into portions, is about 9 g cooked into a tea or taken as a liquid or as a dry extract. A wonderful Chinese patent available from Chinese herbal medicine suppliers is Shou Wu Chich, which is a wine made with hou shou wou and other blood tonic Chinese herbs. It is excellent for making the skin and hair more youthfully lustrous and soft.

Deer antler velvet consists of the antler of the young sika red deer. They are generally raised on farms in the midwestern United States or in New Zealand. The finest quality is carefully harvested from the deer under supervision of a veterinarian to protect the deer from unnecessary suffering and cruelty. Used for over two thousand years, since the time of Confucius in China, for coldness, low metabolism, prevention of osteoporosis, diminished endrocrine production, low libido, and symptoms of menopause, deer antler velvet contains phosphor, glyco-lipids, collagen, and glycoaminoglycans necessary for health. They also have a specific growth factor that is particularly good for the bones and joints. It is commonly used by older people for the treatment of arthritis. Plane-tary formula number 73 (Schizandra Adrenal Complex) has herbs that are specific for the endocrine system's sympathetic and parasympathetic systems. Formula number 67 (Rehmannia Endurance) works more on the sympathetic nervous system, while formula 68 (Rehmannia Vitalizer) has a greater affinity for the sympathetic nervous system. These last two formulas are powerful core formulas and can be taken together. Depending on what endrocrine system one needs to focus more on, one would take two tablets of formula 67 (Rehmannia Endurance) with one formula 68 (Rehmannia Vitalizer) for the parasympathetic nervous system, or two formula 68 with one formula 67 for the sympathetic nervous system, two times daily. To better focus the effects of these tonics, one should take them with warm water to which is added a teaspoon of soy sauce or a pinch of salt. These formulas are good for all illnesses caused by aging and general decrepitude. They will relieve chronic back pain, tiredness, general joint and knee pains, bone weakness, low libido, diabetes, and many other conditions commonly associated with the aging process.

From ancient India a number of tonics are popularly used.

Chyavanprash comes in a delicious paste with approximately fifty herbs in a base of honey, ghee, and raw sugar. Fifty percent of the formula consists of amla fruit. This is one of the most nutrient-dense herbal foods on the planet. It is one of the highest known sources of easily available vitamin C, which comes in a form that is impervious to aging and high heat. This, along with other nutrients in amla, serve as powerful antioxidants against free radicals, known to be the major cause of aging and all degenerative diseases.

Amla is also available in the internal cleansing formula called Triphala. Triphala consists of three related fruits: *Emblic officinalis* (amla), *Terminalia belerica,* and *Terminalia chebula.* Triphala is arguably the greatest of all herbal formulas because it promotes detoxification while not causing any depletion or weakness of vital reserves. It is good for poor digestion, constipation, liver problems, and toxicity and lowers blood lipids and therefore is good for cardiovascular health. It can and should be given on a regular basis weekly or more often to people of all ages.

Guggul is a special type of myrrh resin secreted by certain umbelliferae plants. It is prized in Ayurvedic medicine as a circulatory stimulant that has the ability to raise body metabolism, counteract low thyroid conditions, and lower cholesterol and triglycerides in the blood. This last property makes it especially useful for cardiovascular conditions. It is also used for the increasing stiffness associated with aging. Planetary's Guggul Cholesterol Compound is the traditional Ayurvedic formulation consisting of a number of herbs including triphala that complement as the primary botanical substance. This formula can be considered a special food for the circulatory system.

Ashwagandha *(Withania somnifera)* is also known as "Indian ginseng" because it comes from India. It has adaptogenic properties (helping one to cope with stressful conditions) similar to ginseng, with the difference that it helps to induce a calmer state, thus the term *somnifera,* meaning "to induce sleep." Despite its name, ashwagandha can be taken mornings and evenings along with boiled warm milk for all deficiency, low-energy conditions. It is especially used by older people who wish to increase their vitality. Taken with boiled warm milk, perhaps with the addition of a little honey, the two act synergistically to enhance the tonic effect. Ashwagandha is available from Planetary formulas.

Garlic *(Allium sativum),* as the most popular herb of Mediterranean countries such as Italy, hardly needs any introduction. It is a near-panacea, said to be effective for all diseases except the one it causes (bad breath). Garlic has a wide range of uses for conditions associated with aging. Some of these are circulatory problems, digestive problems, cardiovascular diseases, respiratory diseases, arthritic conditions, and it has antibiotic and antiviral properties. Raw garlic is far more effective for all of these conditions than its cooked counterpart. This is because both aliin and allicin, considered to be the most active constituents of garlic, are destroyed by high heat. They can also be destroyed by stomach acid, so Planetary's enteric-coated garlic tablets are specifically standardized to contain 6,000 mcg of allicin in each tablet, thus preserving the time-proven benefit of this great Mediterranean herb.

AIDS/ARC

DESCRIPTION AND SYMPTOMS: AIDS is a disease of the autoimmune system. One of the viruses commonly associated with this disease is called Human Immunodeficiency Virus (HIV). AIDS or Acquired Immune Deficiency Syndrome is a disease whereby the body can become infected with many different viruses and bacteria that weaken its resistance and eventually expose it to a variety of deadly volunteer infections. ARC is an AIDS-Related Complex also associated with individuals who have tested HIV positive. The symptom complex includes weight loss, fevers, night sweats, diarrhea, and lymph node swelling. ARC is often a preliminary condition leading to AIDS.

CAUSES: Immune resistance is generated by the cell-mediated immune system and the humoral immune system. Both originate from stem cells produced in the bone marrow. Some of the stem cells travel to the thymus gland and become T cells; others are processed in other parts of the body and are called B cells. B cells participate in the more superficial aspects of immunity, involving the lymphatic system, spleen, GI tract, and bone marrow.

T cells specifically are involved with cell-mediated immunity. The particular action of the AIDs virus is to invade and destroy T cells and thus leave the body open to volunteer infections.

AIDS seems to be contracted through direct exposure to blood and possibly other body fluids. Thus male homosexuals who participate in unprotected anal intercourse where there may be a danger of bleeding and damage to the tissues, along with hard-drug users who share hypodermic needles, are at high risk. Individuals who may have accidentally been given a blood transfusion containing HIV virus are also at high risk.

TREATMENT: According to Dr. Richard Bagley in his book *Healing AIDS Naturally,* all long-term survivors are devotees of natural therapies. These include diet and herbal therapy, other vitamin and mineral supplements, exercise, and the development of positive thought patterns. In fact, it can be demonstrated that when any of these factors are lacking, the result more or less is the suppression of the immune system.

Certain herbs are particularly effective in maintaining and stimulating the immune system, which includes B cells and T cells. Herbs that specifically activate T cells are American ginseng, Chinese astragalus root, ganoderma or reishi mushroom, shitake mushroom, Chinese atractylodes alba, ligustrum lucidum, epimedium, and the American echinacea root.

Other herbs and natural substances that have been found to be effective are licorice root, Chinese rehmannia root, South American suma *(Pfaffia paniculatta)*, raw egg yolk, cod and other fish liver oils, human and animal placenta. Most of these also activate the more superficial B cells as well.

Three important formulas that are useful for treating symptoms of AIDS/ARC are the Planetary formula Reishi Mushroom Supreme for the immune system and Echinacea, Golden Seal and Olive Leaf Formula, which has potent antiviral properties. In addition, one should also take a tea of red clover, burdock root, dandelion root, and sarsaparilla three times daily, along with a tablespoon of aloe vera gelatin extract.

The tea should be made by simmering a handful of the herbs in a quart of water for twenty minutes. One cup should be taken three times daily together with three tablets of the two Planetary formulas.

In addition, the following supplements should be taken on a daily basis:

good multivitamin (without iron)

vitamin A	10,000 to 20,000 IU
vitamin C	1,000 to 2,000 mg
vitamin E	400 to 1,200 IU
coenzyme Q10	300 to 600 mg
lipoic acid	200 to 600 mg
zinc	15 to 30 mg
pycnogenol, grape seeds	50 to 300 mg
mixed carotenoids	10,000 to 25,000 IU
essential fatty acids★	1,000 mg daily

Chlorella, green magma, or some other chlorophyll-rich green drink should be taken in water once or twice daily.

Diet should consist of pure wholesome foods following the principles of macrobiotic diet with the addition of about two to eight ounces of organic animal food three times a week. This can include chicken, fish, turkey, and beef. Two or three raw egg yolks or poached eggs should be taken each morning with whole wheat toast or on top of a dish of black beans and brown rice and fried onions.

One should use positive affirmations and visualizations and avoid negative situations. Recreation and exercise are important factors to consider as well.

ALLERGIC RHINITIS

DESCRIPTION: A histaminic reaction in the sinus passages of the nose causing vasodilation and increased permeability of the surrounding capillaries with accompanying swelling of the membranes and acute or chronic mucus secretion.

★I recommend Tyler's Eskimo Oil.

SYMPTOMS: Nasal congestion with mucus discharges. The congestion can be so great as to be accompanied by sinus or temporal headaches. Allergic rhinitis often appears at a particular season and can be traced to high susceptibility to certain plant pollens in the air, dust, animal hair, etc.

CAUSES: Lowered immune system, denatured foods, sugar, consumption of liquids, especially cold, raw fruits and juices; also fats, flour, and dairy products. Poor digestion and assimilation, with subsequent toxins absorbed into the blood and lymphatic system, can cause excess mucus. This in turn can be secreted in various areas of the body including the nasal passages, bronchioles, and lungs as well as the reproductive organs, causing acute or chronic discharges that are usually clear or whitish. If there is inflammation, it will appear yellow.

TREATMENT: It is important to support the immune system as much as possible. If at all possible, consider ways to eliminate life-style stress in terms of job and relationship. If weather and climate is a factor, possibly a change of locality might be important to consider. Certainly for most it would be easier to eliminate dietary stress by limiting or eliminating altogether the following: sugar, flour, and dairy products as well as cold, raw foods including raw fruits, juices, and salads. These cold, raw foods generally lower the body's overall metabolism, further weakening digestion and assimilation, and can cause an exacerbation of the symptoms.

The Ayurvedic formula called Trikatu, meaning "three spicy herbs," is effective for drying mucus and diminishing symptoms of allergic rhinitis. It consists of equal parts black pepper, ginger, and pippli long pepper, and honey.

The powdered herbs are mixed in honey to form a doughy consistency. It can be kept in a closed jar practically indefinitely. A teaspoon is taken two or three times daily with warm water. Trikatu is available in tablet form as Planetary formula number 86 (Three Spices Sinus Complex). Two tablets can be taken three times daily.

Another herb that is known to be effective for allergies is nettles. It is a pleasant, high-vitamin tea that can be taken three times daily, or it is available in various other forms, such as a liquid extract or tablets from reputable manufacturers.

Horseradish is an herb that is used in folk medicine for sinus congestion. A traditional treatment for opening clogged sinuses dramatically is to grate a teaspoon of horseradish root (or one can use the powdered horseradish used as a traditional Japanese condiment) mixed with a tablespoon of apple cider vinegar. This is chewed or kept in the mouth until the flavor is dissipated. It burns, but it will clear out the sinuses. Planetary formula number 77 (Sinus Free) includes horseradish for clearing clogged sinuses. It consists of horseradish root, yarrow, eyebright, and thyme as a liquid extract. It promotes normal health and the movement of mucus secretions and is rich in flavonoids, which help to stabilize mast cells, thereby reducing the release of histamines.

As with all upper respiratory congestion of the lungs and sinuses, Chinese ephedra, also popularly known as mahuang, is very effective. It contains the stimulant alkaloids, epinephrine, and norepinephrine. In general, those who have a tendency toward prostate problems, cardiovascular disease, or high blood pressure should not take this herb. However, for conditions such as allergic rhinitis, asthma, emphysema, and other upper respiratory problems, mahuang works. It can be taken alone or with the addition of a small amount of licorice to help balance and smooth its effect as a stimulant to the adrenal glands. Mullein Lung Complex (formula number 64) contains mahuang in a mild, balanced dose and is effective for allergic rhinitis.

There is an ancient yoga practice called "jal neti," or nasal cleansing. A small pot that contains about a cup of water is filled with a pint of tepid water in which a teaspoon of salt has been dissolved. A small plastic watering pot can be used, or a special jal neti pot. Breathing through the mouth, insert the spout into one nostril while tilting the head to one side over a sink. Allow half a pint of the water to flow up one side of the nostril and it will exit through the opposite nostril. This is then repeated through the reverse nostril. Interestingly enough, a similar practice is used by Scandinavians to prevent colds, relieve allergies, and prevent sinus infections.

Another practice that has worked for many with acute and chronic allergic rhinitis and sinusitis is to sniff five drops of Planetary formula number 9 (Narayana Muscle Oil), which, besides being good for rheumatic pains, will also relieve and cure sinusitis, especially if it is associated with dry sinuses.

Two Chinese formulas that are effective for respiratory allergies are Bi Ming Gan Wan (Allergy Season Pill) and Pe Min Kan Wan.

Herbs to benefit digestion are also a very important consideration. Warm, stimulant, carminative herbs including ginger, pepper, turmeric, cumin seed, coriander seed, fenugreek seed, asafetida, garlic, or any of these forming a suitable combination, can be mixed with the food to create a kind of Indian curry seasoning. For some with an excess condition, cayenne pepper can be taken, two 00-size capsules, three times daily with warm water to remove the congestion and stimulate metabolism. As an acute remedy, a teaspoon of grated horseradish root can be chewed in the mouth until the hot, spicy flavor is completely dissipated.

Specific formulas that will be of benefit include formulas number 1, 19, 20, and 31.

Homeopathic remedies to consider include sabadilla 6th to the 30th potency, which is indicated for spasmodic sneezing with a running nose and redness of the eyes. Another remedy is euphrasia, which is similarly effective for mucus symptoms of the nose and eyes, red eyes, and headaches.

ALZHEIMER'S DISEASE

OTHER NAMES: dementia, senile dementia

DESCRIPTION: Alzheimer's disease (AD) is a progressive brain disorder characterized by rapid cognitive and memory deterioration.

CAUSES: It is difficult to make a definitive diagnosis that would differentiate Alzheimer's from accepted norms of brain deterioration in some seniors. However, through expensive brain scans it is possible to see how in Alzheimer's patients there is an accumulation of amyloid plaques in widespread areas of the brain with a consistent loss of neurons in that part of the limbic pathway that drives the memory process.

Because Alzheimer's is a metabolic degenerative process, it is difficult to attribute to a single cause. Certainly genetics may play a role through an abnormality of the gene that controls the production of apolipoprotein E, a blood protein that transports cholesterol to tissues. It is for this reason that among the newer drugs found to be beneficial for Alzheimer's the anticholesterol statin drugs hold great promise.

Besides genetics, environmental causes also play a role in the development of Alzheimer's. Among these are traumatic head injury, chronic exposure to aluminum or silicon, exposure to environmental toxins, and free-radical damage.

A great deal of attention has been given to the concentration of aluminum in the neurofibrillary tangle, though it is not clear whether this is a cause of or a response to AD. Trying to remove the aluminum through specific chelating agents has seemed to slow the deterioration in some AD patients. Until further evidence is available it seems wise to limit exposure to this metal. Some sources for aluminum include the water supply, food, antacids, deodorants, and preparing food in aluminum containers.

Based on reports published in 1985 and 1986 in respected medical journals, abnormal patterns were associated with both AD and Down's syndrome patients (which is considered similar in some respect to AD).* However in a more recent study conducted in 1992 in France there was no association of particular fingerprint patterns that would distinguish a higher risk for AD patients over normal individuals.†

---

*Fingerprint pattern differences in early- and late-onset primary degenerative dementia. Seltzer B., Sherwin I. *Arch Neurol* 1986 Jul; 43(7):665–8, and Fingerprint patterns in Alzheimer's disease, Weinreb H.J. *Arch Neurol* 1985 Jan; 42(1):50–4.

†Berr C., Okra-Podrabinkek N., Feteanu D., Taurand S., Hervy M.P., Forette F., Piette F., Sebag-Lanoe R., Alperovitch A., Dermatoglyphic patterns in dementia of the Alzheimer type: a case-control study. *J Epidemiol Community Health* 1992 Oct; 46(5):512–6.

As it stands, the most definitive diagnosis of early-stage AD must be conducted by a variety of standard blood tests, together with an EEG test and a CT scan. Once again, these are expensive procedures that may not be available to individuals who are on limited, fixed incomes.

TREATMENT: Recent studies reveal a relationship between AD and high serum cholesterol. Because pharmaceutical statins, naturally occurring in red yeast rice *(Monascus purpureus),* are used to lower serum cholesterol, there is a general perception that statins may be directly beneficial for preventing and slowing the progression of AD. Despite a general agreement involving a possible causal relationship in those patients with high cholesterol and AD, the role of statins in the prevention of AD is controversial.*

There is, however, a common acceptance of the association in individuals with high serum cholesterol with the onset and progression of AD. This is not surprising in view of the fact that patients over the age of sixty who are most at risk for AD display a marked tendency toward elevated serum cholesterol levels. Nevertheless, based in a more recent study from the University of South Florida, Daniel Paris, Ph.D., first author of the study and an assistant professor at the USF Roskamp Institute, was quoted as saying, "These drugs [statins] appear to have anti-inflammatory properties, independent of their benefit in lowering cholesterol, that may help protect against dementia." The conclusion published in *Science Daily* (4/02) is based on research from the University of South Florida at Tampa

---

*Scott, H.D., Laake K. Statins for the prevention of Alzheimer's disease. Updated: 1/1/02, from *Cochrane Review Abstracts.*

that found commonly used cholesterol-lowering drugs, known as statins, to block damage by an Alzheimer's-associated protein in neurons and blood vessels. This and other benefits associated with their use have sparked claims citing statins as the new wonder drugs of the first part of the millennium.

What this demonstrates is that besides genetics, nutrition plays a significant role in the prevention and treatment of AD. Certainly a diet that can be shown to lower serum cholesterol levels, whether it be the low-fat diet for some or the higher protein diets for those who have carbohydrate intolerance, would be beneficial. Even with the higher protein diets it would be prudent to emphasize a lower fat diet utilizing a variety of fish, fowl, and vegetable sources of protein such as soy over the fattier cuts of meat. In addition, a generous amounts of nonstarchy green leafy organic vegetables high in antioxidant vitamins, minerals, and other cholesterol-regulating constituents should be incorporated in the daily diet.

Nutrition for Alzheimer's Patients

Studies have shown that the elderly are often prone to a wide variety of nutritional deficiencies. Among these the B vitamins, especially thiamin and B_{12}, are often low. One of the reasons for B-vitamin deficiencies is lack of positive intestinal flora that tend to manufacture them. Of course, certain B vitamins such as B_{12} must be derived from external sources.

As for thiamin, it is generally unusual for there to be a deficiency, but various studies on the elderly population found that between a third and one half of those tested were low in this crucial vitamin. The B vitamins and thiamin are important for cardiovascular and brain function.

Thiamin in particular mimics acetylcholine, which is an important neurotransmitter involved with memory function and AD. In fact, high-dose thiamin of 3 to 8 g daily seem to produce significant cognitive improvement in Alzheimer's patients.*

The amount of vitamin B_{12} in the body seems to decline with age, and that decline is considered a major nutritional cause of depression in individuals past the age of sixty-five. Regular supplementation with B_{12} has shown tremendous benefits in reversing impaired mental function. Cyanocobalamin is the most common form of B_{12}, but it must be converted to either methylcobalamin or adenosylcobalamin. Unfortunately, with age the conversion process is less, so taking a supplement of 1,000 mcg twice daily of methylcogalamin is recommended as adjunctive treatment for Alzheimer's patients.

Phosphatidylcholine derived from lecithin can increase acetylcholine in the brain in normal patients. However, individuals with Alzheimer's lack the specific enzyme acetylcholine transferase that would combine with choline to form acetylcholine. Assuming that a majority of elderly people worried that they may be developing Alzheimer's because of more frequent memory lapses, which are normal for most people as they age, they might try taking 15 to 25 g of phosphatidylcholine or lecithin for a while to see if it makes a difference. If not, it can be discontinued.

In a number of double blind studies, phosphatidylserine seems to impart significant benefit for those suffering from memory impairment as well as depression in the elderly.

---

*Meador, K. Preliminary Findings of High-Dose Thiamin in Dementia of Alzheimer's Type. *J Geriatr Psychiatry Neuro* 16 (1993): 222–229.

L-acetylcarnitine (LAC) has a direct relationship to the manufacture and activation of the mitochondria, which are the energy-producing molecules in cells. It has been the subject of numerous well-designed Alzheimer's studies, and the results have been very positive. It seems that LAC mimics the neurotransmitting effects of acetylcholine, improving memory function and at the same time acting as an antioxidant to prevent further damage to brain cells. The recommended dose for LAC is about 500 mg three times daily.

HERBS: One herb that has thoroughly impressed itself on mainstream awareness of herbs is ginkgo biloba extract (GBE). This is interesting, because before the extract was pharmaceutically manufactured and tested, the herb was hardly used by herbalists. What use there has been comes from the Chinese herbal tradition; within that system it is the nut that is used to strengthen the lungs. The leaf supposedly barely has a mention in the history of Chinese medicine except for a very short description in a text that is over five hundred years old. So for all practical purposes GBE is an herb that was discovered based on contemporary pharmaceutical research. It works to activate circulation throughout the body, including the brain, and it contains some twenty-four flavoglycosides that in numerous clinical trials have shown significant benefit in the treatment of all forms of senility, including Alzheimer's disease.

It increases normal brain function overall, including increasing cholinergic transmission and acetylcholine receptors. One famous study conducted in six research centers, with the design of the study approved by Harvard Medical School and the New York Institute for Medical Research, was on 202 patients with Alzheimer's disease.* They were given either GBE (120 mg a day) or a placebo for one year. The results were that 64 percent of the patients who were given GBE not only stabilized but actually demonstrated significant improvement, while the placebo group showed no change.

Of all the supplements thus far mentioned, ginkgo is by far the most important for the prevention and treatment of Alzheimer's disease.

Brahmi *(Bacopa monnieri)* is a perennial creeping plant found throughout India in wet, damp, and marshy areas. Its primary use since ancient times is as a potent nerve tonic for rejuvenating mental health and promoting intellect and memory. The first mention of the plant is in the Charaka Samhita, the revered ancient text on Ayurveda, dating from the first century A.D., where brahmi is prescribed as a cure for mental retardation leading to psychosis. One must differentiate the bacopa brahmi from the more popular "gota kola," which is also called brahmi but is far less effective for improving mental function and especially memory. While gota kola may be helpful in "clearing" the mind of unwanted thoughts, bacopa is far more effective for relieving anxiety and improving memory.

Ashwagandha *(Withania somnifera)* is another Ayurvedic herb. It is considered by many as the single most valuable tonic herb in the vast Indian pharmacopoeia. It is widely used for conditions of general debility and as such is made into pills, extracts, and even topical oils for a wide variety

---

*Le Bars P. L., et al., "A Placebo-controlled, Double-Blind, Randomized Trial of Ginkgo biloba for Dementia," *JAMA (Journal of the American Medical Association)* 278, 1997:1327–32.

of conditions associated with the debilities of aging. In the West, ashwagandha is sometimes called Indian ginseng, but unlike ginseng, ashwagandha can be used to restore energy, fertility, and potency while at the same time relieving rheumatic pains and promoting relaxation and sound, restful sleep. It is even given to children to promote good nutrition and strength. For the treatment of Alzheimer's, ashwagandha plays an important foundational role in restoring vitality and nerve strength.

A supplement program that would include the following could make a big difference:

- high-potency multivitamin such as Source Natural's Ultra Multiple
- Ester C: 500–1,000 mg three times daily
- essential fatty acids, derived from fish oils, 300–600 mg daily, or from flaxseed oil, 1 tablespoon once a day
- thiamin: 3–8 g daily
- tyrosine: 500–1,000 mg in the morning or afternoon
- phosphatidylserine: 100 mg three times daily
- methylcobalamin: 1,000 mcg twice daily
- ginkgo biloba extract: 80 mg three times daily. Planetary formula number 7 (Bacopa Brain Strength) combines ginkgo, bacopa, gota kola, ashwagandha, and guggul with other herbs that form a balanced formula to enhance mental acuity.
- Planetary formula number 42 (Guggul Cholesterol Compound)
- Planetary's Ashwagandha Liquid Extract: 30 drops three times daily.

ANAL ITCH

Also known as pruritis ani, it can be one of the most embarrassing symptoms. One must try to rule out many possible causes for this complaint, including pinworm infestation, hemorrhoids, virus, yeast, or bacteria. Stimulating spices and beverages also can cause this condition. Regardless of the cause, the main problem is poor hygiene and the propensity for various pathogenic factors, bacteria, virus, or fungus to infect such areas of the body. Washing the area carefully each day with a germicidal soap and washing the area after each defecation is one of the most effective ways to prevent or treat this condition. This can be combined with washing the area with apple cider vinegar and/or witch hazel extract. In Europe, toilets commonly have a bidet that rinses water over the anus that is effective in preventing anal itch. It is also useful as a treatment to prevent itching of the female reproductive organs.

ANEMIA

OTHER NAMES: Chlorosis, deficiency anemia, iron deficiency anemia, nutritional anemia, pernicious anemia.

DESCRIPTION: Normal blood contains red blood cells, which carry oxygen from our lungs to our tissues; white blood cells, which defend us against bacteria, viruses, and foreign proteins; and blood-clotting factors. Additionally, our blood transports nutrients, hormones, electrolytes, and waste products to and from every cell in the body. A shortage or imbalance in any of these blood constituents will lead to a host of problems, from fatigue to cerebral hemorrhage and death. Eating whole, pure foods, drinking pure water, breathing pure air is vitally important for maintaining rich, healthy blood.

The forms of anemia considered here involve a deficiency in the number or the hemoglobin content of the red blood cells, or a lack of vitamin B_{12}. Anemias and blood disorders involving the other constituents of the blood (such as leukemia, sickle cell anemia, and hemophilia) are beyond the scope of this book.

SYMPTOMS: Anemia involving the red blood cells is characterized by various combinations of fatigue, weakness, headache, dizziness, fainting, thirst, irregular heartbeat, feeling cold, sleepiness, bad memory, paleness, backache, depression, loss of appetite, and constipation. Shock may occur if extreme blood loss is involved. The signs of pernicious anemia may include general weakness, numbness or tingling of the extremities, soreness in the mouth, nausea, vomiting, and diarrhea.

CAUSES: Vitamin, mineral, and protein deficiencies (in other words, poor diet) are the most common causes of anemia. Acute and chronic bleeding are also common causes. Sometimes an anemic condition results from congenital or autoimmune disorders, kidney disease, or blood transfusion. In some of these cases the body may be unable to absorb the required nutrients, even if there are adequate amounts in the diet.

TREATMENT: If you have or suspect that you have anemia, consult your doctor to determine the cause. Common vitamin/mineral deficiencies are vitamins B_2, B_6, B_{12}, and C; pantothenic acid and folic acid; and iron.

This recommendation is useful only for those who

have a high metabolism or are recently detoxing from an overly rich diet of white sugar, processed foods, and red meat. For people more inclined toward vegetarian or infrequent meat eating, a more balanced diet consists of lightly cooked whole grains, beans, vegetables, fruit in moderation as seasonally available, and perhaps a little fish and chicken, once or twice a week. A raw milk, vegetable, and fruit juice diet for two weeks is indicated if you are suffering from anemia; exercise and deep breathing are also important. Raw vegetables, fruits, grains, nuts, seeds, and cultured milk products contain all the vitamins, minerals, proteins, and essential fatty acids necessary to maintain healthy blood. Diets filled with white flour, fried foods, excess fats, refined sugar, excess protein, and preservatives result in toxic, devitalized blood.

Specific foods to aid you in rebuilding your blood are garlic, raisins, prunes, dried apricots, sunflower seeds, leeks, cucumbers, parsley, spinach, carrots, tangerines, oranges, wheat germ, yeast, and raw honey. A tablespoon of crude blackstrap molasses per day is an excellent supplement.

Herbal teas to strengthen the blood are yellow dock, burdock, nettle dandelion, comfrey, alfalfa, red clover, sassafras root, buckthorn, echinacea, kelp, cayenne, and chickweed. In the case of pernicious anemia, if the cause is a simple dietary deficiency of vitamin B_{12} (as may be true of vegetarians), the remedy is to take vitamin supplements that provide an adequate amount. If the cause is an inability to absorb vitamin B_{12} from food, then direct injections of the vitamin are likely to be necessary.

The Chinese herb tang kwai *(Angelica sinensis)* is considered a near specific for anemia as well as B_{12} deficiency. It can be taken daily alone in the dose of three grams two or three times daily. A good tea to make is a combination of nine grams of astragalus and three grams tang kwai root simmered in a covered nonmetallic pot no longer than ten minutes in two cups of boiling water. Have two or three cups daily.

Homeopathic remedies to use are the cell salt ferrum phos or ferrum met, 3rd to 6th potency. Arsenicum is particularly useful for pernicious anemia. Calcarea phos is another cell salt remedy that is particularly useful when there is general weakness, bone weakness, calcium deficiency, coldness, and a general sense of nutritional deficiency. China 30x is useful if there has been a recent loss of fluids from hemorrhage as in childbirth, profuse menses, recovery from an accident or operation, etc.

ANGINA PECTORIS

(*SEE* CARDIOVASCULAR DISEASES)

ANXIETY, STRESS, AND PERFORMANCE ANXIETY

DESCRIPTION AND SYMPTOMS: People with these conditions characteristically exhibit various emotional symptoms of nervousness, irritability, insomnia, and possible physiological symptoms such as skin problems, sweating, digestive upset, sexual impotence, etc.

CAUSES: Just as there are many manifestations of anxiety and stress, there are also many and varied causes, including fear, insecurity, shock, and overwork as well as possible physiological and metabolic imbalances.

TREATMENT: Because there are many causes, there are also many treatments. First, one should ascertain the reason for the anxiety and stress, and if possible change it, or if that is not possible, then try various methods of reframing or changing one's attitude and perspective of the cause of one's stress and anxiety. A psychological counselor may be very helpful in this.

An important condition to consider is getting a balanced diet of protein, complex carbohydrates, vegetables, and fruits. Hypoglycemia (low blood sugar) is often an underlying cause of anxiety and stress. Be sure that you are having sufficient protein at every meal and that you avoid sugar, especially refined sugar, but also an excess of fruit juice.

Meditation, qi gong, tai chi, or yoga are all effective methods to counteract the effects of stress. One should find a qualified teacher.

Alternate nostril breathing is a simple yogic practice used before meditation, helping to achieve a calm, centered state by balancing the sympathetic and parasympathetic nervous systems. Begin by finding a quiet place and sitting in a comfortable position. Next, exhale all air. Then close the right nostril with the thumb of the right hand while inhaling slowly through the left nostril. Next, close the left nostril with the ring finger while slowly exhaling through the right nostril. Repeat the cycle, exhaling and inhaling right, then exhaling and inhaling left. Repeat this cycle at least ten times or more as needed. Usually one will find that at a point of high anxiety and stress one is naturally breathing more from the right nostril. Place cotton in that nostril for an hour or so. Forcing yourself to breathe from the more calming parasympathetic left nostril is a very effective, drug-free way of controlling anxiety and stress.

KAVA Imagine capturing the gentle calming energy of the South Pacific Polynesian islands in an herb. Kava kava

(Piper methysticum) is just that herb, and it has been highly prized by Polynesian people for hundreds of years, especially by people from the island of Fiji, for its ability to almost instantly relieve muscular and psychological tension and anxiety. It is presently one of the most popular herbs on the market because of its highly experiential effect of almost instantly relieving symptoms of nervousness and anxiety. Unlike antianxiety and antidepressive drugs, kava seldom has any side effects, either short- or long-term. Traditionally, the root bark is pulverized and chewed or it can be taken as a powder. It creates an immediate sensation of numbness in the mouth when taken in this way. Many kava products are also available in tablet form and taken that way will not cause this reaction.

It can be taken as needed for either chronic or acute nervousness and anxiety. It is a wonderful herb to use to counteract stage fright, because in moderate dosage it will relieve tension without dulling one's concentration. Kava is also an excellent herb to try for relieving pain ranging from toothache to menstrual cramps. It's the ideal herb to take to counteract a racing mind that impairs concentration and can keep one from a good night's sleep.

One of my favorite ways to take kava is as a simple powder stirred in a little cool water. Kava King manufactures this in different natural flavors. One will find kava extract available in a wide range of prices. Many times this is a case where one gets what one pays for. Planetary Formulas has the highest grade and concentration of kava in both tablet and liquid extract forms, but in this case the price reflects the higher concentration.

Kava works well in formulas for symptoms of stress, nervousness, and insomnia. Two highly effective formulas for these conditions including kava are Planetary formula number 82 (St. Johnswort Kava Compound), which we will talk about under depression, and formula number 50 (Kava Dreams), which is particularly good for insomnia.

Planetary formula number 84 (Stress Free) herbal combination contains a number of antistress herbs, including valerian, skullcap, chamomile, zizyphus seed, hawthorn berry, hops strobile, Siberian ginseng, wood betony, black cohosh, and American ginseng together with calcium and magnesium. All the herbs in this formula work synergistically to induce a state of calm centeredness without drowsiness in normal dosage. However, taken before retiring to bed, Stress Free is very effective for producing a deeper, more restful sleep.

Homeopathic Treatment

- *Arsenicum album.* When anxiety is accompanied by restlessness, fatigue, fastidiousness, clammy skin, and racing pulse, take 6C every half hour for up to ten doses.
- *Culcarea carbonica.* Use this if anxiety is accompanied with forgetfulness, fatigue, obsession with work, and a tendency to complain to others about your ailments.
- *Lycopodium.* If there is apprehensiveness, insomnia caused by worry, decreased appetite, and sweet cravings, take 6C every half hour for ten doses.

ARTHRITIS AND RHEUMATIC PROBLEMS

DESCRIPTION: Painful inflammation of the joints and surrounding tissues. In advanced stages it can lead to deformity of the bones and joints.

SYMPTOMS: Pain and swelling, stiffness, and inflammation of specific joints and areas of the body.

CAUSES: Arthritis is a symptom of the stagnation of the blood, lymphatic and neurological circulation. An imbalanced diet, lack of exercise, and stress are all predisposing factors that can aggravate an arthritic tendency.

TREATMENT: Older individuals are more prone to rheumatic and arthritic conditions. While Western medicine can offer only palliative symptomatic relief, herbal and alternative medicine offers cures for this painfully debilitating condition. Acupuncture, moxibustion, magnet therapy, and herbal medicines are all phenomenally effective for arthritis, and one can only wonder why more patients do not seek out one or a number of these alternatives. In Michael's experience, the key to relief is in diet. Particularly, one must eliminate refined foods, especially the overuse of sugar. A fast on kicharee for four to ten days along with one or a number of the herbal approaches suggested below has been effective for the vast majority of arthritic cases. Of course, some form of regular physical activity is essential for treatment and prevention. Besides some mild form of aerobic activity, one should consider learning yoga, qi gong, or tai chi, which help maintain flexibility and integrate the mind as part of one's workout.

For herbal treatment, the basic strategy is to enhance blood circulation. This can be done a number of ways. The self-application of moxibustion over the affected areas of pain is very effective in relieving arthritic symptoms. Similarly taping the negative polarity of a small acuband magnet to the trigger point will not only relieve the pain but, by enhancing circulation, cure the underlining problem.

There are many herbs and formulas that are effective for arthritic and rheumatic conditions. Michael will present four substances that are particularly useful for preventing and treating this condition:

GLUCOSAMINE SULFATE Glucosamine sulfate and chrondroitin sulfate are purified extracts usually derived from seashell and other sources. Since around 1997 it has become a virtual overnight sensation for the prevention and treatment of pain associated with arthritic and rheumatic complaints. According to Dr. Jason Theodasakis, a leading researcher and author of *The Arthritis Cure* (St. Martin's Press), glucosamine assists in the development of cartilage and "can actually help the body to repair damaged or eroded cartilage." Because of this it is routinely prescribed not only to people who are at risk but also for pets, especially dogs who in later life are prone to crippling arthritis. In fact, there is already a lot of clinical evidence supporting the claims that glucosamine is effective for arthritic pains. Chondroitin sulfate, another derivative of seashells, is often prescribed together with glucosamine, but there is less data to support its efficacy. The recommended adult dose of glucosamine sulfate is up to 500 mg taken three times daily.

There is some suspicion that glucosamine and chondroitin may raise LDL cholesterol (the bad form); some individuals report the increase to be as much as 100 points, which dropped down to normal when the supplements were stopped. At this writing, glucosamine is still regarded as an excellent natural treatment for arthritic pain, but individuals may want to monitor their cholesterol levels. As stated, the original source was seashells; subsequently, other sources such as cow bone may be responsible for the rise in cholesterol in some.

MSM SULFUR Unlike glucosamine, MSM sulfur (methylsulfonylmethane) is a dietary supplement that is found in living tissue, and while it also is fantastically effective for healthy connective tissues such as ligaments, tendons, and muscles and, of course, is a highly effective arthritis treatment, it has much broader therapeutic benefits. Other conditions that have been remedied or improved with the regular use of MSM sulfur include acne, allergies, arthritis, asthma, candida yeast infections, carpal tunnel syndrome, chronic fatigue, constipation, diabetes, digestive disorders, brittle hair and nails, migraine headaches, muscle pain and cramps, parasites, skin damage and aging, toxic buildup, and ulcers.

MSM is derived from DMSO (dimethyl sulfoxide), which was discovered by individuals working in a logging mill who found that when they were around sawdust that had been rained on, their rheumatic aches and pains were alleviated. Since that time there has been extensive research, especially by Dr. Stanley Jacob, director of the DMSO Clinic and professor of surgery at Oregon Health Sciences University, that confirms the efficacy of DMSO as a topical application for the relief of arthritic and rheumatic pains as well as of sprains and bruises. At present the source of MSM is the lignin molecule derived from the cell wall of pine trees.

Unlike sulfur per se, MSM sulfur is safe and possibly even beneficial for asthmatics.

Because sulfur is a compound found in or near osseous structures, muscles, tendons, and ligaments, researchers from Oregon Health Sciences University have conducted numerous studies on both animals and humans and have found that when MSM sulfur is taken as a supplement, those with osteoarthritis, rheumatoid arthritis, and muscle soreness and pain have responded well.

It has been found to be completely safe, and the recommended dose is approximately 1,500 mg three times daily, usually taken in capsule form.

Topical application of DMSO, long used by veterinarians, can safely relieve arthritic and other pains. It is a good idea to apply it to a small patch to determine whether there is any skin sensitivity before using it over an extended area.

BOSWELLIA When the wise men from the East presented their gifts of frankincense and myrrh it may have been for more reasons than for the purifying fragrance of these precious resins. As we have learned, guggul *(Commiphora mukul)* is an ancient remedy for cholesterol and arthritic complaints and is the resinous exudate from a species of plant closely related to myrrh. Similarly, boswellia is a gummy exudate derived from *Boswellia serrata,* a large branching deciduous tree found in India, and it is the source for what is known as olibanum, or frankincense. Both are known to have both antiseptic and insecticide properties, which besides their pleasant fragrance may be one of the reasons they are burned as incense.

Boswellia is highly respected in Ayurvedic medicine for its effective treatment of rheumatic and arthritic pains. In addition, it is good for a number of other conditions, including skin and blood diseases, fevers, cardiovascular diseases, neurologic diseases, mouth sores, vaginal discharges, dysentery, diabetes, and testicular diseases. Like guggul it works by relieving inflammation while promoting circulation. It is effective for both osteo- and rheumatoid arthritis as well as lower back pain, gout, and swollen joints generally. Also like guggul, boswellia has been found to be antihyperlipidemic and antiatherosclerotic, and it has hepatoprotective properties against hepatitis.

The combination of boswellia, guggul, and glucosamine with a few powerful Chinese herbs, including eucommia bark (an herb derived from the latex of the bark of a species of rubber tree) are found in Planetary formula number 41 (Glucosamine–MSM Herbal). It is interesting that this bark that is the source of a highly flexible natural substance is also fantastically effective for joint and lower-back pains. In addition, Glucosamine-MSM Herbal also contains dipsacus root, which is known to regenerate bones and degenerated spinal disks.

DEER ANTLER VELVET Deer antler has been treasured as a tonic since the time of Confucius (551 B.C.). It is humanely harvested under veterinarian supervision from the Sika red deer, which are presently raised on farms in North America, New Zealand, and other parts of the world. Deer antler velvet contains many organic compounds that are integral to the health of bone tissue such as phosphor- and glycolipids, collagen, and glycoaminoglycans. Uniquely, it contains a growth factor similar to human growth hormone, which contributes to the health of bones, muscles, ligaments, and, indeed, to the whole body.

It is known to be effective for a wide variety of problems such as symptoms in children who are failing to thrive, infertility, impotence, coldness, low metabolism, adrenal deficiency, and symptoms associated with menopause, including hot flashes. It is a great supplement to counteract the negative effects of aging, but its most immediate experiential effects (usually after taking it on a daily basis for a month) is for the treatment of arthritic and rheumatic conditions.

It can be taken in many ways. Traditionally, many Chinese people will buy deer antler and soak it in highly alcoholic rice wine. After a couple of weeks one may take it in teaspoonful or tablespoon doses two or three times daily. In this case the small amount of alcohol acts as a carrier and enhances the effect of the antler. Often an alcoholic elixir is made by combining ginseng with high-quality deer antler. It also can be taken as a 250 mg tablet without any of the undesirable effects of the alcohol.

Another Planetary herbal formula that is effective for arthritic and rheumatic problems and assists in promoting general flexibility is number 33 (Flex-Ability). This is a traditional formula used by famous kung fu and tai chi masters to increase joint flexibility and prevent and treat arthritic and rheumatic pains.

TURMERIC There is a tradition in India for those who are practicing yoga to make a preparation with freshly grated turmeric and honey called "golden milk." Taken once daily, this preparation is used to enhance the flexibility of all the joints and thus facilitate the practice of strenuous yogic stretching exercises. There has been a sizable body of research that substantiates the anti-inflammatory effects of turmeric on the muscles and joints throughout the body. Used in Indian and other ethnic cooking to impart flavor and a golden color to food, turmeric has tremendous health benefits assisting digestion, promoting circulation, counteracting inflammation, and protecting the liver.

ASTHMA (AND OTHER SEVERE UPPER-RESPIRATORY AILMENTS)

OTHER NAME: Bronchial asthma.

DESCRIPTION AND SYMPTOMS: Asthma is a disease characterized by extreme difficulty in breathing

caused by localized edema in the walls of the small bronchioles along with the secretion of thick mucus into the
bronchial lumens and accompanying spasm of the smooth
muscle.

CAUSE: Asthma is a disease with a reactivity that is fun-
damentally constitutional in origin. Thus it is an autoimmune disease that particularly affects the lungs and
bronchioles. It can also be caused by an allergic hypersensitivity of the individual to foreign substances in the air,
especially plant pollens. Another cause is exposure to cold
and damp conditions.

TREATMENT: A distinction must be made between the
actual treatment of the asthma attacks as opposed to treatments to prevent the attacks.

Since there is a strong inherited constitutional predisposition to asthma in most patients, the patient must focus
on learning how to control the attacks through diet, life-
style, and psychological factors. Without this approach,
only symptomatic treatment at best can be expected unless the condition is of mild recent onset, which it usually
is not.

During severe attacks, Western medicine resorts to the
use of various bronchodilators such as Bricanyl used in
aerosol dispensers. In particularly severe cases patients are
given cortisone or prednisone therapy.

Since neither of these is satisfactory in the long run, it
is good news for asthma sufferers to discover the many effective approaches to the treatment and management of
asthma with natural therapies.

I would particularly recommend patients to the care of
an acupuncturist skilled in the methods of herbal medicine. If this service is not available, then have someone

apply strong moxa stimulation over the 7th cervical at the base of the neck and the adjoining areas about one to one and one half inches out from the spine between the 2nd and 3rd thoracic and in the lower back between the 2nd and 3rd lumbar vertebrae (*see* Chapter 4, "Acupuncture and Related Therapies").

There are many herbs that are useful for asthma. Some favorites include yerba santa *(Eriodictyon californica)*, mullein *(Verbascum thaspis)*, wild cherry bark *(Prunus virginiana* or *P. serotina)*, and *Lobelia inflata*. Yerba santa helps prevent and eliminate mucus from the bronchioles, while mullein soothes and relaxes them. Both of these have expectorant or mucus-eliminating properties. Wild cherry bark is another effective remedy for the lungs. It is effective for hot, dry, percussive coughs, colds, and all respiratory symptoms. It is both an astringent drying mucus and a bronchial sedative. It can be taken alone or as a tea or made into a syrup or 20 percent alcoholic extract. It contains cyanogenic glycosides and should not be taken during pregnancy. Coltsfoot *(Tussilago farfara)* is a perennial herb that grows on several continents. It has a long history of use for the treatment of asthma, emphysema, and bronchitis. All parts of the plant are used. It is best taken as a tea or in a syrup. *Lobelia inflata* is very effective for controlling asthma episodes. Too much will cause nausea and vomiting, but other than that it exhibits no toxicity when taken in proper dosage. It should be taken as a 20 percent alcoholic extract in ten to fifteen drops three times daily, or more often as needed.

Ma huang *(Ephedra vulgaris)* has been used by the Chinese for the treatment of asthma, colds, emphysema, and other upper respiratory conditions for more than five thousand years. It contains adrenalinelike substances, including ephedrine and norepinephrine, which are used in Western medicine to control asthma.

While any one of the above-mentioned herbs are effective for upper respiratory problems, Michael has had the best experience by combining all of these herbs together with ma huang, licorice, and ginger as follows:

4 parts ma huang
4 parts wild cherry bark
4 parts mullein herb
4 parts yerba santa
72 parts licorice
1 part lobelia herb
2 or 3 slices fresh ginger
(Optional) Add 12 tablespoons of dried garden
   thyme to the brew while it is steeping.

Common garden thyme *(Thymus vulgaris)* also has a beneficial role to play in the treatment of asthma and chronic respiratory complaints. The active ingredients in thyme are its volatile oils, which means that it should not be boiled.

Thyme has many valuable properties including its use as a digestant, carminative (to get rid of gas), diuretic, vermifuge (to get rid of worms and parasites); but most important, it has antispasmodic and expectorant (to bring up phlegm) properties.

Thyme is also good for bronchitis, chronic and acute coughs, and it is the best remedy for whooping cough, especially when combined with ten drops of lobelia tincture.

Steep one teaspoonful of the dried herb in a cup of boiling water, covered. Take three cups daily. Thyme syrup is simply made by steeping one ounce of dried thyme or two ounces of fresh thyme in a pint of boiling water for twenty minutes; strain and add a pint of honey. If it is intended to be used for a long period, keep it refrigerated. Take one or two tablespoons as often as needed.

Vitamin therapy for asthma includes taking 25,000 units of vitamin A, 150 units of B_6, 1,000 mcg of B_{12}, one or two tablespoons of linseed or fish liver oils, 75 mcg of selenium, and raw adrenal extract.

One should follow the balanced macrodiet recommended in this book. Avoid dairy products as well as bananas and avocados and other foods high in acetylcholine and serotonin. Tofu, unless deep-fried, has a cold energy and should also be avoided.

Black beans, onions, black pepper, cardamom, ginger, and garlic are usually beneficial for respiratory conditions. Planetary formula number 57 (Mullein Lung Complex) has helped people suffering from chronic upper respiratory diseases throughout the country reduce or eliminate altogether their drug dependence.

ATHLETE'S FOOT (AND GENERAL EXTERNAL FUNGUS INFECTIONS)

OTHER NAMES: Hong Kong foot, Hong Kong toe, ringworm, tinea pedis.

DESCRIPTION: Athlete's foot is an infection by a form of ringworm, which is not a worm at all but a fungus. It occurs mainly between the toes but also affects the soles of the feet. The name comes from its association with warm, moist places, such as athletes' locker rooms, where it thrives.

SYMPTOMS: Athlete's foot first will call itself to your attention with mild itching and burning sensations. If these are ignored, it goes on to produce reddening, cracking, and scaling of the skin, small blisters, and softening of the tissue in the affected area.

CAUSES: The spores of the ringworm fungus, which attach themselves to the skin, are everywhere, not just in locker rooms or saunas. Whether an active infection occurs or not depends partly on individual susceptibility, which in turn is determined by the health of one's skin and by one's habits of foot care. Even with the most conscientious care, though, ringworm may find the warm, moist hospitality of a foot in a closed shoe irresistible.

TREATMENT: There are various effective treatments for athlete's foot, but prevention is the best remedy. Considering that one's feet can pump up to a gallon of sweat each week, drying one's feet carefully, and wearing natural-fiber socks to absorb unwanted foot moisture and being sure to change them daily, are good preventive measures. Many people have found that using a hair dryer on the feet is very good both for treatment and prevention. Another step is to use Gold Bond medicated powder on one's feet daily. For more stubborn cases, try soaking the feet for twenty minutes daily in a gallon of hot water to which two tablespoons of Epsom salts or baking soda have been added. Antifungals can be applied topically. Different ones seem to work better for some than others. Michael has had varied success with the topical application of any one of the following: garlic oil, blood root, black walnut tincture, or tea tree oil. For particularly stinky feet, some people have found that urinating on one's feet in the shower has been effective.

BAD BREATH

OTHER NAMES: Halitosis

CAUSES: There are many possible causes for bad breath, and one should go through the list to discover what may be the particular cause in your case. Some causes are:

- Poor dental hygiene.
- Diet with strong, spicy foods such as garlic and onions and too much meat, coffee, alcohol, or tobacco. Once the chemicals from these foods get into one's blood, no amount of breath sprays or mint lozenges will cover it up.
- "Hunger breath" occurs as a result of skipped meals. This is also noticed with individuals when they fast. When the body is not receiving outside nutrients it begins to break down its own reserves, which causes a strong breath odor.
- Insufficient amounts of water.
- Drugs such as those used in chemotherapy, DMSO, antidepressants, diuretics, and antihypertensives are all known to be possible causes for bad breath.

TREATMENT: Obviously with the above as a guideline, one should be able to sort out what to do in most cases. In general one would want to consume more vegetables, which help to alkalinize the blood and counteract putrefaction. Probiotics such as acidophilus are also very beneficial for fighting bad breath.

There are a few simple herbal aids that are beneficial. One is oil of parsley *(Petroselinum crispum)*, sold in small capsules; it is a good emergency treatment for bad breath. Another simple herb to prevent bad breath is green tea.

Besides fighting cancer, green tea also fights harmful mouth bacteria that may cause cavities, plaque, and bad breath. In this case green tea is more useful than black. Black tea is simply tea that has been fermented to concentrate and release more caffeine. To make the best green tea do not boil the herb but simply allow it to steep in water that has come near the boiling point. The leaves should only be steeped for two or three minutes or to taste.

BALDNESS

OTHER NAMES: Alopecia, alopecia areata.

DESCRIPTION, SYMPTOMS, AND CAUSES: Loss of hair. It can have an inherited constitutional cause or it can be caused by general debility and anemia.

TREATMENT: Alopecia is treated with herbs that stimulate the scalp and thus encourage the growth of hair. Usually, stimulating volatile oils are used. These include a combination of thuja (cedar) oil and sesame oil, eucalyptus oil, and sesame or olive oil. These are massaged once or twice daily directly into the scalp where hair loss is occurring. A combination of thuja, eucalyptus, and olive oils can be used together.

Using a Chinese dermal hammer (*see* Chapter 4, "Acupuncture and Related Therapies"), one should tap the scalp around and within the periphery of the affected area of the scalp after applying the oil. The oil is then massaged again so as to penetrate the scalp better.

One should use a hair shampoo with a base of jojoba or aloe vera. A hair rinse of sage, yarrow, and nettles is good to use daily after showering or shampooing.

One study in Scotland tested the use of essential oils

on people with alopecia areata, a condition where the hair comes out in patches. It was found that those who used the essential oil mixture experienced a 44 percent improvement in hair growth, and the others who used only the "carrier" oils (i.e., jojoba or grapeseed) only had a 15 percent improvement.

You can make your own by mixing some two drops of thyme oil, three drops of rosemary oil, three drops of lavender oil, and two drops of cedarwood oil into 3ml of jojoba oil. This is thoroughly blended and massaged into the scalp for two minutes each night. Wrap a warm towel around the head to help the skin absorb the oils.

Internally, one should take supplemental lecithin, fish liver oils, and the Chinese herb Ho Shou Wou *(Polygonum multiflorum)*. This remarkable herb is well-known in Traditional Chinese Medicine as a blood tonic for anemia and liver weakness. It also has an esteemed reputation for benefiting the hair, i.e., restoring hair color and growth in those who have become prematurely gray and/or bald. This herb is easily obtained in herb stores and Chinese pharmacies throughout the world. One should take a good dose of 900 mg three times a day of the powdered herb. Another fine liqueur made with Ho Shou Wou and other Chinese herbs for the blood is called "Shou Wou Chih. It is commonly available from familiar sources.

A Chinese patent formula specifically used for alopecia is called Sheng Fa capsules.

The following supplements are also useful for hair loss: 2,000 units vitamin E, niacin and B_6 for circulation, pantothenic acid and B-complex, 150 mg zinc, 200 mcg selenium, 15 mg B_{15}. Glandular extracts of thyroid, pituitary, and adrenal.

BEDSORES

DESCRIPTION AND CAUSE: This is a painful condition that results from being confined to lying in one position in bed over a prolonged period.

TREATMENT: Remarkable relief and healing of chronic bedsores can be achieved with a poultice of powdered comfrey root, slippery elm, and echinacea root directly applied and bandaged onto the affected area. This can be changed once or twice daily as needed.

BED-WETTING

OTHER NAME: Enuresis.

DESCRIPTION, SYMPTOMS, AND CAUSES: Bed-wetting is usually a result of neurologic weakness. It is important to realize that only 3 percent to 5 percent of cases have any organic cause. These include physiologic urological abnormality, renal disease, chronic retention, dribbling incontinence, spina bifida occulta, urinary infection, and emotional problems. Thus many diuretic herbs that strengthen the urinary system along with nervine herbs have often been effective.

TREATMENT: Refrain from drinking fluids at least two to three hours before retiring to bed. One of the most effective herbs for bed-wetting is a tincture made from the bark of sweet sumac (Rhus aromatica), which is a North American shrub. Five to twenty drops of the tincture or fluid extract is taken three times daily.

St. Johnswort (Hypericum perforatum) is also a good general tonic for the nervous system and therefore useful in the treatment of bed-wetting and enuresis generally. Finally, a combined tincture or tea of linden flowers and valerian in equal parts has been useful for many to help overcome this problem. Planetary formula number 84 (Stress Free) together with formula number 77 (Uva Ursi Diurite) is useful to inhibit bed-wetting. These should be taken three times daily.

BITES

DESCRIPTION: Various bites by rabid dogs, poisonous snakes, and other venomous animals and insects.

SYMPTOMS: Various symptoms ranging from severe pain, swelling, convulsions, coma and sometimes death, depending upon the toxicity and severity of the bite.

TREATMENT: For most bites, try to wash the area with warm water and apply a suction cup to draw out as much of the venom and infectious matter as possible. In an emergency, this can be done by mouth; otherwise, make a superficial crosscut with a razor and apply a suction cup immediately (see Chapter 4, "Acupuncture and Related Therapies").

Immediately give twenty to thirty drops of tincture of echinacea every half hour for at least six doses and then every hour or two. Externally keep the area open and draining with Epsom salts soaked in a towel. Otherwise, a poultice of plaintain leaf with a sprinkle of cayenne pepper will also be very effective.

Use echinacea along with formula number 14 every two hours with a tea of red clover, chapparal, and burdock root.

For more superficial bites such as bee stings and such,

chew a leaf or two of plaintain or a wad of tobacco and apply topically.

Homeopathically, give ledum 6th to 30th potency.

BLADDER AND KIDNEY INFECTIONS

OTHER NAMES: Bladder infection: cystitis; Kidney infection: honeymoon disease, nephritis.

DESCRIPTION AND SYMPTOMS: An infection in the bladder or kidney, characterized by burning discomfort, sometimes dark-colored and scanty urine.

CAUSES: Many causes including an infection transmitted through improper hygiene, excessive irritation from sexual intercourse, an overly acid condition, overeating of sweets, coffee, and other denatured foods, emotional upset, and anger.

TREATMENT: Parsley *(Petroselinum crispum)* is a reliable herbal remedy for urinary infections. It is high in chlorophyll, which itself will build the body's resistance to infections. Both the leaf and the root may be used. Simply steep a large handful of fresh parsley leaves or a smaller handful of the dried leaves in two cups of boiling water for twenty minutes. Strain and drink three to four cups daily until symptoms abate.

Cranberry *(Vaccinium macrocarpon* or *V. oxycoccus)* is effective in preventing urinary tract infections. For mild cases they are also effective for treatment. Ideally they should be taken unsweetened, but lightly sweetened cranberry juice will impart some therapeutic benefit. They work by increasing the natural acidity of the urine, which prevents bacteria from invading. Cranberry juice also has been shown to have significant antioxidant properties, making it useful for preventing many other diseases, including serious diseases such as cancer.

Uva ursi *(Arctostaphylos uva-ursi)* has antimicrobial effects against *Escherichia coli, Proteus vulgaris, Enterobacter aerogenes, Streptococcus faecalis, Staphylococcus aureus, Salmonella typhi,* and *Candida albicans.* In addition, it is an effective diuretic for the treatment of urinary tract infections. In fact, it is considered to be an overall potent urinary disinfective. One of the active biochemical constituents in urva ursi is arbutin. The dose for the tea should be 1 tablespoon steeped in a cup of boiling water. This is allowed to stand until cool enough to drink. A cup should be taken two or three times daily.

Planetary formulas number 90 (Uva Ursi Diurite) or 21 (Cranberry Bladder Defense) are both useful for the treatment of many cases of urinary tract infections. They can be taken four times daily with warm water or a half cup of parsley tea. Again, if symptoms don't improve within a couple of days, one should seek qualified medical intervention.

Avoid the intake of all forms of sugar, including that of honey, fruit, and sweet fruit juices. Diet should be very simple, emphasizing drinking the juice of Japanese azuki beans and/or up to a quart or two of cranberry juice a day. It is also a good idea, especially if there is any constipation or bowel sluggishness, to take triphala each evening.

Homeopathic treatment for cystitis:

• Cantharis. When there is a strong frequent urge to urinate, sharp burning pains, lower-back ache, and a sense of incomplete urination, take 30C dose every half hour for up to ten doses.

- Nux Vomica. When there is a painful need to urinate, with chills and wanting to be alone, take 6C every half hour, up to ten doses.
- Staphysagria. When there is a continual burning sensation in the urinary tract with a sense that there is a trickling through the urethra and accompanying anger, take 6C doses every thirty minutes, up to ten doses.

BREAST LUMPS

DESCRIPTION AND SYMPTOMS: Malignant or nonmalignant lumps in the breasts of women.

CAUSE: The breasts are related to the liver and reproductive organs so that imbalances in these systems will cause lumps to form. Make sure to have regular medical check-ups.

TREATMENT. Fibrocystic breasts can be caused by stagnation in the liver. These often are associated with excess fat in the diet and/or emotional stress. One of the best formulas is Planetary formula number 10 (Bupleurum Calmative), which is based on a traditional Chinese formula called "Xiao Yao Wan." It contains among other herbs the Chinese herb bupleurum that helps release stored toxins from the liver. Either benign or malignant breast lumps are not an easy condition to treat, so that anyone with these symptoms should seek qualified medical advice immediately. Another herb that has been shown to be effective for this condition is vitex agnus-castus. The ingestion of soy in the form of soybeans, tempeh, or tofu is associated with a much lower incidence of cancers of the breast, prostate, and colon. Genistein, one of the isoflavones in soy, has been found to decrease the growth of tumors implanted in mice, and Asian women, who regularly ingest soy as part of their weekly diet, have a statistically lower incidence of these diseases, which changes when the same population lives in the United States. The isoflavones and other chemical constituents in soy seem to act as estrogen precursors and interfere with the transformation of excess estrogen, which would tend to promote tumor growth, by converting it to an inactive form. Another herb commonly used in Chinese medicine for all breast problems, including benign and malignant growths and lumps, is dandelion. An ounce of the entire herb (aerial and root portions) should be simmered in three cups of water for twenty minutes. Allow to cool, and drink three cups daily. Poke root (Phytolacca americana) has a well-deserved reputation as an herb that purifies the glands, including the breasts. However, taken in high dosage, the root can be toxic. It is safe to take a 20 percent extract of poke root tincture, about five to ten drops only four times daily. In addition, one can chop and simmer the fresh root in olive oil. Strain and use this to rub on the breasts regularly. Another herb to use for breast cancer is red clover (Trifolium pratense). A tea can be made by combining the following:

4 parts dandelion root
4 parts red clover
4 parts burdock root
1 part chaparral
½ part Lobelia herb
1 or 2 slices ginger

Purchase each of these in quantity and combine accordingly. Simmer two handfuls of the first five herbs for thirty minutes in a covered container, and then add the ginger when steeping. Drink a half cup four times daily and take with twelve tablets each of Planetary formula number 29 (Echinacea–Goldenseal and Olive Combination) and 66 (Red Clover Cleanser). In addition, to strengthen the body's immune system, two tablets of Planetary formula number 70 (Reishi Mushroom Supreme) should be taken three times daily.

Such a treatment protocol is for both prevention and treatment and should be followed for many months, with a break each week of one day without any supplements, and after a couple of months, there should be a week without taking the herbs. The standard anticancer diet consists of whole grains, beans (all beans contain cancer-fighting isoflavones), and cooked vegetables and the regular intake of shiitake mushrooms (at least five a day) as well as soups and whole grains made with a stock from boiling 9 ounces of astragalus in a quart of water.

BRONCHITIS

OTHER NAMES: Bronchial catarrh, chest cold, pulmonary catarrh.

DESCRIPTION: The trachea, or windpipe, divides into two main stem bronchi, or branches, one for each lung. These bronchi further divide into smaller branches (bronchioles), finally ending in the air cells (alveoli) of the lungs. The purpose of this system is to bring air into the lungs so that oxygen can be transported to the rest of the body. All these passages are lined with mucous membrane, and bronchitis is inflammation of this membrane. The resulting catarrhal discharge and swelling make it more difficult for air to pass through the bronchial tubes. Coughing is the body's attempt to rid itself of this catarrh. Bronchitis can be acute or chronic.

SYMPTOMS: Bronchitis is accompanied by fever, sore throat, backache, headache, hoarseness, and rapid pulse and breathing. Coughing is likely to be painful; the cough may or may not produce mucus, and it may be paroxysmal. Symptoms of acute bronchitis generally last from one to two weeks.

CAUSES: Bronchitis arises in two main ways. First, it can be a complication of another illness or condition, such as viral diseases (colds or the flu), asthma, tuberculosis, measles (in children), constipation, excess mucus in the system, sudden chill, overwork, or fatigue. Second, it can result from exposure to injurious substances, either environmentally or in the diet. Cigarette smoking is particularly likely to be involved in mild, chronic bronchitis. Environmental pollutants (dust, smoke, chemicals, gases) also tend to irritate the bronchial lining. Misuse of alcohol and consumption of excess refined sugar and starch will weaken the body's resistance to all forms of disease, including bronchitis.

TREATMENT: Acute bronchitis requires rest, a liquid diet of fruit and vegetable juices (perhaps only water for the first day or two), and enemas or colonics to cleanse the system. Hot fomentations and mustard poultices can be used on the chest to help decongest it. Steam inhalation—whether plain or with various aromatic herbs, such as chamomile, eucalyptus, balsam, pine, wintergreen, or tincture of benzoin—helps loosen the mucus, as does vigorous massage of the chest. A hot bath enhanced with lots of fresh pine needles can also be beneficial; nightly hot Epsom salt baths are recommended for the acute stage. A hot pack on the back will help relieve a hacking cough. Follow this with a massage of the back and the abdomen, some hot lemon juice taken in water, and a hot mustard footbath before retiring. This treatment is best when done every other night.

Drinking water after every time you cough will eventually soothe the irritated membranes. Teas of thyme, chickweed, slippery elm, sanicle, maidenhair, marshmallow, and mullein are also soothing to inflamed bronchi. Linden, lobelia, coltsfoot, red clover, licorice, horehound, and wild cherry bark help to quiet a spasmodic cough (but do not use these herbs to treat a productive cough that helps to clear the system). Lungwort, pleurisy root, cubeb berries, and goldenseal are other healing herbs for the lungs. A cough syrup made of honey in which chopped raw onion or garlic has been kept for twelve hours is very effective and healing. An increase in the intake of vitamins A and C is recommended to strengthen the system.

Take rosemary baths twice a week to help with elimination; take enemas nightly for three or four days and as necessary after that. Deep breathing exercises are important; combine a daily chest massage if possible with deep breathing. Outdoor sports in fresh, clean air are very beneficial. Above all, try to identify the cause and eliminate it.

Diet for the more acute stage of bronchitis should consist of thin porridge, vegetable soup, and, most beneficial for all inflammatory conditions, black bean soup, cooked with onions and/or garlic. Meals should be very light and can be supplemented with diluted fruit juice and water, about half and half, served at room temperature. Avoid dairy products; although for strength, boiled warm milk with a teaspoon of honey is all right. Later, the diet can broaden out to the more balanced macrodiet recommended in the diet and therapeutic foods section of this book. Of course one should avoid refined foods, sugar, coffee, alcohol, and smoking.

Herbs for treating bronchitis:

Garlic *(Allium sativum)* is one of the most effective remedies for the upper respiratory tract. Macerate several cloves of crushed garlic in olive oil. Have the patient dip bread into the oil and eat it freely.

Eucalyptus *(Eucalyptus globules)* is an old-fashioned herb whose volatile oils have antiseptic properties. It is the primary ingredient in the propriety Vicks VapoRub sold in pharmacies. It is put into inhalers and a kind of tent is made over the patient's head so he can inhale the vapors from the hot steam. If one doesn't have an inhaler, simply put a tablespoon of the ointment into a pot of boiling hot water, put a towel over the patient's head, and have him inhale the steam.

Mullein *(Verbascum thapsus)* is excellent for coughs and all upper respiratory complaints. It can be taken as a tea by simmering an ounce of the dried or two ounces of the fresh herb in a pint of boiling water for twenty minutes. If you have mullein root available, chop it finely and add it to the tea as well. Allow to cool and sweeten with honey to taste. Take a cup three or four times daily.

Yerba santa *(Eriodictyon californica)* is an old-time remedy of the Pacific Northwest that has a longtime, cherished reputation for the treatment of all upper respiratory complaints, including bronchitis. It can be made into a tea by steeping an ounce of the dried or 12 ounces of the fresh leaves in a pint of boiling water in a covered pot.

Allow to steep for twenty to thirty minutes or until cool enough to drink. Take a cupful mixed with honey three times daily. It combines very well with other upper respiratory herbs such as mullein.

Wild cherry bark *(Prunus virginiana)* is a popular old-time remedy for coughs of all kinds, including bronchitis. Like the previous mentioned herbs it has expectorant properties, will help loosen phlegm from the throat and chest and lessen the frequency and severity of most coughs. Simply steep an ounce of the ground bark in a pint of boiling water in a covered pot for twenty minutes. Strain, add honey to taste, and allow to cool. Take one-half to one cupful at least three or more times daily. Keep it covered. Again, as mentioned, it can be combined with any or all of the above-mentioned herbs for broader effect.

Red clover blossoms *(Trifolium pratense)* is a versatile herb that is usually thought of as a blood purifier. However, it has an esteemed reputation for fevers and lung complaints. I have used it successfully to help patients overcome longstanding bouts of bronchitis when all else has failed. It needs to be made strong, one ounce to a pint of water. It can be taken sweetened or unsweetened if preferred.

Licorice *(Glycyrrhiza* species) is a famous remedy for lung and bronchial infections, including bronchitis. Simmer an ounce in a pint of boiling water for twenty to thirty minutes. Allow to cool and take a half cup every hour or two.

Lobelia inflata should be taken as a 20 percent alcoholic extract or it can be taken as an extract in apple cider vinegar. The dose should be ten to fifteen drops taken alone or with any of the above-mentioned herbs to enhance their effect. It has antispasmodic and expectorant properties. In higher doses it is emetic.

As stated, all the above herbs can be taken singly or will combine very well as a formula. To make any of the above teas more palatable, one can add a drop or two of pure anise extract to each cup of tea. Anise seed is also effective for bronchitis.

Planetary formula number 61 (Old Indian Cough Syrup) can be used as well as number 57 (Mullein Lung Complex), which contains many of the herbs mentioned.

Er Chen Tang, a Chinese patent, is very effective. A variation of this is Er Chan He San Zi Yang Qing Wan (Clear Phlegm Formula pill).

Homeopathic remedies that are useful for laryngitis as well as bronchitis are aconite 6x at the very beginning, belladonna 6x when there is a dry cough with fever and headache, hepar sulph 6x when there is profuse expectoration, arsenicum 6x for the aged and weak, and byronia 6th to 30th when there is a wheezing sound associated with fear of suffocation.

BUNIONS

OTHER NAMES: Hallux valgus, hallux varus.

DESCRIPTION, SYMPTOMS, AND CAUSES: Bunions are painful swellings or protrusions on the side of the foot, at the joint where the big toe is connected to the rest of the foot. Bunions are caused when a shoe rubs or presses against the bony spur of that joint causing the big toe to be pushed toward the opposite side of the foot. This generally results from habitual wearing of shoes that are too tight or too short. (In some people, such a misalignment of the big toe is an inherited condition; the result is the same.) The continuous pressure and irritation cause a chronic inflammation of a fluid-filled sac in the toe, resulting in formation of the bunion.

TREATMENT: Once a bunion has formed, relief from the pain can be obtained by wearing comfortable, roomy shoes with supportive inserts and by shielding the bunion from friction. Epsom salts footbaths are also said to help relieve pain from bunions. To correct the condition permanently requires surgery for removal of the bone spur on the toe joint or for realignment of the bones, if necessary.

Footbaths will soften the bunion and ease the problem. For a splendid herbal antiseptic foot powder, mix equal parts of dried and finely powdered slippery elm bark, bayberry bark, and goldenseal. Sprinkle a small quantity of the mixture into stockings and shoes.

Rubbing daily with a combination of olive and castor oils will help to soften and dissolve the bunion. Follow by taping a thin slice of garlic over it each evening before going to bed. Other effective treatments include dabbing lemon juice or spirits of turpentine—do not use synthetic turpentine—each morning and evening.

BURNS

DESCRIPTION: Burns are injuries or tissue damage caused by heat, electricity, chemical agents, or radiation. Severity can range from mild sunburn to charring and destruction of the skin. First-degree burns are those in which the outer layer of skin (the epidermis) is damaged; these are generally not serious unless they are extensive. Second-degree burns, in which the inner layer of skin (the dermis) is also damaged, are more serious. These should be seen by a physician, particularly if the hands, face, feet, or genitals are affected. Third-degree burns, in which both layers of skin are destroyed, should be seen by a physician immediately, unless only a very small, noncritical area is affected.

SYMPTOMS: First-degree burns will produce redness, warmth, tenderness, pain, and sometimes swelling. With second-degree burns, the same symptoms are accompanied by blisters filled with a clear fluid. With third-degree burns, the surface may appear charred, white, blistered, and lifeless or coagulated. When nerves are damaged, there will be little or no pain.

Note: Extensive burns over the body can cause shock. The symptoms of shock are pallor, shortness of breath, sweating, and confusion or combativeness. A shock victim should be taken to a hospital immediately.

CAUSES: Burns obviously are caused by excessive exposure to or contact with sunlight, flames, hot objects, hot water, electricity, radiation, and chemicals such as acids and alkalis. Accidents and carelessness account for the great majority of all burns.

TREATMENT: The first and principal treatment for all burns is to apply cold water or wet compresses (but not ice water or ice) to the affected area. If chemicals or other damaging substances are still present on the area, it is best to flush thoroughly (for ten to thirty minutes) with running cold water. The following are supplemental or follow-up treatments.

First Degree: Wet liniments made from comfrey, sage, nettle, blueberry, marigold, burdock slippery elm bark, red raspberry leaves, chickweed, or elder flowers can be applied. Aloe vera gel, cucumber juice, or potato juice applications also help decrease inflammation. To promote recovery, cold-pressed oils in the diet, with only natural foods and supplementation with extra vitamins A, B-complex, C, and E, as well as the minerals zinc, manganese, magnesium, and copper, will help.

Second Degree: Treat like a first-degree burn, but also apply vitamin E (from wheat germ oil) directly over the burned area. Although it was common in the past to recommend breaking burn blisters, this is now considered inadvisable because it increases the risk of infection. When the blisters eventually rupture or dry up on their own, they often become caked, brittle, and painful. Emollient salves with oil bases will help at this stage; olive, linseed, and sesame oils, as well as lanolin and honey, have all been used successfully.

Third Degree: If the burn is very small and in a noncritical area, treat like a second-degree burn. Otherwise, see a physician immediately. Application of vitamin E during recovery has been shown to decrease scarring.

The following burn paste is said to heal third-degree burns: Make a paste of 3 parts of comfrey root or leaves, 1 part lobelia, ½ part wheat germ oil, ½ part honey. (Use powdered herbs.) Cleanse the burned area and apply the paste thickly for three days.

For all burns, whenever it is necessary to protect the area from contamination, cover with clean or sterile dressings or with cold, wet compresses. Exposure to the air, however, is most effective in promoting healing. Aloe vera gel—preferably obtained fresh from the live plant—can be beneficial in all types of burns.

Homeopathic ointment of calendula is one of the best

remedies to use for burns. For electrical burns use phosphorous 6th to 30th potency. Applying fresh-squeezed ginger juice can be a very effective treatment for burns.

BURSITIS

OTHER NAMES: Housemaid's knee, miner's elbow, tennis elbow.

DESCRIPTION: Bursitis is inflammation of the bursae, which are small sacs that contain a lubricating fluid. They absorb shock and reduce friction between bones, muscles, tendons, and other tissues that rub against each other. They are found mostly in the vicinity of joints, and the ones that most often become inflamed are those associated with the shoulder, elbow, knee, ankle, heel, and big toe (a bunion is bursitis at the big toe; *see* BUNIONS).

SYMPTOMS: In acute bursitis there is localized pain, swelling, and tenderness. The skin in the area becomes red and hot. Moving the joint may be difficult and painful, particularly if calcium deposits are present.

CAUSES: Trauma or continual irritation of the bursa from rubbing, bumping, stretching, or pressure is the most common cause for bursitis. Others are acute or chronic infection, allergies, rheumatoid or inflammatory arthritis, and gout. Occasionally, bursitis occurs without any obvious cause.

TREATMENT: If possible, of course, the cause should be eliminated (for example, tight shoes that cause bunions or activities causing heavy wear on the shoulders, elbows, or knees).

Acute bursitis should be treated as follows (in addition

to treating any infection that may be involved). Apply three wet, cold towels to the affected area and cover with two dry towels. Leave on for one hour and keep the joint immobilized. Give the area a friction rub until it becomes warm. This sequence can be done twice a day and an additional wet cold pack applied overnight. The following herbs can be used in compresses, bath additives, or liniments for external application: arnica, eucalyptus, ginger, and apple cider vinegar. These can also be used for chronic bursitis. Teas made from meadowsweet, pansy, poplar, or willow can be taken to help reduce inflammation and pain. Fasting with fruit or vegetable juices helps the healing process. Supplementing the diet with vitamins B_{12}, C, and E, as well as with two tablespoons of molasses daily, is recommended.

With chronic bursitis, or when an attack of acute bursitis has subsided, it is useful to exercise the affected joint in order to restore its freedom of motion. It may be helpful to apply heat before starting each session. Start with short sessions and use only simple motions appropriate to the natural movement of the joint (like leaning forward and gently swinging the arm in a circular manner for bursitis in the shoulder). Progressively increase the duration and vigor of the exercise as freedom of movement improves, but never continue in a session if acute pain occurs.

A tea or tablet of willow bark can be taken to relieve pain and promote healing. It has the same properties as aspirin but will not be so injurious to the digestion. The tea is made by simmering one teaspoon in a cup of boiling water for ten minutes; two or three cups should be taken per day. Another more pleasant tea that has similar properties is made from equal parts comfrey, nettles, and rosemary. Steep one teaspoon in a cup of boiling water for five minutes. Cod liver oil taken daily will also help to strengthen the joints and counteract stiffness; it also helps reduce cracking noises in the joints.

Parsley tea, made by boiling one packed cup of fresh leaves in a quart of boiling water for five or ten minutes, reduces pains caused by acid accumulations in the joints. Cherries and cherry juice are a near specific for such pains; take frequently for four days, abstain for four days, and repeat as needed. All of these approaches are equally useful for the treatment of rheumatic and arthritic pains as well.

(For homeopathic treatment, see ARTHRITIS.)

Certainly the universally safe and beneficial products known to relieve pain are the various naturally derived pain-relieving liniments and ointments. Two that are particularly effective are the Chinese Possum Oil and Tiger Balm. Internally, Planetary formula number 96 (Willow Aid) contains willow bark extract, corydalis root (related to the poppy family), dong quai root to aid circulation, valerian root to relieve pain, and resins of guggul and boswellia, which promote circulation and help relieve pain. Two or more tablets of this pain-relieving formula should be taken as often as needed. Externally, number 59 (Narayana Oil) is the most popular Indian Ayurvedic oil for relieving stiffness, aches, and pains anywhere in the body.

CANCER

OTHER NAMES: Carcinoma, malignant neoplasm, malignant tumor, sarcoma.

DESCRIPTION: In simple terms, cancer occurs when a normal cell in the body loses its "intelligence" and becomes undifferentiated; that is, it no longer performs its original function but rather begins to divide in an uncontrolled way. As cancerous cells and growths overgrow into other surrounding normal tissues, they cause obstruction and compression of ducts, organs, vessels, and nerves; decrease the number of normally functioning cells; and decrease the amount of nutrients available to healthy, normally functioning cells.

There are many different types of cancer. Some spread quickly from their origin, traveling through the bloodstream and the lymphatic system and establishing new tumors in other parts of the body; others grow slowly and stay more or less in one place. The prognosis for a given case depends on the type of cancer, the overall health of the person's body and immune system, and the promptness and thoroughness of treatment.

The most common cancers in men are cancers of the lung, prostate, colon and rectum, urinary tract, and blood and lymph system. Women suffer most often from cancers of the breast, colon and rectum, lung, uterus, and blood and lymph system.

SYMPTOMS: The symptoms vary greatly, depending on the type and location of the cancer. Weight loss, fatigue, pain, loss of bodily functions, anemia, and deformity are all common. More specific signs that may indicate cancer include refusal of a sore to heal, persistent indigestion or lack of appetite for which no cause can be found, difficulty in swallowing, noticeable change in a mole or wart, a hard lump (especially in the breast), a chronic cough or hoarseness, unusual bleeding (such as blood in the urine or the stool, or in a nonmenstrual vaginal discharge), changes in bowel habits that last more than a few days, persistent unexplained fever, and unusual susceptibility to bruising. More often than not, these symptoms are indicative of something other than cancer; but when they occur, it is only prudent to get a competent professional diagnosis.

CAUSES: Much research has been and is being done on the biochemical and molecular mechanisms by which the many forms of cancer begin and spread. But for our purposes, these mechanisms are not the main concern. The basic causes of cancer are those environmental, dietary, and psychological factors that allow apparently normal cellular processes to get out of control and develop into cancer. The situation is so complex that no single theory can hope to provide a complete explanation, but the following are some of the more plausible attempts.

Hans Selye's theory of the General Adaptation Syndrome states that chronic or local stress on an organism or tissue will weaken that tissue and set up conditions in which the cells under this strain become undifferentiated. The assault of cigarette smoke on the lungs is an excellent example of such stress. It is thought, though, that even in healthy individuals' cells are always becoming undifferentiated, but they are quickly identified as foreign bodies and scavenged up by the immune system. This is known as the surveillance theory. Cancer is believed to develop when the immune system's functioning is compromised by excessive stress so that its surveillance cannot keep up with the rate of release of undifferentiated cells.

According to the "tissue damage syndrome hypothesis" of Ling and Gersen, when the ratio of sodium to potassium in the body becomes higher than normal, cells swell with water; the extra water in the cells damages intracellular proteins, causing the cells to become undifferentiated.

The "catalase and antioxidant hypothesis" states that we are routinely deficient in catalase and antioxidants. These are molecules that neutralize or prevent the formation of "free radicals," which are very reactive molecules that disrupt the "intelligence" of the normally functioning cell and cause it to become undifferentiated. Catalase, an enzyme manufactured in the body, is destroyed by ingested drugs, inhaled toxins, radiation, canned and devitalized foods with preservatives, and other environmental, stress-related, and dietary factors. Specific antioxidants that we are deficient in are vitamins C and E, and selenium.

Emotional stress deserves to be mentioned separately as a cause of cancer. Many studies indicate that loss of a significant other, frustration over an important life situation or goal, or a tendency toward feelings of despair, hopelessness, and grief is common to over 75 percent of the individuals who develop cancer. As already mentioned, the stress of such situations impairs the ability of the immune system to cope with the amounts of undifferentiated cells produced in the body.

The fact is that there are many causes for cancer, including hereditary factors, and there are many forms of cancer. Given this, it seems that even seemingly healthy individuals who are predisposed can develop cancer. Certainly people who function in optimum health, eating pure food, breathing pure air, drinking pure water, and are not overly exposed to the many carcinogens in the environment stand a much better chance of never contracting cancer. If they do, they would have a much better chance of either recovering or living a long life with it in a relative slow-growing state.

Whatever the claims, most cancers are not easy to cure, so that there simply is not a single treatment that one can rely on as equally effective for everyone. At present, treating cancer is too often like trying to choose between a rock and a hard place where none of the available options are desirable. Nevertheless, one needs to choose, and before doing so, it is always wise to consider all possible options. Obviously one should seek out qualified and expert medical advice, ideally from more than one source. Michael always suggests that cancer patients begin by going online to cancer researcher Ralph Moss's Web site and purchase the selected *Moss Report* that pertains to the particular cancer you may have. It is one of the best investments a cancer patient can make, since it will inform them of the type of cancer they may have, the prognosis, and possible treatments using both conventional and/or alternative medicine. I would also direct the reader to my books, *The Treatment of Cancer with Herbs: An Integrated Approach* (Lotus Press) and *The Way of Herbs* (Pocket Books) and to other books on alternative medicine cancer treatments listed in the bibliography of this book.

TREATMENT: Unfortunately, it's a rare person that functions at an optimum level of health all the time. For the great majority of people, cancer is an ever-present risk. If you find that you have a form of cancer, seek help from a qualified naturopath or physician who believes in the principles of natural medicine. After consultation with this person, you will have to make a choice about your treatment. Some cancers are treated very effectively with surgery, radiation, chemotherapy, or a combination of these methods. If your physician tells you that the success rate is from 80 percent to 100 percent with these techniques, and the side effects of the treatment are not worse than the cure, you might do well to try them. Furthermore, if your cancer is removable with these treatments, you can have it removed and then change your life-style to try to prevent a recurrence.

Nonmetastatic forms of skin cancer, prostate cancer, and cervical dysplasias are good candidates for early self-treatment. However, regardless of what form of treatment chosen, the reader is advised to have all cancers monitored by a licensed, qualified health practitioner.

If the cancer has not spread and is localized appropriately for topical treatment, the regular application of vitamin A oil applied to the area has been shown to be very effective. Open a capsule containing oil-based vitamin A and place the oil over the cancer. Apply twice daily until the cancer disappears or falls off.

For other forms of cancer, the following regimen is excellent and has saved many people; but, of course, nothing can be guaranteed. Its success depends greatly on your level of participation, including careful monitoring of your own condition. Professional supervision is strongly advised.

1. Exercise: This is vitally important. Your immune system, circulation, and overall health are dependent on movement. Daily brisk walks, stretching, aerobics, and muscle toning are all excellent. However, never exercise to the point of exhaustion. Bouncing on a small trampoline or rebounder is a good, nontraumatic way to increase tone and oxygenation for every cell in your body. If you are debilitated, start with range-of-motion exercises in bed. Rebuild your strength gradually. You must believe that you are going to get well, and act accordingly. Exercising is taking a giant step toward improvement.

2. Diet: There are a number of therapeutic diets that have been proven effective in many cases.

For many types of cancers, the macrobiotic vegetarian diet based upon the use of 40% to 50% whole grains (especially brown rice and barley), about 10 percent fish and 20% beans (including soy, black beans, and red azuki beans), 20% to 30% lightly steamed vegetables, 2% to 5% sea vegetables, and 5% to 10% seasonally available fruits has proven phenomenally effective in ameliorating many forms of cancer. (See *The Book of Macrobiotics* by Michio Kushi in the Bibliography.)

For cancers in strong individuals who have previously consumed an excess of denatured foods, overly rich foods, meats, dairy, sugar, alcohol and coffee, a raw fruit and vegetable diet can be followed. Along with this diet, drink each day: four seven-ounce glasses of green-leaf vegetable juice, five seven-ounce glasses of apple or carrot juice, one seven-ounce glass of orange or grapefruit juice. One glass of juice should be taken each hour, alternating until all ten portions have been consumed. Follow this program for twenty-one days, along with the recommended herbal tea and supplements. After twenty-one days, continue to eat a high-fiber fruit, vegetable, and light-grain and bean diet, including only those foods you know you are not allergic to. Ask your naturopath or physician about the cytotoxic test.

3. Medication: This aspect of treatment should be supervised very closely by your naturopath or physician. Recent research has shown that beta carotene, a substance that the body converts into vitamin A, is excellent to protect against respiratory, stomach, bladder, skin, and breast cancer. Carrots are high in beta carotene; other sources are apricots, cantaloupe, sweet potatoes, tomatoes, spinach, cabbage, broccoli, cauliflower, and brussels sprouts. Beta carotene has the advantage that it does not cause the liver toxicity associated with megadoses of vitamin A. In large doses, it may turn your skin yellow, but the effect is harmless and disappears when the intake is reduced.

4. *Hydrotherapy:* Daily hydrotherapy is a must so that blood circulation can be optimized and toxins eliminated. The following should be done: a) contrast baths (*see* Part Three); b) warm poultices to any involved area, using equal parts of the following herbs: comfrey, plantain, slippery elm, white oak bark, mullein, prickly ash bark, lobelia (¼ part), walnut leaves, and skullcap; cover the poultice and keep it in place for one hour; c) see Part Three for other beneficial treatments.

5. *Meditation/Yoga/Prayer:* Our belief system plays a very powerful role in our lives and especially in our health. Prayer is not to be underestimated: it does have the power to heal you, and it certainly offers comfort and hope. Visualizing your cancer diminishing and your immune system strengthening is extremely important. Carl Simonton has clearly demonstrated that, even without a change in diet or life-style, our beliefs and imagination can eliminate life-threatening cancers. Meditation and yoga also promote mental states that support the natural healing mechanisms of the body.

6. *Play:* This may be very difficult to do, but you must try to have a lighter attitude and outlook. Enjoying your family, friends, work, and activities is important. Believing that you will live is essential.

7. *Counseling:* Resentment is the one emotion most often associated with individuals who have cancer. Practicing forgiveness is necessary if you are to allow yourself to be

rid of your disease. Talking over your fears, emotions, worries, and problems is helpful and supportive. Don't hold anything back. Your cancer is not just a physical event.

8. *Purpose:* Although feelings of loss, grief, hopelessness, and despair are closely linked to the cancer personality, they are not irreversible states. Having something to live for has long been recognized as a vital component in survival and longevity. Seeking help from others is very important at these times. Look to your family and friends; explore your hobbies and interests. Look toward life.

9. *Other Therapies:* Four other aspects of treatment deserve separate mention: hyperthermia, the grape diet, enemas, and new herbal drugs.

Hyperthermia, consisting of slowly raising the body temperature for a sustained period of time, is effective in selectively killing cancer cells that are especially sensitive to higher temperatures. This has been known for some time, but as reported by Reuters on November 6, 2001, a specialist from the Siberian city of Novosibirsk reports that heating the body to 43.5° or 44°C confirmed that cancer cells die at around 42.5°C, or 108.5°F.

Patients were placed in a bath of water heated to 46°C (118.5°F) for forty-five minutes to an hour once or twice a week. They were administered drugs to increase the tolerance of tissues and organs to heat and to support heart function. This included a general anesthetic and a modified lung ventilator to assist breathing. After this their body temperatures were returned to normal under supervision. The center's director claimed that this treatment was successfully applied to 180 out of 500 cancer patients with all major types of cancer. Hyperthermy alone was found to be effective and increased the beneficial effects of chemotherapy while greatly reducing adverse effects such as hair loss. Besides killing cancer cells, hyperthermy reduced the tolerance of cancer cells to chemotherapy.

Herbal oil enemas every four to six hours may be necessary at the outset of the treatment program. Regular bowel habits should be maintained (*see* CONSTIPATION).

To aid liver detoxification and speed the healing process, a daily coffee-retention enemy may be added. In extreme cases, this may be administered twice a day.

Prepare the coffee by drip or percolation; do not use instant coffee. The enema consists of an eight-ounce cup of coffee to one quart of water. This is injected into the colon at room temperature and retained for fifteen to thirty minutes. To ease bowel cramping and aid longer retention, have the enema bag no more than six inches above the body. During the retention period the bowel should be massaged and the patient gently turned to allow the solution to reach all parts of the intestines.

The liver is the key to detoxification, and the coffee enema, along with the recommended herbs, is an effective method used by many metabolic therapists. Liver detoxification must be accomplished before one can rebuild the immune system. Caffeine stimulates bile secretion, thus cleansing the liver and restoring an alkaline condition to the small intestines.

Extracts of a tropical species of periwinkle (*Vinca rosea,* Madagascar periwinkle) have shown specific activity against some forms of cancer. Two drugs derived from the plant are in medical use: vincristine for leukemia and vinblastine for Hodgkin's disease. This treatment is strictly for use under medical supervision.

One should purify the blood, lymphatic system, and liver with formulas 14 and 15, suma, and a tea of Planetary

Bitters. This consists of 10 parts chaparral leaves, 6 parts each of red clover blossoms and hawthorn berries, dandelion root, burdock root, sarsaparilla root, poke root, American ginseng, sassafras bark, Oregon grape root or barberry root, echinacea root, angelica root, yellow dock root, gravel root, prickly ash bark, and 2 parts licorice root.

To prepare, simmer four tablespoons in a quart of boiling water for ten minutes. For cancer treatment, take one-half cup every two hours for twenty-one days, then three or four cups daily. This is also an excellent healthful tea to take once each morning or more often during the day if needed. It is also an excellent treatment for the prevention and treatment of arthritis and rheumatic problems.

Homeopathic remedies to consider are as follows: Carcinosim 30 to 200th potency—one dose taken once or twice monthly. Arsenicum 30 to 200th potency—for burning pains, tumors. Lachesis to the 6th potency—for tumors that appear scarlet, deep blue, or ash-colored. Sulphur to 6th potency—when there is exhaustion in the morning, cold extremities with the head warm and face flushed, aggravated at bed time. Calcium fluoride to the 6th potency—when there are stony hard lumps.

Other homeopathic remedies to consider include Phytolacca, Sanguinaria, and Hydrastis—all in 6th to 30th potency.

Although it may appear overwhelming at first, the program, as outlined, can be accomplished at home with the help of one person. Keep your spirits up. An old saying among natural healers is that there are no incurable diseases, only incurable patients.

CANDIDA ALBICANS

OTHER NAMES: Systemic thrush, thrush.

DESCRIPTION: This disease is caused by an overgrowth of candida albicans yeast. It is normally present in small amounts in the body, but when it is at the stage of overgrowth, it is commonly found as thrush in the mouth. Only recently has it been considered that an overgrowth of the yeast systemically can give rise to the plethora of symptoms.

SYMPTOMS: Moodiness, extreme food sensitivities with gas and bloating after meals, depression, low energy, weakness, extreme PMS symptoms in women.

CAUSES: Generally this condition is caused by the suppression of acute diseases such as colds, fevers, and other inflammatory diseases with excessive use of antibiotics. In point of fact, even taking so-called natural anti-inflammatories such as ascorbic acid in high doses can predispose one to this condition.

One of the more serious causes is an unbalanced diet. Essentially this condition is characterized in Traditional Chinese Medicine as a liver, spleen, and digestive system disorder. The liver and pancreas regulate the smooth flow of important digestive enzymes which, if lacking, will cause gas and bloating. Specifically, the accumulation of abdominal fluid and gas will put pressure on the sensitive nerves and meridians in the gastrointestinal tract, giving rise to a number of paradoxical emotional reactions ranging from anger and anxiety to depression. Thus there is a strong connection with hypoglycemic reactions in such individuals.

One who overindulges in cold, raw foods, and lacks in proper protein balance can give rise to the candida overgrowth condition. Another cause is eating too many rich or denatured foods.

TREATMENT: The major issue is to first restore digestion by correcting the dietary imbalance. The problem is that many foods that would normally be good for one to use, such as whole grains, beans, and so forth, may prove to aggravate the symptoms. One must have great patience to gradually restore the digestive fire. One way is to soak all grains and legumes a day before cooking. They should be served with a curry-like mixture made up of the following spices: coriander, turmeric, cumin seed, ginger, and asafetida. These herbs are freshly powdered and first sautéed in a tablespoon of ghee (clarified butter) until the flavor begins to become apparent. Then stir in the precooked legumes or grains. A pinch of saffron is also good to add to rice and grains when cooking because it has powerful circulating properties. All food must be well cooked, not raw; avoid cold foods, fruits, juices, dairy, alcohol, and most drugs.

One of the most important treatments for candida patients is to restore normal intestinal flora by taking large doses of acidophilus and bifidus cultures daily. Michael uses Metagenics brand in our clinic and, in addition, we recommend another product with soil-based organisms manufactured by Ganeden called Primal Defense.

Specific symptoms may vary and should be treated accordingly. However, Planetary formulas number 7 (Triphala) and 15 (Digestive Grape Bitters) taken before and after meals (about thirty drops), and formula number 16 (Candida Digest), are very beneficial for restoring digestive strength.

In many cases the candida overgrowth is so endemic that patients may have to consider seeing a medical doctor and using anticandida drugs such as nystatin or diflucan. After the yeast is under control they should strictly follow the candida diet and use herbal digestive aids described above.

CARDIOVASCULAR CONDITIONS
(INCLUDING ANGINA AND HEART ATTACK)

While we cannot specifically address all cardiovascular conditions, the following, including angina pectoris, arteriosclerosis, congestive heart failure, and hypertension, is a representative range. Heart disease is potentially a serious condition, and while in many cases it has proven amenable to alternative treatment, it should nevertheless be carefully monitored by a qualified medical doctor.

DESCRIPTION: Angina is a condition that causes moderate to severe chest pain. There are two forms: Stable angina occurs when a person is at rest, while unstable angina occurs during or after some form of moderate exercise. The worst form is unstable angina, and it indicates risk of a heart attack. The cause is atherosclerosis, which occurs when the vascular system becomes narrowed with the deposit of cholesterol-rich plaque on the walls of the arteries. This results in a lack of nourishment and oxygen to the heart, which triggers angina or a full-blown heart attack.

Arteriosclerosis is a blocking of the coronary arteries due to a buildup of plaque on its walls as a result of prolonged elevated cholesterol and triglycerides. In general, it is better that one's total cholesterol is close to or under

200. More important, however, is a good ratio between the HDL (so-called "good cholesterol") and the LDL (the so-called "bad cholesterol").

Hypertension, or high blood pressure, is an increase in peripheral resistance caused by a vasoconstriction or narrowing of the peripheral blood vessels.

Congestive heart failure is a condition accompanied by symptoms of weakness, breathlessness, abdominal discomfort, and edema in the lower parts of the body caused by congestion and reduced outflow of blood from the left side of the heart.

Cardiac arrest, or myocardial infarction, occurs when the heart muscle doesn't receive an adequate supply of blood. This is usually a result of previous, untreated arteriosclerosis and often, though not always, cardiac arrest is preceded by angina symptoms. In the actual case of a heart attack, one should administer CPR and call for assistance.

CAUSES: The risks associated with cardiovascular diseases include arteriosclerosis (hardening of the arteries) and/or atherosclerosis (blocking of the arteries with plaque). Heart attacks can be triggered by sudden shock, fear, and overexertion. Other causes are smoking tobacco, diabetes, hereditary predisposition, and an imbalanced diet that is too high in carbohydrates, saturated fats, and salt.

TREATMENT: Anyone with these life-threatening symptoms should be monitored by a medical doctor. However, many herbs and supplements have proven to be effective for this condition. Since heart disease is a major killer in the western world, we will offer a number of supplements and herbal remedies that have been found to be effective.

Hawthorn *(Crataegus laevigata* or *C. Monogyna).* This is

one of the most popular and effective herbs and is widely prescribed by doctors in Germany for the treatment of angina, hypertension, and the early stages of congestive heart failure. The berries, leaves, and flowers are used. The berries, flowers, and leaves are rich in flavonoids considered important for the herb's therapeutic effects. They also contain from 1 to 3 percent oligomeric compounds also known as pycnogenols or procyanidans. These have the ability to dilate the smooth vessels of the coronary arteries. The daily dose ranges from 160 to 900 mg of hawthorn extract. A tablespoon of the crushed berries, together with the leaves and flowers, can be simmered in a cup of boiling water and steeped for twenty minutes. A cup of this tea can be taken once or twice daily for angina, hypertension, or early stages of congestive heart failure. Again, heart symptoms can be serious and one should seek proper medical assistance. Furthermore, the use of hawthorn in conjunction with other cardiac tonics such as digitalis or Lanoxin should be monitored carefully as hawthorn may increase the activity of these drugs. Hawthorn also should be carefully monitored if one is taking anticoagulants such as aspirin or coumadin, although Michael has not seen or known of any problems with the use of hawthorn in normal dosage with these drugs. In general, one should monitor the use of hawthorn over the course of two months to determine whether it is having any beneficial effect.

Dan shen, or Chinese red sage root *(Salvia milthiorizum),* a member of the mint family, is another great herb. It is particularly useful for angina pectoris and coronary heart disease and will also relieve other symptoms that are often associated with or precede heart problems, including insomnia, palpitations, and irritability.

Red sage root, called "dan shen" by the Chinese, has also been well researched and seems to improve microcirculation of the capillaries throughout the body, dilate the coronary artery, and increase blood flow, improving myocardial contraction and adjusting the heart rate. Thus it is most commonly used by the Chinese for coronary heart disease either as a single agent or in compound formulas.

Besides its value for the heart and in the treatment of heart diseases, dan shen promotes the regeneration and repair of tissues and inhibits the excessive growth of fibroblasts and tumor cells. It also inhibits the coagulation of blood and excessive active fibronolysis, and is antibacterial, being effective against *Pseudomonas, E. coli, Vibrio proteus, B. tyhi, Shigella dysenteriae, Shigella flexneri,* staph, aureus, and other bacteria; lowers blood cholesterol; reduces enlarged liver and spleen; has mild sedative and tranquilizing effects; and reduces blood sugar levels. Because of its effects on vascular circulation, dan shen is frequently used in gynecology for dysmenorrhea (painful menses) and amenorrhea (stopped menses).

Arjuna: wonder herb for the heart. One of the most effective herbs for angina and other heart problems is the Ayurvedic herb called arjuna *(Terminalia arjuna)*. The pulverized bark is astringent and a cardiac stimulant and tonic. Arjuna has been used in India for heart disease since the sixth century. It is one of the most effective herbs for a wide variety of heart diseases, including angina, endocarditis, mitral regurgitation, pericarditis, and congestive heart failure with symptoms of abdominal swelling (dropsy). Double-blind short- and long-term studies have been conducted comparing arjuna extract for congestive heart failure on patients taking 500 mg capsules once every eight hours. While the mechanism of its action could not be determined, it was found to be very effective both long- and short-term compared with conventional therapy and placebos. The cardiotonic activity of arjuna may be due to either or both its glycoside content or the free-radical scavenging actions of the plant's tannins and flavones.* Arjuna is a coronary vasodilator. Take one half teaspoon of the powdered bark with some honey and warm water. Arjuna is available both as a single herb but works with even greater efficacy in a clinically tried formula from Planetary formulas.

Garlic *(Allium sativum)*. It has been shown that a regular increase in the use of onions and garlic as part of one's diet significantly lowers blood fibrinogen levels, which if not lowered tend to lead toward elevated cholesterol and congestive heart failure. The versatile "wonder herb," garlic can also be taken as a supplement.

Guggul *(Commiphora mukul)*. Guggul is a resin from an herb growing in India. It is closely related to myrrh. It is used in special formulas in Ayurvedic medicine to promote circulation, relieve arthritic pains, treat hypothyroids, and treat cardiovascular disease associated with elevated cholesterol and triglycerides in the blood. It contains essential oils and guggulsterones known to lower blood lipids. In studies guggulsterones are known to bind with the bad LDL cholesterol and remove it from circulation. Three-month studies in humans found that guggul low-

---

*Bharani A., Ganguly A., and Bhargava K.D. Salutary effect of *Terminalia arjuna* in patients with severe refractory heart failure. *Internal Journal of Cardiology*, Vol. 49, 1995–99. Reichert, R. *Terminalia arjuna* for congestive heart failure. *Quarterly Review of Natural Medicine,* Fall 1996, 177–78. Lad, Vasant, *The Complete Book of Ayurvedic Home Remedies* (Harmony Books, 1998).

ered total cholesterol on average about 24 percent and serum triglycerides about 23 percent. A double-blind study compared guggul to the cholesterol-lowering drug clofibrate and found that both had similar cholesterol- and triglyceride-lowering effects, but guggul uniquely had the ability to raise the ratio of HDL (the good cholesterol) compared to LDL (the bad form). The average dose is 500 mg of the standardized 25 mg guggulsterones, taken in tablets three times daily. The traditional Ayurvedic preparation known as Yogaraj guggul is available in Planetary formula number 42 (Guggul Cholesterol Compound).

Chinese red yeast rice (Chinese: hong qu). Red yeast rice has been used by Chinese cooks over a thousand years to flavor and color meat and fish and to preserve food and make rice wine. It is still used in China and Japan to improve blood circulation. Various studies have shown that red yeast can lower significantly LDL cholesterol and triglycerides while raising HDL cholesterol. One of the constituents of red yeast is lovastatin, which is the same cholesterol-lowering drug called Mevacor manufactured by Merck, the pharmaceutical giant. Despite its proven cholesterol-lowering efficacy, Merck succeeded in getting the FDA to ban products based on the use of red yeast as a dietary supplement for lowering cholesterol. While the drug only contains lovastatin, red yeast contains other "statins," which gives it a milder but wider cholesterol-lowering effect.

One study found that for individuals taking 600 mg of red yeast rice twice daily compared to 1,200 mg of another Chinese herb the red yeast reduced total cholesterol on average 22 percent while the other Chinese herb only reduced it 7 percent. For many a 22 percent reduction of total cholesterol is adequate to get their cholesterol levels down to normal. Compared to the price of the various statin drugs, it is no wonder that there has been such a concerted effort to ban the use of this natural substance from therapeutic use. Red yeast is available in Chinese markets and pharmacies throughout the world. While it may not be standardized, the dose can be adjusted in the same way that it is for statin drugs, based on blood tests that measure cholesterol levels after taking the drug for a month.

Historically there have been no serious side effects reported from the use of red yeast, while there are many from the use of the various statin drugs. Nevertheless, one should be on the watch for symptoms such as elevated liver enzymes (which will revert back to normal soon after quitting the drug and presumably the red yeast). Statin drugs are known to have anticoagulant properties, which should be considered for those who have a tendency to bleed or are about to undergo surgery. Other symptoms caused by statin drugs include inexplicable pain and weakness in the joints (especially the knees, ankles, and legs). These should be reported to one's doctor.

The drug manufacturers claim that these symptoms only occur in a small percentage of people taking these drugs, and considering the benefit for some in preventing a heart attack they claim it to be a worthwhile risk. Personally, Michael has found a considerable number of elderly individuals who have stopped their cholesterol-lowering statin drugs in favor of being able to walk. It has never been studied, but it is worth a try substituting a modest dose of approximately 1,200 mg of red yeast twice daily to be a worthwhile compromise.

Recently, the statin drugs, having also shown other benefits ranging from the treatment of acne, allergies, arthritis, and Alzheimer's, are being touted as the new wonder drugs. A good question is whether red yeast is a good alternative for these conditions as well.

For many, elevated cholesterol levels are a matter of constitution and heredity. Considering that a significant number of people with normal or low cholesterol nevertheless die of heart failure and a significant number with elevated cholesterol seem to live a normal life span, there is something to consider in all of this as well. Regardless of what supplement one chooses, it is always preferable to try to use diet and lifestyle modification and supplements such as guggul, L-tyrosine (also known to lower cholesterol), niacin, and garlic.

Gold water. Saying that one may have a "heart of gold" may have more significance than one may think. Gold is a metal that is healing for the heart and may gradually reduce cholesterol and relieve angina and arrhythmias. To make gold water, simply boil a piece of pure 24-carat gold in 12 cups of water until 1 cup evaporates. One teaspoon of this can be taken twelve or thirteen times daily, according to Ayurvedic physician Dr. Vasant Lad, "to energize the heart, strengthen mental faculties and awaken pure awareness." Boiling the gold in this way will not damage it.

Tienchi ginseng (*Panax pseudoginseng*; also known as "san qi" ginseng). This is a plant that is a close relative of the more popular Asian or American ginsengs and is one of the most valuable and important herbs known. It improves energy and vitality, strengthens blood circulation, dissolves clots, and promotes healing. Imagine an herb that can stop bleeding and promote healthy blood circulation at the same time. Tienchi is the key ingredient in a famous Chinese wound-healing formula known as yunnan bai yao, first developed for serious knife and gunshot wounds during Mao's Communist revolution. Indeed, it will stop serious hemorrhages and at the same time dissolve harmful blood clots. It is an important herb in Planetary formula number 44 (Hawthorn Heart Formula). If one is taking tienchi as a separate herb, the recommended dose of the powdered herb is about 4 g twice daily with warm water and a little rice wine to act as a carrier. Otherwise, one can make an alcoholic extract by macerating 60 g of the freshly ground root powder in a pint of vodka or brandy. Allow this to stand for a few days and then take one teaspoon once or twice daily.

Night-blooming cereus *(Selenicereus grandiflorus)*. This herb has been found growing throughout the tropics of North America. Both the flowers (which bloom only once a year) and the stems are used. It is used to treat a wide variety of cardiovascular conditions including angina, endocarditis, myocarditis, and palpitations as well as urinary tract problems such as cystitis, irritable bladder, and edema. It also has been successfully used to treat symptoms of hyperthyroidism and benign prostatic hypertrophy. The best form to take it in is as an alcoholic fluid extract, about 5 to 10 drops taken 3 or 4 times daily.

Vitamin E, EPA/DHA (omega-3 fatty acids), coenzyme Q10, carnitine, and taurine. All of these food supplements have shown conclusively positive effects in relieving many cardiovascular problems. The first two work by inhibiting platelet aggregation, reducing blood pressure, strengthening the heart, and improving circulation. Co-Q10 improves cellular oxygen utilization in the heart, reducing cardiac stress and relieving symptoms. Carnitine and taurine have been shown to improve cardiac function and reduce angina in multiple studies.

Life-style, diet, vegetables, and garlic for angina and other heart problems. Life-style issues that contribute to cardiovascular diseases include stress, sedentary life-style, smoking, alcohol, high-fat diet, obesity, caffeine, and a low-fiber diet. While a diet emphasizing vegetables, whole grains, and beans are good for reducing cholesterol and treating heart disease, together with moderate exercise, garlic and onions have been found to be of specific benefit. These members of the lily family seem to slow blood-clotting, reduce the oxidation of LDL cholesterol (the bad kind), and have other known cardioprotective effects.

CARIES

OTHER NAMES: Tooth decay.

DESCRIPTION, SYMPTOMS, AND CAUSES: Caries is the rotting of the teeth. This is usually caused by the action of *Streptococcus mutans* bacteria. Caries begins with the deposit of plaque in the teeth. The bacteria inhabit this plaque and are therefore available to cause tooth decay. Bacteria depend largely on carbohydrates, which stimulate their metabolic systems and cause them to multiply. This increases acids, particularly lactic acid and proteolytic enzymes. Acids also aid in the breakdown of calcium salts of the teeth, furthering their decay.

TREATMENT: Eliminate or limit all refined foods with white sugar. Brush and floss the teeth after eating. A good herbal tooth powder to prevent tooth decay as well as gum disease (pyorrhea) is a combination of powders of cinnamon, bayberry bark, peppermint leaf, and oak bark.

CARPAL TUNNEL

OTHER NAMES: CTS, repetitive stress injury of the wrist.

DESCRIPTION, SYMPTOMS, AND CAUSES: Carpal tunnel is a common painful condition caused by compression of the nerve that passes between the bones and ligaments of the wrist. Painful symptoms may be occasional or constant. Often it is most aggravated at night. There is pain with a sensation of tingling or burning radiating from the wrist to the forearm and shoulder. It is usually caused by some repetitive stress, i.e., from typing, carpentry, etc.

TREATMENT: The first thing is to try to find a way to lessen the repetitive stress on a particular joint or muscle. Alternating hot- and cold-water treatments often will relieve the pain. Periods of stretching the hand and arms are also important. Acupuncture and moxibustion are very effective for this condition.

Magnet Therapy for Carpal Tunnel, Pain, and Inflammation

Michael has personally found magnet therapy to be the quickest and most effective in practically all cases. The single most important thing is to select the correct magnet polarity, which is the negative or north polarity. This is determined by placing a small compass next to one side of the magnet. The side that attracts the north point end of the needle should be marked with nail polish or some means as biomagnetic north. This is not true north but the side that magnet therapists universally call north. This is very important, because in most cases the biomagnetic south side can aggravate the condition for which it is applied. Next, select an appropriate magnet with the highest gauss (strength) rating possible. Take time to carefully palpate as precisely as possible the area from which the pain seems to radiate. Apply the magnet over the area with the north or negative pole facing against the skin. Now, lightly tap on it with a finger for thirty to fifty times in succession. Usually this is enough to relieve the pain significantly. It's quite amazing in most cases for patients to discover their repetitive stress pains nearly or completely gone in less than two minutes.

Michael specifically uses small, 6,000 to 9,000 gauss strength, "acuband" magnets (see Resources). These are the most economical and the most convenient and effective magnets in my clinical experience. They are sold in sheets of twelve fastened to a specially manufactured Band-Aid. The proper polarity is already with the north or negative side, having a small indentation on the side that faces outward. I recommend that patients buy extra Band-Aids, since the magnets can be reused practically indefinitely.

I use them for pain of the back, wrists, knees, shoulders, neck, elbows, and ankles. Magnets are not 100 percent effective; sometimes the polarity needs to be reversed on some individual, with the south or positive side against the skin; sometimes the pain is simply too deep or there is too much deterioration of underlying tissue. They are cheap and always worth a try. In practice Michael finds them to be approximately 80 percent effective for most pains and inflammations.

CATARACTS

OTHER NAME: Lens opacity.

DESCRIPTION: A cataract is a progressive clouding of the normally transparent, crystal-like lens or the lens capsule in the eye. This degenerative process most commonly occurs in the elderly, in which case it is referred to as "senile cataract." Various diseases or eye injuries, however, can cause cataracts to form at any age. One eye or both eyes may be affected.

SYMPTOMS: Cataracts generally develop gradually, causing a painless progressive loss of vision that may or may not eventually lead to blindness. Both blurring of vision and difficulty in focusing may occur. An eye examination will show gray opacities in the lens, their size depending on the stage to which the cataract has progressed.

CAUSES: Trauma to the eye, diabetes mellitus, gout, rickets, hereditary disease (galactosemia), certain toxic agents, eye inflammation and infection, X rays, microwaves, heat, and drugs have all been known to cause cataracts. An infant whose mother contracts rubella early in pregnancy may be born with cataracts. The main cause, however, is the degeneration of the lens with age as it gradually becomes less efficient at taking up nutrients from the liquid that surrounds it.

TREATMENT: First, proper diet and health habits will help prevent or slow down the formation of cataracts. In particular, vitamin C, riboflavin, and calcium have been noted to be necessary for proper lens metabolism and functioning.

If cataracts have developed and have progressed to the point of near blindness or severely reduced vision, the lens cannot be restored and will have to be partly or entirely removed by one of several surgical means. In some cases, a substitute lens can be placed into the eye; otherwise, glasses or contact lenses will have to provide the focusing function that is lost when the lens is removed. Follow this operation with a cleansing and rebuilding diet (see Chapter 3).

If there is clouding of the lens but vision is not yet seriously affected, the following program may help to restore normal vision.

If you are debilitated, change your diet to 80 percent raw green, leafy vegetables and fruits, and 20 percent complex carbohydrates, unsaturated fats (like safflower or sunflower oils), and protein in the form of fish, cultured milk products, or nuts and seeds, and follow the recommendations listed below.

If you are not debilitated, begin with a three- to five-day diet of diluted fruit juices. Then, follow the diet suggested for the debilitated for up to one month. Afterward, switch to the diet recommended under HEART ATTACK, *Treatment*. Take daily warm-water enemas, hot and cold showers. The following treatments are recommended for all cases:

- Herbal baths, three times a week.
- Epsom salts baths. Keeping the eye closed, bathe it for ten minutes with a solution of one teaspoon Epsom salts in a pan of warm water.
- Hydrotherapy. Using pure water at 82°F, irrigate the eye directly with a syringe and irrigate the forehead with water at 60°F. Do this for three to five days, every three hours. Footbaths in 68°F water, taken at the same time, will be helpful.
- Color therapy with green, yellow, and red light. This is very regenerative. Rotate for five to twenty minutes every twelve hours; the light does not have to be bright. Daily sunning is also a *must* (see EYE STRAIN).
- Poultices of carrot, raw potato, or clay are healing, as

are fomentations of eyebright, hyssop, fennel, dandelion, comfrey, or chamomile.

- Extra dietary supplements should include vitamins A, B-complex (especially B_2), C, D, and E, as well calcium, multiple vitamin/mineral tablets, bee pollen, raw honey, silica, and pangamic acid (vitamin B_{15}). B_{15} drops into the eyes are also useful.

HERBAL EYEWASH: Equal parts eyebright herb, bayberry bark, goldenseal and a half part cayenne pepper. Steep one teaspoon in a cup of boiling water for ten minutes. Strain through a fine cloth to remove any particles. Rinse each eye two or three times daily using an eyecup obtained at a local pharmacy. Because of the pepper, the eyewash will sting somewhat but this only indicates an increase of blood circulation through the eye and it is this that will ultimately help dissolve the cataracts.

Another treatment is to use drops of the juice of cineraria maritima. This is a traditional treatment for most eye disorders in Middle Eastern countries as it is very effective to help remove cataracts as well as strengthen the eyesight.

In India, triphala is made into a tea and is used to rinse the eyes several times daily to clear the vision. This is followed with a drop of honey in each eye.

To make triphala eyewash, dissolve four triphala tablets in 1 cup of boiling water. Allow to stand overnight or approximately for four hours. Strain through a fine cloth. Place in a covered jar. Rinse each eye 20 to 30 seconds using an eyecup purchased from a pharmacy. After three days prepare a new batch. This is good for all eye conditions, including cataracts, glaucoma, itchy eyes and conjunctivitis, and to improve vision.

Internally, one should use herbs that open the liver, such as dandelion root, Oregon grape root, or bayberry bark. Formula number 13 (Bupleurum Liver Cleanse) is a very useful formula. Taking triphala complex each night is also very beneficial. An excellent herb for clearing the eyes in Chinese medicine is chrysanthemum flower tea, which also benefits the liver.

One of the finest eye drops useful for most conditions is made from cineraria maritima. One drop is instilled into the affected eye three times daily for six months.

Homeopathic remedies include calcarea fluoride 6th, also cannabis Ind. 3rd.

In conditions of cold stagnation, the diet based on cooked foods using whole grains, legumes, vegetables, and fruit is more appropriate.

CATARRH

OTHER NAMES: Cold, cough, hay fever, postnasal drip, rhinitis.

DESCRIPTION: *Catarrh* is an old term for inflammation of the mucous membranes, especially those that line the throat and nose, and for the resulting increased mucus flow.

SYMPTOMS: The well-known symptoms include nasal congestion, postnasal drip, runny nose, headache, sometimes fever, and runny eyes (if it's an allergic reaction, as in hay fever).

CAUSES: Catarrh may result from bacterial or viral infection, or from allergic irritation of the mucous membranes. Underlying one's sensitivity to these can be habitual overeating, not chewing food properly, a poor diet high in starchy foods and milk, habitual shallow breathing, lack of exercise, poor circulation, stress, and harmful habits like smoking or excessive drinking. Living in a polluted environment can also contribute.

TREATMENT: See the treatments recommended under COLDS. Additional treatments include treatment of allergies with selenium, ascorbic acid (vitamin C), pyridoxine (vitamin B_6), and bioflavonoids; also, eating local raw honey produced by bees that pollinated the flowers of plants that you are allergic to. Taking a teaspoon of fresh radish juice every four hours is helpful for catarrh. For infants, breast-feeding is preferable to cow's milk; otherwise, goat's milk is relatively nonallergenic. To minimize the production of mucus, mothers should not drink more than two cups of milk a day if breast-feeding. Other specific remedies are cherry stalk tea, black currant juice, and almond oil. Whole-body steam baths and foot steam baths are also helpful (see Part Three).

At the first sign of catarrhal conditions with chill and fever, the local application of spirits or oil of camphor over the chest and/or nose, externally, is very helpful.

Planetary formulas number 25 (Three Spices Sinus Support) and number 21 (Mullein Breathe Free) should be taken with a tea made by steeping three or four slices of fresh ginger in a covered cup of hot water. The ginger tea can be made with a part of the skin of an organic orange, tangerine, or grapefruit. It can then be sweetened with a teaspoon of honey. One should take two or three cups of this tea daily for three or four days to dry excess mucus.

Homeopathic remedies to consider are bryonia 6th to

30th when there is burning sensation, cough, phlegm, nasal congestion; arsenicum alb. 6th for profuse acrid discharges with frequent sneezing, simultaneous affection of eyes, nose and throat; pulsatilla 6th when there are putrid discharges, ear pains, and loss of taste, smell and sensations; allium cepa 6th for frequent sneezing, profuse watery discharges.

For chronic catarrh, pulsatilla 6th to 30th or, if this fails, kali sulph 6th to 12th will be effective.

CHILBLAIN

OTHER NAMES: Exposure, frostnip, pernio.

DESCRIPTION: A chilblain is the swelling and inflammation of body tissue as a result of exposure to cold temperatures. It usually affects the feet, hands, nose, and ears. Chilblain is not as severe as frostbite, in which the tissue actually freezes.

SYMPTOMS. Chilblains cause swelling, redness, itching or stinging, especially when the affected area is exposed to heat. If some freezing of tissue has occurred, the area will initially be cold and white. Thawing and warming will restore the normal color but may also result in blistering, followed by scab formation and healing.

CAUSES: Prolonged exposure to cold (not necessarily freezing weather), especially with humidity and wind, is likely to produce chilblains in the extremities or in inadequately protected body parts. Susceptibility depends greatly on the ability of the body to maintain its internal temperature and therefore is closely linked to the functioning of the circulatory system. Anything that impedes the circulation of the blood—including tight clothing, cardiovascular disease injury, or certain drugs—will make one more susceptible to the effects of cold. Susceptibility is also increased under conditions that produce an unusual loss of body heat—for example, wearing wet clothing, overexercising, or having too much alcohol (which dilates the capillaries and increases heat loss). Susceptibility is also related to physical conditions that reduce the body's normal resistance to cold, particularly dietary deficiencies, fatigue, and dehydration.

TREATMENT: If the affected part is still cold, the first treatment is to warm it up and restore normal circulation. This can be done by placing the part in warm water or by covering it with another part of the body (for example, placing a hand in the armpit to warm it). Don't rub the area because the skin can be easily damaged. Hot, stimulating (nonalcoholic) drinks, such as coffee or herbal teas made from ginger, dandelion root, rosemary, yellow dock root, linden flowers, damiana leaves, angelica root, elder flower, and fennel, are useful for restoring circulation and normal body functioning. A pinch of cayenne pepper can be added to almost any tea to increase its stimulant properties.

For follow-up treatment during the recovery period, a number of external applications have been recommended. Poultices for unbroken chilblains can be made from raw onion, grated horseradish, or garlic pulp; an ointment made from a turnip or with oil of wintergreen can also be applied. If the skin is broken, use a roasted onion rather than a raw one for a poultice. Epsom salt baths and washes with herbal teas can also be beneficial for chilblains with blistered or broken skin; use teas made from calendula, chamomile, oak bark, European mistletoe, lady's mantle, yarrow, oat straw, St. Benedict thistle, or eucalyptus. Extra vitamins A, C, and E, as well as calcium and zinc, are also needed to promote recovery.

The best treatment, as always, is to prevent chilblains in the first place. When going out into the cold, wear loose, layered clothing and be sure the susceptible parts of the body are well protected. (Sprinkling cayenne powder in your socks will help keep the feet warm.) Of course, following a healthful diet and life-style is important for strengthening the body's resistance against cold.

CHILDREN'S AILMENTS

Included are some effective natural treatments for some of the more common diseases of children. While these are not intended to supplant proper medical attention, they offer some uncomplicated alternatives that are usually effective and certainly without harmful side effects.

For fevers, give chamomile tea and/or diluted lemon water or fruit juice (especially berry). To reduce fevers in babies and small children, give a bath in which a strong pot of willow or white poplar bark tea has been poured. An enema using a cool tea of red raspberry leaf is also effective. Use a small bulb syringe to slowly and gently insert the fluid (up to four ounces maximum) into the rectum of the child. Reduce somewhat the child's intake of milk and other proteinaceous foods for a while.

For infant diarrhea, have them abstain from food for twenty-four hours, giving diluted lemon water. If the diarrhea persists, give rice or barley water spiced with a pinch of cinnamon, nutmeg, and ginger. Cook one cup of barley or rice in one and a half cups of water. Strain through a fine mesh screen or cloth and add a pinch of each of the above-mentioned herbs.

For most gastrointestinal problems, including diarrhea, dysentery, colicky stomachache, have them fast for twenty-four to forty-eight hours, giving them only tepid dill water. This is made by steeping one ounce of dill herb or seed in a quart of boiling water. Allow to cool. Give frequently throughout the day. This is one of the best remedies for colic and all digestive complaints of infants and small children.

An excellent herbal food for all infants with gastrointestinal complaints including diarrhea and vomiting is slippery elm gruel made from the finely powdered bark of the slippery elm tree *(Ulmus fulva)*. Make a small well of slippery elm powder and slowly add warm water, mixing until the desired consistency is attained. This can be flavored with a little honey, a pinch of cinnamon, nutmeg, and ginger and fed as a food with or without a little warm milk.

Syrup of garlic is made by blending several cloves of fresh garlic with honey to a syrupy consistency. This can be given in quarter- to half-teaspoon doses for any acute infectious diseases, including coughs, colds, flus, and fevers. It is antibiotic, antiviral, antiparasitical, aids digestion and promotes internal warmth and circulation. It is very useful for bronchitis and coughs and prevents bacterial complications from developing as a result of one of these diseases.

To prevent children from catching infectious diseases, sew some pure camphor crystals into a small pouch and pin it to the upper part of their undergarment. A clove of peeled garlic will also work quite well. These substances actually help to repel and destroy contagious pathogenic factors from the atmosphere surrounding the child.

Planetary formula number 94 (Well Child Echinacea-

Elderberry Syrup) is specifically intended for children to protect them from common colds and flus. It contains echinacea root, elderberry syrup, honeysuckle blossoms, lemon balm, chamomile, catnip, cinnamon, and licorice.

It's always wise to have a good salve or ointment for minor cuts, scrapes, bruises, stings, and bites. Planetary's Comfrey Care Salve contains comfrey leaf and calendula. Plantain, St. Johnswort, yarrow, echinacea, barberry, lavender, and essential oils of lavender and chamomile are ideal for this purpose.

Tincture of echinacea *(Echinacea* species*)* is very useful for a variety of possible inflammatory conditions. Approximately ten drops at a time can be given hourly for severe acute infections, tapering off as symptoms subside. This should be given without fail at the first sign of colds, fevers, injuries, infections, bites, and so forth to promote healing and help prevent further complications.

For sore throats, have the child chew on a leaf of sage *(Salvia off.)* or make a tea of sage leaves. Give a teaspoon or more frequently until the problem is cleared up.

For earaches, make garlic olive oil by crushing one or two cloves of fresh garlic *(Allium sativum)* in a quarter cup of olive oil. Allow to stand in a warm place for two or three days and strain by squeezing through a cloth. This can be made more quickly by heating the garlic in the olive oil, allowing it to cool and then immediately squeezing it through a cloth. The resultant oil will keep a few months. One or two drops can be placed in each ear along with three to five drops of echinacea tincture. Another effective remedy is oil of rue, made by steeping an ounce of rue *(Ruta graveolens)* in a pint of olive oil and storing in a dark warm place for three to five days. It is then press-strained for use.

For eruptive diseases, make a tea of elder flowers *(Sambucus nigra)*, lemon balm *(Melissa off.)* and/or calendula flowers *(Calendula off.)*. Use equal parts and steep one ounce covered in a pint of water. Give an appropriate dose at least three times a day. This will help the measles ripen and come to completion sooner.

For worms and parasites, homeopathic Cina 1x is very effective. Give a few tablets four times a day for four days to a week. Garlic oil can be taken as well as refraining from the use of any sweets or refined foods.

Roman chamomile *(Anthemis nobilis)* or the milder German chamomile *(Matricaria chamomila)* are generally the best herbs to give to children for most inflammatory diseases as well as fevers, colds, flus, and gastrointestinal complaints. It is specific for irritability, peevishness, and hyperactivity of infants and children generally.

Lemon balm *(Melissa off.)* is another herb that seems specific for infants and children. Besides being the best and most pleasant-tasting herb to give for fevers, it has soothing and calming properties that make it useful for infants and childhood nervousness and anxiety.

Both chamomile and lemon balm are contained in Planetary formula numbers 13 and 14 (Calm Child). This formula has proved to be very successful for whining and needy children of all ages (including infants past the age of 6 months), hyperactive children, and children diagnosed with ADD or ADHD.

Homeopathic treatments are usually very effective for children. Because of their pleasant milk sugar base they are readily taken and even relished by them. Use the same indications as listed for specific diseases. Probably the single most useful remedy is chamomile 30th potency because this is useful for many diseases associated with peevishness and irritability. It is used for teething children, colic, colds, and fevers. Belladonna 10th potency is also very commonly indicated for those kinds of acute high fevers, colds, and sore throat, convulsions as well as eczema with intense redness. Ledum 10th to 30th potency is useful for puncture wounds from stepping on nails and needles. Thuja 30th potency is good for treating warts and to give to ameliorate the side effects of vaccinations. In all of these a dose of the remedy is given four times daily for four days.

CHRONIC FATIGUE

OTHER NAMES: CFS.

SYMPTOMS: Severe exhaustion and fatigue are the primary symptoms with, after ruling out other causes, at least a 50 percent reduction in activity for six months. Other symptoms include: low-grade fever, sore throat, and palpable or tender lymph nodes. In addition there may be mild fever, muscle weakness or pain, prolonged fatigue after exercise, recurrent headaches, migratory joint pains, hypersensitivity, increased sensitivity to light, confusion, forgetfulness, poor concentration, depression, sleep disturbance (hyperinsomnia or insomnia), and sudden onset of symptoms.

CAUSES: There are many possible causes for CFS. These range from viruses, allergies, food sensitivities, emotional problems, stress, drug reactions, yeast infections, and Epstein-Barr virus (EPV, which is known to be the cause of mononucleosis). Patients commonly report that their chronic fatigue seemed to set in after a strange cold or flu. This gives strong support to chronic fatigue being of viral origin. In fact, because viruses even more than other pathogens have a well-known propensity to mutate and alter rapidly, based on a number of factors. Like EBV, CFS causes transient immune deficiency by depleting pathogenic killer B cells and depleting levels of immune potentiating immunoglobulins. This will cause the immune system to react by increasing certain T-cells. With AIDS, the virus (presumably HIV) shifts its identity so quickly that the immune system is worn down beyond recovery in its efforts to recognize it. With CFS-type viruses, the viral form does not change, so that if one is given support by first eliminating known stress factors, including worry, overwork, lack of sleep, and a diet high in stimulants, coffee, alcohol, carbohydrates, and refined foods, and then supplied with those kinds of foods and herbs that naturally increase immune function, this will result in a faster recovery.

TREATMENT: Treatment needs to be individually tailored to the needs of the patient based on their symptomatology. In most cases response will be gradual, with periods of ups and downs as the body is able to mobilize its immune capabilities to fight the virus.

The first thing is to realize that in order to recover you will have to limit stress in all forms, giving your body plenty of time to rest. Considering that many who come down with CFS were previously known as type A overachievers, the disease dictates that, at least during its course, the patient will have to come to terms with much less stimulation to say the least. Michael has known some CFS patients who after months into the disease hardly had enough energy to pick up the telephone.

CFS patients seem to respond best to a low-carbohydrate, high-protein, high cooked-vegetables diet. Food must be easily digestible and wholesome. Soups with hearty meat and vegetable stock are a very good choice. These can be prepared with Chinese herbs including 3 ounces each of codonopsis (an energy tonic), 9 ounces of astragalus (an immune system tonic), 6 ounces of poria mushroom (to relieve damp stagnation), 3 ounces of atractylodes (tonifies energy and improves assimilation), and 2 ounces of licorice (peacemaker herb). This is the basic formula without astragalus that is Planetary formula number 38 (Ginseng Classic).

These herbs, and especially astragalus and reishi mushroom, should be purchased by the pound from a Chinese pharmacy so the herbs are always on hand to be cooked into tea or to make into a stock for soups or cooking rice. Rice is the only grain that should be eaten on a daily basis. If digestion will permit, one should use short-grain brown rice. If digestion is weak, use white rice or a mixture with a little brown rice.

To aid digestion one should take a bitters before meals, about a tablespoon or two. If the small amount of alcohol causes a problem, put this in boiling water and allow it to stand in order to evaporate most of the alcohol away. Two beneficial digestive liqueurs are the Ayurvedic formula called "draksha," available from Indian import stores; another is Planetary's formula number 24 (Digestive Grape Bitters).

For the immune system one should use reishi mushrooms (Ganoderma lucidum). Of all herbs this is the most powerful immune tonic known. Michael uses Planetary formula number 70 (Reishi Mushroom Supreme).

Guggul should be taken to clear the channels and enhance metabolism and circulation (Planetary formula number 42). Triphala should be taken each evening to promote balanced elimination.

Besides tonification and circulation, one should also attend to reducing the viral load in the body by the use of Planetary formula number 18 (Complete Cat's Claw Complex).

If insomnia is a problem, take Planetary formula number 84 (Stress Free) each evening with the PM mineral supplement.

In addition, one should take chlorella, which is a single-celled algae that is loaded with easily assimilable vitamins, minerals, and antioxidants. It is a very important adjunctive nutritional therapy for chronic fatigue patients.

Nutritional supplementation for CFS patients should be as follows:

1. a high-potency multiple vitamin
2. a high-quality multimineral supplement taken each evening
3. esther C, 500 to 1,000 mg three times daily
4. myelized vitamin E, 400 to 800 IUs daily
5. thymus extract, 750 mg
6. magnesium, 300 mg
7. pantothenic acid, 250 mg daily

CHRONIC PAIN

TREATMENT: Where Western medicine tends to use drugging therapy to relieve pain, natural therapists consider pain to be a symptom of blockage and use therapies that promote circulation in the affected area(s). This does not mean that for certain severe pains one should refuse appropriate medical intervention. The purpose of this book is to provide a simple first line of treatment before resorting to more Western medical intervention, which can have detrimental side effects that herbs and hydrotherapy and other therapies described in this book simply do not have.

There are many ways both internally and externally to facilitate the necessary movement of blood and energy that will relieve pain. Many of them are presented elsewhere throughout this book. I will list a few approaches one can try:

1. The use of hot- and cold-water baths, mustard plasters, and liniments.
2. Applying oil over the affected surface and taking the edge of a glass Chinese soup spoon and scraping vigorously in one direction until there is a general rubefacient (reddening) of the surface of the skin. This is very effective for neck, back, and limb pains. When the skin is made red on the surface, the congested blood underneath is drawn up, and new, oxygenated blood is allowed to circulate into the area to feed oxygen-deprived cells literally agonizing over the lack of nutrients and oxygen. This and some of the following methods are probably best done by one experienced in their practice, usually a licensed TCM practitioner.
3. A similar method to skin scraping is to apply suction cups over the area of pain. This is done by temporarily creating a vacuum in a small glass or cup so it will fasten over the affected painful area.
4. Michael has been able to provide nearly miracu-

lous pain relief and healing by pricking a specifically painful site and using the suction cups to
draw a teaspoon to a tablespoon of blood out.
He has even been able to provide lasting relief
for patients with degenerative spinal discs or
knees. Again, this is a method that should be administered by one experienced in this mode of
therapy.

5. Acupuncture is very effective for pain.

6. Internally, herbs that move congested blood and
energy are very effective for relieving pain.
Herbs such as corydalis, myrrh, and boswellia are
in this category. Planetary formula number 96
(Willow Aid) contains some of these and other
herbs to relieve pain. In general, anyone who is
pregnant should avoid using herbs with strong
moving properties. For gastrointestinal and chest
pains, different herbs are used. Planetary formula
number 23 in a one-time double to triple dose
with warm water is effective for those kinds of
pains.

7. Magnets are a wonderful way to relieve pain. I
have described their use under carpal tunnel and
in my book *Biomagnetic and Herbal Therapy* (published by Lotus Press).

CIRCULATORY PROBLEMS

OTHER NAMES: Arteriosclerosis, cold extremities,
hardening of the arteries.

DESCRIPTION: Circulatory problems, which deprive a
part of the body of enough blood to provide proper nutri-

tion and oxygen for the cells. Arteries, the carriers of our blood, can undergo many abnormal changes that reduce their carrying capacity. These include clogging, constriction, hardening, obstruction, compression, and general deterioration. It is only after menopause that women become as susceptible as men to arteriosclerosis. The risk also generally increases with age.

SYMPTOMS: Cold hands and feet are characteristic of blood vessel problems. Hands or legs may become pale or even white; numbness, tingling, and loss of function may also occur. There may be cramplike pains, especially in the legs, after exertion or exercise.

CAUSES: Poor diet is the number one cause: specifically, a diet low in fiber and high in fats, refined sugars, and refined foods. Smoking, alcohol, stimulants, and many drugs contribute to arteriosclerosis. High blood pressure and diabetes greatly increase the risk and should be treated under the supervision of your doctor. Stress not only causes generalized deterioration but can also cause muscle spasms or contractions that misalign and compress the arteries, thereby impeding circulation.

TREATMENT: Hydrotherapy (see Part Three) is one of the principal tools used to increase circulation to the extremities. Hot and cold water should be applied to the chest, back, and extremities at least three times a week. If a healing crisis (that is, headache, depression, fatigue, or other acute symptoms) occurs during your hydrotherapy treatments, do not take drugs to suppress the symptoms. Rather, fast with fruit juices for three to five days until the crisis is over. If you are too weak or debilitated to fast, consult your physician immediately for help in getting through the crisis. Massage and gradually increasing daily exercise are excellent measures to help restore lost circulation. The recommendations under HEART ATTACK apply equally to the treatment of arteriosclerosis.

Circulation is benefitted by the use of bitter herbs such as gentian or goldenseal root, to unblock the veins and arteries, but more directly by using warm, stimulating herbs such as a combination of the following: cinnamon bark, ginger root, angelica root, prickly ash, black pepper, anise seed and a half part of licorice to help smooth out the formula. One teaspoon to a tablespoon is taken in a tea with a little honey, or the powder can be mixed with boiled warm milk to be used more as a tonic.

In addition, the Ayurvedic formula Trikatu taken daily is very beneficial.

CIRRHOSIS OF THE LIVER

DESCRIPTION: Cirrhosis of the liver occurs when the liver cells gradually lose their function and are replaced by hard connective, fibrous tissues while the organ itself shrinks.

There are two major diseases of the liver, cirrhosis and hepatitis. Because of the importance of the liver, we will here outline some of the more important functions.

No one knows for sure about all the functions of the liver, but there are some five hundred that have been recognized. As a gland it secretes bile and stores it in the gallbladder until necessary for digestion. The liver inspects and processes all broken-down food particles, fatty acids, and glycerol, following which it sorts and assimilates them into compounds that the body can use.

The liver produces important enzymes and performs

other chemical functions that enable organic substances to alter their structures for utilization or elimination by the body. Since it produces these catalytic enzymes at an incredible speed, it can work on the amino acids and sugars as soon as they enter the intestines through capillaries and the great portal vein. One of the causes of hemorrhoids is congestion of this portal vein.

The liver also produces the blood clotting agent prothrombin as well as two anticoagulants, heparin and antithrombin. It converts and stores energy in the form of glycogen which is released for emergencies and after exercising. Red blood cells that have served their purpose (at the approximate rate of 10 million per second!) are broken down by the liver and provide the raw materials used for building new blood cells and other organic tissues. Those wastes that cannot be used are converted into bile and the nitrogen waste of protein is turned into urea and sent to the kidneys for elimination.

Regulating the balance of salt and water in the body is accomplished by the liver through the building of amino acids into albumin. The growth hormone thyroxin is controlled by the liver as well as other sex and mood hormones which regulate sexual urge and certain important vitamins such as A, D, B-complex, and minerals such as iron, zinc, and copper.

One of the most important jobs for the liver in our time is the removal of various toxins from the blood. These include the toxins of industrial poisons, sprays, solvents, drugs, alcohol, nicotine, and caffeine.

The liver also helps to protect the heart, receiving both fresh arterial blood through the capillaries and, after cleansing it of toxins, returning it to the heart through the veins. Since the human liver weighs five to eight pounds, it has the ability to store up to one-fourth of the blood, thus further protecting the heart from overflooding and taxing.

SYMPTOMS: Cirrhosis of the liver is of gradual onset as the scar tissue that forms gradually impairs circulation and function within the liver. In advanced cases, the liver develops a hobnailed appearance because of the proliferation of this scar tissue.

There are many outward symptoms: head—thin hair, bulging eyes, jaundice, reddish areas on the face caused by dilated capillaries, spider nevi or pinhead red dots caused by tiny ruptured veins and capillaries; trunk—spider nevi of the collarbone region, breast enlargement in the male, swollen liver, the presence of collateral veins formed when the main blood vessels are broken, small testes and absent or reduced pubic hair; limbs—wasting of the muscles, club fingers, opaqueness and other abnormalities of the fingernails, edema, purpura (bluish skin caused by hemorrhage and poor circulation). There is also general fatigue, nausea, and gastric weakness, swollen and dropsical abdomen, and pain and tightness under the right subcostal region (right front ribs).

Cirrhosis of the liver is one of the ten major causes of death in the United States and one of the third or fourth leading causes of death among individuals between the ages of 25 and 65 in the city of New York (Dr. Charles S. Lieber, chief liver specialist at Bronx Veterans Hospital, published in the *Evening Chronicle*, September 9, 1974). Despite all of this, there must be a considerable amount of destroyed or damaged liver tissue for it to be detected as an abnormality in laboratory tests.

The effect upon the mood and personality of an individual with an abnormal liver function is so profound as to give rise to a variety of psychological disorders ranging from moodiness and premenstrual syndrome, disorders associated with the climacteric and menopause, schizophrenia and depression. This is because the liver is primarily responsible for neutralizing excess hormones secreted as a result of stress and other factors. When these are not sufficiently eliminated, the result is that they continue to circulate in the blood, conjuring up inappropriately old moods and feelings that may be no longer appropriate.

Liver symptoms being so variable and so much involved with the emotions and personality of the patient, it is no wonder that these patients are most often the bane and source of frustration (the emotion of the liver) of doctors and other health practitioners. Characteristically, the liver patient experiences pain just below the ribs of the right side of the abdomen, an area commonly called the hypochondrium, and liver patients are often unwittingly labeled as chronic "hypochondriacs."

Despite the abuse and damage the liver receives in our time, it has tremendous capability of regeneration. Further, it has been established that an individual can function with as much as 80 percent of the liver removed or destroyed.

It is interesting to note how liver dysfunction is implicated in many lesser imbalances such as dyspepsia, indigestion, gas, heartburn, hyperacidity, premenstrual tension, white-coated tongue, and depression and moodiness. Imagine if you will, the overburdened liver with the accumulation of exogenous toxins from the environment and food and endogenous toxins in the form of the excessive secretion of certain hormones, all ganged up waiting for detoxification in an organ that is often lacking in essential nutrients. The result is that the blood and lymphatic systems are overwhelmed with these unprocessed sugars, amino acids, and hormones generated from stress and undetoxified chemicals.

It is no wonder that one of the last stages of terminal illness is liver failure and that most of the harmful side effects of Western drug medicine are against the liver. Some countries such as France recognize as part of folk wisdom daily episodes of liver crises affecting the digestion and personality. Among many European rural people a familiar greeting is "How is your liver today?"

CAUSES: Among the causes of liver cirrhosis are alcoholism, malnutrition, protein deficiency, severe hepatitis, prolonged bile obstruction, congestive heart failure and syphilis. At least according to one article published in *The New England Journal of Medicine*, written by Drs. Charles S. Davidson and George F. Gabusda, cirrhosis of the liver is most common where people eat largely high-carbohydrate diets lacking in animal protein. The article also points out that it does not seem to matter how high or good the quality of animal protein. Liver cirrhosis is most common when there is a lack. Thus there seems to be a scientific basis for the need of at least some people to include animal protein in their diet on a regular basis. It should be borne in mind that animal protein for a vegetarian could include small amounts of dairy products, good-quality milk such as raw goat's milk, cheese, or yogurt.

TREATMENT: The liver is considered by the Chinese as part of the wood element; this identifies its natural affinity with the plant kingdom and green vegetables particularly. Aside from attending to getting the necessary levels of protein so the liver can regenerate itself, the most important foods that help the liver in its cleansing and detoxifying process are carrots and green vegetables.

To get good-quality protein one should include brewer's yeast, about three to five tablespoons per day; raw goat's or cow's milk—also cheese or yogurt made from these; sprouted seeds and grains; raw nuts; and tahini. Only organic meats and animal proteins should be used, as all others are loaded with drugs and hormones that are injurious to the liver. Greens in the form of endive, dandelion roots and greens, artichokes, beets and beet tops, carrots and carrot tops (used in soups), celery, black radish, burdock root, and steamed nettles should be used once or twice daily. Garlic, cucumber, and the juice of beets, carrots, and lemons are all very good.

Foods that should be restricted include all refined foods, white sugar, foods that are high in fats, fried foods, coffee, canned foods, foods with artificial chemicals, coloring, or preservatives, and alcohol and drugs of all kinds.

Herbs can have a powerful healing effect on the liver and these include milk thistle seeds. *(Silybum marianum),* a powerful regenerator of the liver, blessed thistle, dandelion root, Oregon grape or barberry root, artichokes and artichoke leaf tea, boldo *(Peumus bodus),* yellow dock root *(Rumex crispus),* and Chinese bupleurum root. Stronger liver-purging herbs include cascara sagrada, chebulic myrobalan (called haritaki, one of the three substances in triphala), culver's root, and American mandrake root.

Most of these herbs are contained in Planetary formula number 11 (Bupleurum Liver Cleanse), which can be taken with formula number 89 (Triphala) and dandelion root tea to treat liver cirrhosis. In addition, if one is attempting to regenerate the liver, add extra amounts of silybum extract or powder to your daily program. Also use

Chinese lycii berries, which are delicious cooked like raisins and added to the morning cereal or simply taken as a tea. These are very good for improving vision, are extremely high in easily assimilated beta carotene, and have the added benefit of being quite delicious. Dandelion root and chamomile with a small amount of crushed fennel seeds is an herbal combination to take for occasional or chronic liver disorders. Triphala should be taken at least once a week or once each evening before retiring.

A good liver flush is a combination of two ounces of olive oil, lemon, water, and garlic, blended together. One eight-once glass is taken each morning for four days to a week at a time. This can be accompanied with a coffee enema (one cup of freshly brewed coffee) each morning and evening, retained at least twenty minutes.

COLDNESS

DESCRIPTION AND SYMPTOMS: Feelings of coldness and numbness in the extremities or other parts of the body.

CAUSES: The underlying cause is some metabolic imbalance, low thyroid or adrenal function, poor circulation. It can have partially hereditary causes as well as be acquired through overeating a diet of cold, raw foods, juices, improperly prepared food, and exposure to cold.

TREATMENT: Try to protect yourself from cold drafts and dietary and life-style causes, and take measures to keep the body warm. It is most important for well-being and longevity to keep one's lower back and waist warm. The Japanese have traditionally used an article of clothing called a "harimaki," or what I call a kidney-adrenal warmer. This is worn around the lower back and abdomen, below the navel, and will help tremendously if used at night or during cold winter months.

Strictly limit raw fruits and vegetables, at least during the cold seasons. Individuals living in severe cold climates should protect themselves from the cold and damp and also regularly consume some red meat. Such climates are not good places for practicing a vegetarian diet.

Foods can be combined with curry spices such as turmeric, coriander, cumin seed, asafetida, ginger, fenugreek, and whole red chili peppers sautéed in ghee (clarified butter). Other warm spices such as ginger and cinnamon can also be used regularly.

A good spice tea is made with a teaspoon of cinnamon bark, three or four slices of fresh ginger root (dried ginger powder can also be used), and a pinch of cloves, nutmeg, and black pepper. Add honey to taste. If desired, some angelica root, licorice root, sarsaparilla, and sassafras bark can be added to this tea. Steep about a tablespoon of the ingredients in a covered cup of just-boiled water, and take when cool enough to drink.

Another good combination to take regularly is Trikatu, which is made with powdered ginger, black pepper, pippli long pepper, and honey. These are mixed into the honey to form a thick paste, and a half to one teaspoon is taken one to three times daily.

For cold feet, sprinkling a bit of cayenne pepper in the socks will be quite effective.

Planetary formula number 36 (Ginger Warming Compound) and number 86 (Three Spices Sinus Complex) are specifically indicated for coldness.

There are several homeopathic remedies to choose from: ferrum phos 6x and calcarea phos 6x as general remedies, then consider carbo veg 6th to 30th if there is weak digestion, a tendency to bloat, and flatulence. Arsenicum 6th to 30th is always indicated, no matter what the other symptoms may be. Calcarea carbonic 6th to 30th is used when the individual is weak both physically and mentally, tires easily, and has a tendency to sweat upon the slightest exertion; such individuals may tend toward plumpness, with poor muscle tone, and have an extreme aversion to cold, the open air, or damp environments.

COLDS

OTHER NAMES: Acute rhinitis, catarrh, coryza, upper-respiratory infection.

DESCRIPTION: The common cold is an acute viral infection that affects the mucosal membranes lining the nose, throat, and larynx, and often those of the trachea and bronchi, producing generalized catarrhal inflammation. More than a hundred rhinoviruses (*rhino* = pertaining to the nose) have been identified and implicated as causes of colds. The common cold can also be complicated by a secondary bacterial infection affecting the ears and sinuses.

SYMPTOMS: One to two days after contact with the virus, the symptoms of a cold begin with a sensation of a scratchy throat, followed by sneezing, nasal discharge, and malaise. In adults there is usually no fever, whereas infants and small children often have a fever of 100° to 102°F. Various combinations of laryngitis, hacking cough, tracheal inflammation, headache, chills, watery eyes, muscular aches, and temporary loss of smell and taste may be present to some degree. Normally, the mucus discharge thickens throughout the course of a cold, but if the ears or sinuses begin to hurt and the mucus discharge is very thick, a secondary bacterial infection may be involved. The common cold usually ends in four to ten days.

CAUSES: Since the viruses that cause colds are always present in our environment, susceptibility is the key to whether you catch a cold or not. The main causes of increased susceptibility are a weakening of the natural immune system due to poor dietary and living habits, and accumulation of toxins. Susceptibility increases in the winter months when people eat heavier foods, exercise less, and spend more time indoors in poorly ventilated spaces with inadequate humidity and oxygen. In addition, the body's natural defenses can be weakened by fatigue, stress, inhalation of noxious substances in the air, nasal allergies, and menstruation.

TREATMENT: The best time to treat a cold is at the very first sign. If this is not done, chances are that subsequent care will be directed to enhancing the detoxification process that such an acute disease represents as well as relieving the symptoms and hastening recovery.

There are many effective first-line natural treatments for colds and flus and all involve some form of metabolic stimulation, light diet, sleep, and bed rest. Usually one considers first the use of diaphoretic teas to promote perspiration, such as lemon balm *(Melissa officinalis)*, yarrow *(Achillea millefolium)*, mint *(Menta* species), elder flowers *(Sambucus nigra)* used singly or in combination in a tea. Other warming stimulants that can also be used include cayenne pepper, garlic, and ginger taken as a tea or powder.

An important stimulant combination with antibiotic and antiviral properties is the old-time North American doctor's composition powder, which was widely used for the first stages of colds, flus, and fevers. Its primary ingredients are herbal stimulants such as bayberry bark *(Myrica cerifera)*, cayenne pepper *(Capsicum annuum)*, ginger *(Zingiberis off.)*, white pine bark *(Pinus silvestris)*, cloves *(Caryophyllus aromaticus)* and various other herbs, according to the preference of the herb doctor. A variation on this old-time remedy, in which I incorporate cinnamon bark because of its flavor and antiviral properties, is called Ginger Warming Compound (formula number 36). This should be taken one to two grams every hour or two as needed at the first sign of a cold or flu.

Among the most common herbal remedies for colds and flus is a tea comprising equal parts yarrow, elder flowers, and mint. One ounce of the mixture is steeped in a pint of boiling water covered for twenty minutes or until cool enough to drink. Honey may be added if desired. Another common remedy is a tea made by steeping four to six slices of fresh ginger root in a cup of boiling water. Still one more is to use the white part of scallions or garlic steeped in a cup of water. Use about six scallions or one or two cloves of crushed garlic.

After drinking one or two cups of this tea, the patient should go to bed, covered with several blankets and lying motionless until perspiration ensues. Allow the patient to sweat for a while but not to exhaustion. Follow with a cool-water sponge bath from head to foot, taking no longer than one minute for the entire operation. Change the bedding and let the patient retire to bed to rest.

Echinacea *(E. angustifolia et species)* and boneset *(Eupatorium perfoliatum)* have a long history of effectiveness in the treatment of colds, flus, and viruses. Echinacea has recognized immunostimulant properties with no generally recognized side effects at even large doses. Nevertheless, it is wise to begin with a small dose of any strange substance to determine whether there is an allergic sensitivity. After this, to be of optimum effectiveness during acute disease, an appropriate dose of echinacea according to whether it is a tea, powder, tincture, or tablet should be taken every two hours. The cool-water sponge bath and cold sheet treatment is one of the most effective treatments for overcoming colds and fevers. It is administered as follows: After giving a good dose of either the composition powder and/or one of the teas described above, wrap the patient with a sheet that has been wrung out in cold water. Have him retire to bed with several blankets and a cold towel on his forehead and a hot-water bottle (or a hot brick wrapped with a towel) near his feet. Cover the bedding with rubber or plastic to protect it from dampness. Again, after allowing the patient to sweat for a while, sponge him off with cool water and let him retire to bed with fresh covers.

For small children or infants, sponging with cool water or alcohol will help bring down the fever accompanying a cold or flu. Babies respond very well to warm baths in which a tea of willow or white poplar bark has been put into the bathwater. Of course if there is any constipation or bowel sluggishness, a mild laxative formula such as triphala can be given in the evening. Alternatives might be taking an extract of cascara bark *(C. sagrada)* or rhubarb *(Rheum palmatum)* with some ginger root to prevent abdominal gripping.

During a cold or fever, one should eat very simply if at all. Usually a light vegetable soup, thin porridge, or diluted fruit juice are all good. One particular food that will actually help in overcoming the virus or bacteria is a soup made from either black beans or green mung beans. This latter can be made Indian style with a little ghee, a pinch of salt and a small amount of ginger, cumin, coriander, and turmeric spices.

Many acclaim the benefits of taking large doses of vitamin C at the first sign of a cold. It should be kept in mind that the body hardly needs such large doses of vitamin C and that probably the way that it works is by pushing the body metabolically. This approach works well for some (especially those who are more disposed to eating red meat, dairy, and refined foods with sugar) and not at all for those who have a more sensitive yin constitution or are strict vegetarians. Homeopathic treatments: For colds with flulike symptoms and fevers, use gelsemium 30th potency. For the beginning stages of colds—headache or feeling of heat in the face and head, achiness of the muscles—use aconite 3rd to 30th potency. For colds with profuse mucus discharge, dryness of the mouth, chilliness, restlessness, and prostration, use arsenicum 10th to 30th potency. For colds with severe high fever, throbbing headache, dry and sore throat, use belladonna 10th to 30th potency. One dose of the selected remedy is taken four times daily for four days.

Michael also recommends that an individual with a severe cold take plenty of garlic in the form of mashed garlic cloves and olive oil. This should be taken hourly throughout the day by dipping whole wheat bread in the oil. Planetary formula number 101 (Yin Chiao Echinacea Complex) is also effective for colds and should be taken every two hours.

Vitamin C is also useful both for the prevention and to shorten the duration of colds. I recommend that one take from 2,000 to 5,000 mg divided into three daily doses. The best form of vitamin C to take is the nonacidic ester C.

COLIC

OTHER NAMES: Biliary colic, intestinal colic, renal colic.

DESCRIPTION: Colic is the painful spasm of a duct or other tubular organ in the body. An inconsolable baby is the first image that the term *colic* may bring to mind. Adults can also have colicky pain, however.

SYMPTOMS: Colic produces severe pain, usually in the abdominal area or in the kidneys. The pain of intestinal colic comes in waves; biliary and renal colic produce a steady pain. Pressure on the affected area tends to relieve the pain; passing gas relieves the pain of intestinal colic. Nausea, vomiting, and either diarrhea or constipation may occur. The abdomen becomes hard and distended; the feet are cold. The patient will tend to draw up the legs and double over because of the pain. Since the symptoms may resemble those of apprendicitis, ruptured spleen, or ectopic pregnancy, consult your physician if they do occur.

CAUSES. Intestinal colic can result from many causes: faulty digestion, food allergies, roundworms, foreign bodies in the intestinal tract, overfeeding, obstruction of the intestines, poor diet of a nursing mother, or a poor emotional state when eating. Gallstones and kidney stones can cause colic when they pass into ducts.

TREATMENT: Consult your physician for the treatment of stones and to diagnose the cause of the colic.

For infantile colic, which usually results from food intolerance, a small enema of soap suds, chamomile tea, catnip tea, or plain water is very helpful. Give gentle abdominal massage after the enema, in a right-to-left circular motion. Warm water in a hot-water bottle can be placed on the abdomen to help provide relief. Chamomile and/or dillweed tea is specifically useful for infant colic. Nursing mothers should avoid eating cabbage, garlic, legumes, and onions. If other symptoms appear (such as eczema or asthma), the child should be tested for food allergies. Colic usually disappears after the child is about three months old.

For intestinal colic in adults, use large enemas of the types described above. Warm baths (not sitz baths), linseed poultices, and hot abdominal compresses are also beneficial. Internally, drink chamomile or peppermint tea; to relieve gas, also drink tea made from ginger, cloves, fennel, coriander, thyme, cayenne, caraway, or rosemary. Wild cherry and quince, eaten as fresh fruits, are also useful.

CONSTIPATION

OTHER NAMES: Atonic constipation, colon stasis, lazy colon, psychogenic constipation.

DESCRIPTION: Constipation is the infrequent or difficult passage of feces because peristalsis—the involuntary contraction of the intestines that moves the waste matter through—is weak or does not occur. With this condition, the time it takes for matter to pass through the bowels is variable at best. Cultures that eat vegetarian diets can have complete evacuation of a day's meals within eighteen to twenty-four hours. Times for Americans and other "advanced" peoples vary from forty-eight to seventy-two hours. Hard stools or the incomplete passage of the food ingested is also referred to as constipation.

SYMPTOMS: Hard feces, the absence of defecation for three days or more, a small quantity of feces compared with the food ingested over the preceding three days, and straining at the stool are the most common symptoms. Other symptoms that may be present include cramping, abdominal fullness, excessive gas, a desire to defecate with inability to release a stool, no desire to defecate, and watery diarrhea around the impacted fecal mass. Headaches, bad breath, coated tongue, mental sluggishness, paleness, and dizziness are also associated symptoms.

CAUSES: Most causes of acute constipation are fairly serious: obstruction of the bowel, insufficient bile secretion by the liver, lack of peristalsis due to nerve paralysis, drug toxicity (such as from morphine), and infection. Eating concentrated food with little or no water intake can also result in acute constipation.

Chronic constipation most commonly results from a diet high in unrefined flour products, meats, sugar, and fried foods, and lacking in liquid and in fiber from fresh fruits and vegetables, whole grains, and seeds. Poor muscle tone due to lack of exercise, being overweight, and habitual use of laxatives can also lead to chronic constipation. The elderly can have atonic constipation secondary to nerve dysfunction that reduces or halts peristalsis. Psychogenic constipation is due to the belief that one must defecate at least once a day to rid oneself of "impure" substances. The result is anxiety and overuse of laxatives. (Normal bowel elimination patterns vary widely from one person to the next, ranging from three times a day to three times a week.) In adults, irritable-bowel syndrome can cause spasms and result in constipation.

Children can develop constipation from overconsumption of milk. Breast-fed infants can have highly variable bowel patterns, and a lack of defecation for one to two days is not necessarily constipation. Infants less than a month old who have constipation should be seen by a physician to rule out megacolon, a condition in which peristalsis does not occur.

TREATMENT: The key to curing constipation is to treat the underlying cause. If the problem results from dietary habits and a detrimental life-style, this seven-point program will help establish regular bowel habits:

1. Begin by eating a fiber-rich diet high in bran, fresh vegetables, fruits, whole grains, and seeds. Drink six to eight glasses of spring water, juices, or herbal tea per day. Avoid refined carbohydrates (especially sugar), salted meats, and fried or fatty foods. Some good foods that promote natural elimination are prunes, figs, tomatoes, rhubarb, buttermilk, flaxseed, bee pollen, honey, wheat and oat bran (always take bran with liquid), apples, whey powder, sunflower and pumpkin seeds, yogurt, apricots, lemons, and comfrey root mucilage. Healthy adults should consume six to eight grams of fiber per day. To avoid getting intestinal gas and bloat, increase the amount of fiber in the diet gradually rather than adding a large amount all at once.

2. Exercise. Walking is excellent. A simple and effective exercise is to hop on one foot while raising the other knee to the chest; keep this up as long as you can, alternating between the right and left foot. Use of a slant board or inversion of the body changes the direction of the gravitational pull and allows the bowels to rest. Do exercises that strengthen the muscles of the abdominal wall, and twisting and stretching exercises to increase bowel tone. Cold sitz baths and hot and cold gushes to the abdomen and anal orifice are also helpful (see Part Three).

3. Always respond *promptly* to nature's call to move the bowels.

4. Try to establish a regular time for a relaxed trip to the bathroom.

5. Maintain regular sleeping, eating, and relaxation habits. Do deep breathing exercises to promote relaxation and internal massage.

6. Avoid all harmful habits and work on eliminating as much destructive stress as possible from your life.

7. Use enemas, colonic irrigations, or herbal laxatives *only* to get things going; their extended use can cause dependency and have the opposite of the intended effect. Herbal laxatives that also help to nourish and restore tone to the colon are psyllium seed, fennel seed, fenugreek seed, carbo pods (St. John's bread), senna, cascara sagrada, buckthorn bar, and rhubarb.

When constipation is due to a specific underlying health problem, treatment should be medically supervised. But most constipation is due to faulty dietary habits and lack of exercise. *Don't make this simple issue complex.* Remember the above seven rules and you will be free of constipation.

Triphala (formula number 89) is an excellent formula to take for helping to regulate the bowels and clean the digestive tract so as to improve digestion. Unlike harsher laxatives, it contains three important tropical fruits, one of which is called amla or Indian gooseberry *(Chebulic myrobalan),* which is very high in vitamin C. One small amla fruit is equal in vitamin C to eight lemons. Further, the vitamin C in amla is bound up in a unique form with harmless vegetable tannins that will preserve the C content when subjected to heat. Triphala, the mildest and safest of internal cleansing agents, is not at all depleting. Some people undergoing treatment in India take it each evening, while others may use it regularly only once a week. Anywhere from two to six grams can be taken in a single dose.

Psyllium seed husk can also be taken in the evening with dark grape juice or warm honey-water.

Planetary formula number 87 (Tri-cleanse Bulking Compound) contains a combination of psyllium seed husks with triphala and other carminative herbs useful for dry constipation.

Homeopathic remedies to consider include nux vomica 6th to 30th when there is frequent but ineffectual desire to ease oneself; natrum mur. 6th to 12th; bryonia 6th to 30th when there is no desire; lycopodium 30th when there is difficulty passing stools, tendency toward bloating, and gas after meals; and sulphur 30th when there are lower abdominal feelings of heat and heaviness with burning and itching of the anus.

CORNS AND CALLUSES

OTHER NAMES: Clavus, heloma, keratoderma.

DESCRIPTION: Calluses, of which corns are the most troublesome type, are localized thickenings of the horny outer layer of the skin. They most commonly occur on the feet and the hands. Corns usually take the form of hard bumps on the tops of toes.

SYMPTOMS: Hardening and thickening of the skin is the obvious symptom. There may be discomfort or pain if the affected area is subjected to friction or pressure.

CAUSES: Calluses are the body's defensive response if a specific area of the skin is exposed to extended or repeated pressure or friction. Hands can become callused from hard physical labor, and the bottoms of most people's feet naturally become more or less callused from walking. But corns on the toes result from unnatural pressure or friction due to tight, ill-fitting, or poorly made shoes.

TREATMENT: One way to treat corns and other problem calluses is with patience: If the cause is removed, they will eventually disappear. For corns caused by shoe problems, for example, it makes sense to put the comfort and health of your feet ahead of vanity—in other words, forget the latest pointy-toed faddish style, buy the proper size for your feet (they should fit comfortably without slipping from the time you buy them), and spend enough to get shoes with high-quality materials and workmanship. If necessary, corns can be protected from physical irritation by using unmedicated corn pads, foam rubber, or a simple bandage around the toe. Going barefoot as much as possible not only eliminates the source of irritation, it also benefits the whole foot by letting it breathe and flex naturally.

If you can't wait for corns and calluses to go away, you can help their departure along—but carefully. It used to be common to take a knife or razor blade to corns, but that's unnecessarily risky. The key is to soften the horny tissue thoroughly so it can be removed easily. Before going to bed, simply wrap the toe or toes in a strip of wet cloth and put on one or two socks to help keep the cloth in place and retain moisture. The next morning, soak your foot in hot water for ten to fifteen minutes. It should then be easy to remove the corn, or at least part of it, with your fingers. For stubborn corns it may be neces- sary to repeat the treatment. Plain water will work, but some people prefer to use an herbal wrap or footbath. Sage, calendula, sweet gum bark, olive oil, castor oil, and lemon juice are sometimes recommended; any emollient herb (such as aloe vera, comfrey root, slippery elm, or mallow) is helpful.

These softening treatments can also be used to reduce calluses other than corns. Rubbing the softened area with a pumice stone will abrade the callus, but this should be done only a little at a time.

Once your feet are in good condition, you can keep them that way by giving them the proper footwear, as much unconfined time as possible, two footbaths a day, a daily alcohol rub, and a daily massage with Junipcrosan, a foot oil made from juniper berries.

COUGH

DESCRIPTION AND SYMPTOMS: There are many types of coughs, including spasmodic coughs such as whooping cough and coughs caused by phlegm. Coughs that have a thick yellow phlegm are inflammatory or hot natured; coughs that have clear or white phlegm are cold natured.

CAUSES: Coughs can be caused by accompanying colds or flus in which mucus and phlegm drip down into the bronchioles and lungs. This commonly can set up a sec- ondary infection in the lungs, which gives rise to a cough. Other types of coughs, such as asthmatic or whooping coughs, also have spasmodic factors that affect the bronchioles.

TREATMENT: Coughs can be treated with thyme tea and syrup, or with teas and/or syrups of coltsfoot,* mullein, loquat leaves, elecampane root and flowers, and wild cherry bark.*

Other native American herbs that serve as expectorants include yerba santa *(Eriodictyon californica)*, grindelia grandiflora, balm of Gilead *(Populus balsamifera* and *P. candicans)*, polygala senega, sundew *(Drosera rotundiflora)*, lobelia seed or leaf tincture *(L. inflata)*, boneset *(Eupatorium perfoliatum)* and pleurisy root *(Asclepias tuberosa)*. Many of these are to be found in formula number 1, which is very good for all upper respiratory ailments.

Give echinacea pills or extract every hour or two to help overcome any infection and to stimulate the body's immune system. When there is a lot of accompanying heat and fever, take goldenseal *(Hydrastis canadensis)* and garlic along with the echinacea every two hours. Slippery elm bark *(Ulmus fulva)* is very good to take as a pill mixed with honey or a little water to soothe the throat.

A tea of eucalyptus leaves can be brewed and used for chronic coughs. To help break up congestion in the lungs and sinuses, place several eucalyptus leaves or a teaspoon of eucalyptus oil or the commercial products called Vicks in a bowl of very hot water. Have the individual hold his head over the bowl and place a towel over his head, allowing him to breathe in the volatile oils that are emitted. Another effective treatment is to steam several chopped raw onions and wrap them in a towel and apply to the chest or back as hot as possible.

---

*There is some controversial research associating liver-damaging pyrolizidine alkaloids in comfrey and coltsfoot. Occasional use is fine, but pregnant women, infants, and children should avoid use of these herbs until further studies are available.

Apply camphorated oil or spirits on the chest and back and a eucalyptus ointment such as Vicks to give further relief. Finally, make syrup of garlic by blending several cloves of garlic in honey and give a teaspoon or more every hour or two. This has antibiotic properties and will have a definite effect, at least in preventing further complications or a secondary infection.

For spasmodic coughs and whooping coughs, thyme is very effective as well, but it can be enhanced by giving five drops of tincture of lobelia, which is a powerful antipasmodic.

Planetary formula number 57 (Mullein Lung Complex) combines mullein, ephedra, wild cherry bark, licorice, and other herbs useful for most upper respiratory problems. Formula number 61 (Old Indian Cough Syrup) combines yerba santa, echinacea, osh, grindelia, wild cherry bark, elecampane, and many other herbs in a pleasant-tasting syrup.

(See also ASTHMA.)

DANDRUFF

OTHER NAMES: Scurf, seborrhea.

DESCRIPTION: This unsightly and often uncomfortable condition results when epidermal cells are produced and die at different rates at different places on the skin. Dandruff flakes or scales are clumped clusters of dead skin cells that formed and died abnormally quickly. The scalp is the most common site, but other areas of skin can also be affected. Strangely, dandruff can be associated with oily, dry, or normal skin.

SYMPTOMS: The main visible evidence of dandruff is the appearance of loose skin flakes in and around the affected area. Depending on the condition of the skin, they may range from oily to dry and from yellow-gray to gray-white. The other main symptom is itching, which usually accompanies the flaking.

CAUSES: Opinions on the causes of dandruff differ. Suggested causes have included simple bacterial infection, hormonal imbalance, indigestion and constipation, and imbalance in the nervous system resulting from the stress and tension of modern life. The most likely answer is that stress, diet, hormonal activity, hygiene, and bacterial infection are all more or less involved in creating the conditions that lead to dandruff.

TREATMENT: There is general agreement that daily brushing or thorough combing of the hair is important to clean the hair and stimulate the scalp. Don't forget to clean the brush or comb daily as well. Massaging the scalp with the fingers for five to ten minutes a day is also recommended. Be sure the fingers and fingernails are clean.

Many shampoos and rinses can be both effective against dandruff and good for your hair; alkaline shampoos are the best. Frequent shampooing with herbal shampoos or castile soap can be used as a treatment by itself or as an adjunct to other treatments. Scalp treatments that have been recommended include cider vinegar diluted with water or with an aromatic herb water; diluted nettle juice or strong nettle tea; lemon juice; warm olive oil or linseed oil; strong birch bark, chamomile, chaparral, rosemary, sage, willow bark, or witch hazel tea; the juice or sap of the century plant (American agave), extracted with water; and juice from fresh grated ginger, mixed with olive or sesame oil. These are usually applied by massaging with the fingers and then left on for fifteen minutes to a half hour. Finish each non-oily treatment with a thorough clear-water rinse and each oily treatment with a good shampooing. In India, an herbal oil called "Brahmi Oil" is made by macerating gotu kola herb in sesame oil. It is rubbed into the scalp daily and can be left on or applied for an hour or so before showering.

In general, try to determine what may be causing dandruff to appear. If appropriate, cut down on or eliminate hot-air drying and chemical applications like hair sprays, tints, and perms.

Homeopathic remedies to use internally include sulphur 30th, calc, car. 6th to 30th, lycopodium 6th to 30th.

DEPRESSION

OTHER NAMES: Boredom, manic depression, melancholia, moodiness.

DESCRIPTION: Depression is a state of mind that ranges from mild, temporary sadness over some disappointment or loss to a psychotic sense of worthlessness and futility that may lead to suicide. In manic depression, the person's moods alternate between extremes of depression and euphoria. Short-term, occasional depression resulting from a specific cause is normal. Only when it occurs repeatedly for no apparent reason or lasts longer than about two weeks is there real cause for concern.

Depression is becoming more and more common in children and teenagers, often even leading to suicide. Do not take lightly any threats your child may make about "ending it all."

SYMPTOMS: The moody behavior we commonly associate with depression may not be the most obvious symptom. According to the American Psychiatric Association, depression involves "loss of interest or pleasure in all or almost all usual activities and pastimes." For a clinical diagnosis of depression, at least four of the following eight symptoms have to be present for at least two weeks (children under six must show at least three of the first four):

1. Either increased or decreased appetite with noticeable change in weight.
2. Excessive sleepiness or sleeplessness (insomnia).
3. Either hyperactivity or a slowed pace of activity.
4. Having no interest or pleasure in one's usual activities, or having a reduced sex drive.
5. Fatigue or lack of energy.
6. Feelings of guilt, self-reproach, or lack of personal worth.
7. Impaired mental abilities.
8. Preoccupation with thoughts of death or suicide; attempted suicide.

These characteristics may express themselves outwardly or physically in various forms, including unusual irritability, withdrawal from contact with others, crying spells, nervousness and anxiety, sudden changes of mood, and unwillingness to get out of bed in the morning. Psychological symptoms may include tiredness, insomnia, headache, intestinal gas, constipation, chest pain, muscle pains, heart palpitations, and ringing in the ears. Children suffering from depression may have headaches or cramps without any apparent cause and may become violent, destructive, or antisocial.

CAUSES: Aside from a genetic susceptibility to depression (which runs in some families), the cause is probably an interaction between external stress and the physical and psychological condition of the person. Of course, all of us face innumerable external stresses, the most serious of which are the death of a person one is close to, divorce, loss of a job, financial collapse, neglect or abuse, childbirth, menopause or mid-life crisis, and the realization that one is not likely to achieve significant life goals. These and even less severe stresses can trigger depression, particularly in persons who are psychologically weakened by chronic or acute disease, vitamin or mineral deficiencies, too much water in the system, overexertion, allergies, and abuse of drugs or alcohol.

TREATMENT: In many cases of depression, especially the more severe ones, counseling by a trained therapist can be very helpful and may be necessary. But at the same time it's important to take charge of yourself and do what you can to promote your own recovery.

Rest and exercise are important, especially when life stresses are involved. Outside motivation and emotional support can be very helpful, but not if they provide more psychological "strokes" for being depressed than for being cheerful and involved with life. Whole-body massage and deep breathing are very therapeutic (see Part Three). Dietary supplements of vitamins A, B-complex (particularly folic acid), C, and E, as well as calcium and magnesium, may be indicated.

Herb teas to lift the spirits include sage, ginseng, peppermint, cayenne, St. Johnswort, borage, and balm. Cloves added to any herbal tea or clove tea by itself is excellent. If the problem involves too much water in the body, diuretic herbs such as dandelion, cleavers, pipsissewa, buchu, fresh cornsilk, barberry, and juniper berries should help. Also, consult your physician to find out why you are retaining water.

Whenever depression is chronic, an elimination and cleansing program is indicated. Start with three to four days on an all-fruit diet, eating only ripe, raw fruits (except bananas) and drinking two cups a day of hot water containing a half teaspoon brewer's yeast and a half teaspoon of a vegetable extract flavoring. For four days after that, add raw salads made from combinations of lettuce, raw cabbage, celery, tomato, carrot, onion, watercress, and raw beetroot, as well as a serving of cottage cheese. Then, for one month, follow this diet:

- Breakfast: Whole-grain cereal with a heaping teaspoon of wheat germ and with raisins or prunes; then ripe, raw fruit.
- Lunch: Steamed vegetables, one leafy and one root vegetable; one and a half ounces cheese.
- Supper: Raw salad as above with a sprinkling of grated cheese or some cottage cheese; then yogurt or ripe, raw fruit if desired.
- Drink two cups of the vegetable extract and brewer's yeast both (described above) each day before meals and small quantities of pure fruit juices whenever desired.
- Eat two lightly boiled or poached eggs per week.
- Eat no more than two slices of whole wheat bread with butter per day.

When the month is up, repeat the program, beginning with the all-fruit diet. After the second session, be conscientious about permanently maintaining a nutritionally sound, healthful diet.

During a cleansing diet like this, it is possible that a "healing crisis" will occur—that is, there may be fever, a localized inflammation, a rash or boils, a cold, or diarrhea. The proper response is to fast for a few days, taking only diluted pure fruit juices until the symptoms are gone. At the end of the fast, take one day on the all-fruit diet before resuming the program where it was interrupted.

Do not resort to drugs of any kind during this treatment because they can be more dangerous than usual during this time. Pep pills and the like are decidedly harmful at any time and should be avoided at all costs if you truly want to get well.

Herbal combinations useful for depression include Planetary formula number 10 (Bupleurum Calmative) and formula number 82 (St. Johnswort–Kava Compound). St. Johnswort has been clinically found to be effective for mild to moderate clinical depression. While it has many other uses as an anti-inflammatory and an analgesic for nerve pains. St. Johnswort *(Hypericum perfoliatum)* has become the primary herb used for depression in both Europe and North America. Kava *(Piper methysticum)* originating from the Pacific South Sea islands is a wonderful herb to use either in formula or occasionally to impart near immediate relief from anxiety. The herb lemon balm makes a pleasant tea that has been used for centuries to treat depression. Finally, as if their beauty were not enough to relieve our melancholic states, red rose petal honey, made by blending freshly dried red rose petals from an older heritage rose (that has scent) with honey, makes a good-tasting jamlike spread that can be eaten as is or spread on a piece of toast.

Homeopathic treatments for chronic emotional symptoms are many and probably require expert opinion. Some remedies that frequently come up include lycopodium, arsenicum, sepia, and apis, but these are usually taken in extremely high potencies and should be professionally prescribed.

DIABETES

OTHER NAMES: Diabetes insipidus and diabetes mellitus.

DESCRIPTION AND SYMPTOMS: The most extreme symptoms of diabetes include excessive thirst, urination, hunger, weight loss, fatigue, and weakness. However, in most instances, a simple blood test can determine whether or not there is excessive sugar in the urine and will provide a diagnosis of diabetes. If diabetes is not satisfactorily controlled, severe dehydration and acidosis may result. Further, if the body pH drops below 7.0 the diabetic will develop coma.

Because of a tendency toward narrowing of the arteries, there is a gradual impairment of circulation, especially to the legs and feet, so that in advanced stages of diabetes, there is a danger of gangrene of the feet. Another side effect of advanced stages of diabetes is a rupturing of the capillaries of the eyes. This can result in blindness, but fortunately, modern medicine has developed the ability to perform delicate laser surgery on the eyes and save the sight of diabetics.

CAUSE: A lack of insulin to metabolize and regulate blood sugar (glucose) levels. Insulin and protein are secreted from the "Islets of Langerhans" cells of the pancreas. When there are insufficient amounts, the result is poor carbohydrate and sugar metabolism. Excess sugar from the blood spills over into the urine, making it possible to perform a simple test for diabetes by checking the amount of sugar in the urine. When there is a lack of carbohydrate metabolism, the result is the symptoms of diabetes.

The difference between diabetes mellitus and diabetes insipidus is that the latter is caused by a pituitary malfunction and tends to be constitutional and genetic in origin. Diabetes mellitus, although often precipitated by an inherited weak pancreas, is most often acquired later in life because of overconsumption of sugar and refined carbohydrates and is thus more amenable to natural treatment. It is interesting to note that an overworked pancreas, which at one stage in life would cause hypoglycemia or low blood sugar, can later change to hyperglycemia or diabetes.

TREATMENT: Central to the treatment of diabetes is to eliminate simple sugars and limit calorie intake according to weight and activity. Overly concentrated intake of sugar, fried foods, and foods high in fats will overtax the diabetic's insulin levels, causing blood glucose to rise dangerously. This can result in coma and the blood glucose level must be quickly lowered with insulin. Further, diabetics seem particularly inclined toward atherosclerosis, and saturated fats and oils are definitely contraindicated.

Diabetics must learn to substitute fresh fruit for rich, sugary desserts. While refined sugar and carbohydrates such as white flour are bad, diabetics seem to do well on unprocessed and unrefined complex carbohydrates high in fiber. This includes all whole grains, beans, a little organic fish or fowl, and steamed vegetables. Vegetables both steamed and raw seem to be particularly good for diabetics and can be freely eaten.

One may wonder why complex carbohydrates seem to be beneficial when simple sugar and refined carbohydrates are so harmful to diabetics. The reason is in the speed of absorption. While refined sugars and carbohydrates flood the blood with sugar, unrefined carbohydrates including whole grains, cereals, fruits, honey, maple syrup, and vegetables break down more gradually and release sugar slowly over a prolonged period of time and do not upset blood glucose levels.

One of the most important supplements is the trace mineral GTF chromium. This explains why brewer's yeast, which is particularly high in this trace mineral, also seems to be so beneficial for diabetics. A diabetic should take three to five tablespoons of brewer's yeast daily. It has been discovered that diabetics often have normal amounts of insulin but, with a deficiency of chromium, are not able to utilize it. Thus, according to a press release from the FDA (April 6, 1966), malnourished infants made overnight recovery in their bodies' ability to utilize sugar when given small amounts of chromium in their diet. Another study reported in *Medical World News* (May 19, 1972), by Dr. K. Michael Hambidge, stated that most elderly persons have impaired glucose tolerance. Clinical trials were conducted and "as many as 50% of such patients have been restored to normal glucose tolerance on daily doses of 150 mcg. of trivalent chromium."

To prevent gangrene of the feet, diabetics must stop smoking, as tobacco is known to further constrict the arteries; never wear garters, nylon stockings, elastic tights or tight-fitting socks; wear colorfast socks, ideally white, and change the socks daily; wear pliable shoes; do not sit with legs crossed or with pressure on the femoral artery; wash the feet twice a day with a hypoallergenic soap and warm water. Do not attempt to remove calluses or corns either with chemicals or cutting.

The direct application of the ash of mugwort *(Artemisia vulgaris)*, used by herbalists and in moxibustion, can be mixed with water and directly applied to stop infections or bleeding on the feet. For this reason, many acupuncturists save the ash from their moxa.

Walking and regular exercise are very beneficial for circulation and seem to decrease the need for insulin. Diabetics should try to avoid stress and anything that stimulates adrenal activity, which in turn will increase blood sugar levels. Other supplements that are of benefit to diabetics are vitamin C, 1,000 mg three times daily; vitamin E, 400 units one to three times daily; B-complex, 100 mg formula one to three times daily; vitamin A, 25,000 units once daily; niacin, 100 mg one to three times daily; magnesium, 200 mg once daily; manganese, 100 mg one to three times daily; potassium, 300 mg one to three times daily; zinc, 50 mg one to three times daily. Arginine should also be taken, as it has been found to help release stored insulin.

The same diet is necessary for both types of diabetes but diabetes insipidus should include glandular extracts of the posterior pituitary, hypothalamus, and renal organs.

There are a whole range of plants that contain insulin-like action and are useful for the treatment of diabetes. While not as strong as pancreatic insulin, these plant substances are called glukinins. Thus diabetics with less severe cases can be effectively treated with herbs, including the leaves of huckleberry or whortleberry leaf *(Vaccinium myrtillus)*, bean pods, cedar berries *(Juniperus monospermum)*, jambul *(Syzguym jambolana)*, onions *(Allium cepa)*, and trillium root *(T. pendulum)*, In Traditional Chinese Medicine, chronic diabetes is treated with a formula called "Liu wei" or "Rehmannia Six Combination"; this is the basis of formula number 67.

The late Dr. Christopher discovered the use of cedar berries in reducing blood sugar. As a result, the following formula was developed: equal parts cedar berries, licorice root, uva ursi, goldenseal root, mullein, and cayenne. These herbs are all powdered and two 00-size capsules are taken three times daily.

For less serious diabetes, huckleberry leaf tea using one ounce of huckleberry leaves steeped in a pint of boiling water is very beneficial. It is ideal to take any of the above herbal supplements with this tea.

Gymnema leaf *(Gymnema sylvestre)* is a treat native to Africa and India. It has the unique effect of temporarily blocking one's sense of the sweet flavor when chewed. Granulated sucrose will taste like sand after chewing on gymnema and will remain so for approximately one to two hours. Because of its ability to block sweet cravings it has a reputation for the treatment of diabetes. In fact, clinical studies has shown that it is able to lower blood sugar. The hypoglycemic properties of gymnema are related to gymnemin and a group of bitter compounds, and while its exact mechanism of action is yet unknown, it is thought that it works by increasing the efficiency with which insulin is released as well as by making cells more sensitive to insulin.

A Chinese patent formula that is effective for helping to regulate blood sugar for many with adult-onset diabetes is called yu quan wan or jade spring pill (*see* appendix).

DIARRHEA AND DYSENTERY

DESCRIPTION, SYMPTOMS, AND CAUSES: An inflammation of the intestines with symptoms including abdominal pain, severe diarrhea and bloody, mucous feces. The cause can be either bacterial or amoebic. Diarrhea can be caused from a chill, food sensitivity, or bowel toxicity. Dysentery is most often contracted from infected food or water.

TREATMENT: One effective folk remedy to stop diarrhea is to boil milk in an iron pot down to half its volume of liquid. Steep a teaspoon of cinnamon and/or three or four slices of fresh ginger in one cup of the milk and let stand until cool enough to drink. Take three cups a day before meals.

A tea of the following is also good for the treatment of diarrhea: equal parts cinnamon bark, bayberry bark or oak bark, and blackberry or raspberry leaves. Steep one teaspoon of the mixture in a cup of boiling water until cool enough to drink. Take three times daily before meals until normal.

Another good remedy for diarrhea is to simmer an ounce of blackberry root in a pint of boiling water for twenty minutes. Take one cup three times daily.

For bacterial or amoebic dysentery, make a powder of three parts goldenseal and two parts each of chaparral, garlic, bayberry bark, and wormwood. Take two 00-size capsules every two hours. Avoid sweets and fruits, and emphasize eating whole grains with a small amount of beans or legumes for protein.

Blackberry leaf, raspberry leaf, and yarrow are all good to use as a tea for either diarrhea or dysentery. Kudzu root

(Pueraria thunbergiana) with fresh ginger or cinnamon is also good for most intestinal complaints. If there is intestinal bleeding, give an enema with marshmallow root *(Althaea officinalis)* tea.

DIZZINESS

OTHER NAMES: Giddiness, orthostatic hypotension, postural hypotension, vertigo.

DESCRIPTION: Dizziness is a general term for a variety of sensations ranging from momentary vague light-headedness to a prolonged sensation of spinning around (vertigo). Light-headedness is a common feeling that people get when standing up from a sitting or lying position, especially if the movement is rapid. A more serious form of dizziness is characterized by temporary general disorientation and a sense of loss of balance. In vertigo, the most severe form, the sensation of movement and loss of balance can be frightening and can last for hours.

SYMPTOMS: Dizziness in all its forms involves some feeling of giddiness or light-headedness. The more severe forms involve various combinations and degrees of unsteadiness (floors seem to rise and fall, surroundings appear to spin), nausea, vomiting, headache, sweating, loss of balance and hearing, and possibly fainting.

CAUSES: The brief dizziness associated with standing up suddenly (orthostatic or postural hypotension) is probably due to an associated reduction in the blood flow to the brain. Low blood pressure and certain medications (especially drugs for high blood pressure) can have a similar effect. So can a startling experience (like the sight of blood), which may briefly lower the blood pressure by causing the heart to slow down.

The more severe forms of dizziness have a variety of causes, including injuries or infections that affect the inner ear; excessive use of drugs, alcohol, or tobacco; severe eyestrain; anemia; atherosclerosis; high blood pressure; and misalignment of the cervical spine.

TREATMENT: There is no direct treatment for dizziness; the underlying cause must be eliminated. If a medical checkup shows that you have anemia, atherosclerosis, high blood pressure, or low blood pressure, treat these conditions as described under the corresponding entries in this book.

To remedy nutritional deficiencies, supplement the diet with B-complex vitamins (especially choline, pantothenic acid, and inositol), vitamins C and E, iron, calcium, magnesium, and bioflavonoids. Discontinue or minimize the use of drugs, alcohol, and tobacco. (If you are taking any prescription drugs, ask your physician about the possibility that they are causing the symptoms.) Make sure your eyeglass prescription is correct. See a naturopathic physician trained in spinal adjustment, or a chiropractic physician, to determine whether your cervical spine is in alignment. Follow the general recommendations in this book for cleansing a toxic system.

In Chinese medicine dizziness is said to be a condition of "liver wind" and is treated with a whole category of herbs appropriate to this condition. Perhaps the most effective of all is one called *Gastrodia elata* or in Chinese "Tian Ma." Specific formulas incorporating this and other herbs are available from herb stores and Chinese pharmacies. One in pill form is called "Tian Ma Wan."

Homeopathic remedies to consider include aconite 6th, especially if there is accompanying darkness around the eyes; belladonna 6th if there is flushed face and a throbbing headache; nux vomica 30th if there are sudden twinges of pain in the head.

EARWAX

OTHER NAME: Cerumen.

DESCRIPTION, SYMPTOMS, AND CAUSES: Earwax, or cerumen, is a natural secretion of the thousand or more sweat glands located in the ear. It is a yellowish substance composed of water, fats, fatty acids, lecithin, and cholesterin. It has the very important functions of lubricating the ear, warding off infections, and aiding hearing. One of its obvious functions is to trap dust that would otherwise lodge itself on the eardrum and cause hearing distortion. Ceruminosis, which is an inordinate increase in earwax, can cause tinnitus or noises in the ear, deafness, and earache; if the wax gets lodged behind the isthmus of the ear, it can cause a cough.

Despite the fact that earwax serves a positive function, an accumulation or impaction of it can actually foster the proliferation of bacteria and other pathogenic factors in the substance. Anyone, young or old, who has hearing loss should definitely investigate the possibility that it may be caused by an impaction of earwax.

Normally, chewing naturally dislodges earwax; however, with the overeating of refined and overly rich foods, it can accumulate faster than it can be eliminated.

TREATMENT: Eliminate the cause by changing to a more wholesome balanced diet. Switching to foods such as whole grains that require more chewing is very beneficial.

EAR CANDLES: One method of drawing out earwax is to dip an 8½-by-11-inch piece of paper or linen cloth in melted paraffin or beeswax, allow to dry, and roll lengthwise into the shape of a conical tube so that one end is small enough to fit snugly into the inner opening of the ear. Have someone assist by holding the cone in place and lighting one end. Allow it to burn down to within a few inches of the ear, then quickly remove and snuff out in a small bowl of water. The wax will be found at the base of the cone.

Another method of dissolving and eliminating earwax is to take a piece of 8½-by-11-inch paper and roll it into a small tube. This should be taped or fastened together in some way and one end shallowly but firmly inserted into the ear of the patient. Set fire to the outer end of the paper and allow it to burn down to a safe distance away from the head and hair of the patient. It should then be quickly extinguished. The heat forms a vacuum, which serves both to dislodge and draw out the earwax.

ECCHYMOSES

DESCRIPTION AND SYMPTOMS: This is a condition associated with discoloration under the skin, such as a black and blue mark.

CAUSES: While it is usually an acute condition, it is also found as part of a chronic deficiency causing blood stagnation, flooding and rupturing of fine veins and capillaries. It is quite typical of those who consume too much alcohol and spices.

TREATMENT: First one should go on a balanced diet, eliminating strong spices, alcohol, and coffee. Next, one would use blood-moving herbs such as motherwort *(Leonurus cardiaca)*, angelica, hyssop, hawthorn berries, and rose hips. Topically, one can apply a fomentation of witch hazel, a liniment of cayenne, myrrh, goldenseal, hyssop, and oak bark decoction.

ECZEMA

OTHER NAMES: Adult eczema, infantile eczema, weeping eczema.

DESCRIPTION AND SYMPTOMS: Eczema is a superficial skin disease that has various stages and forms. It can be dry or weeping or a combination of both. It is always characterized by a rash with severe itching and burning.

CAUSES: Allergies to certain foods, dairy products and foods with saturated fats, bottle-feeding of babies (infantile eczema seems to be rare in breast-fed babies), stress and nervous tension, and other potential toxic environmental factors can all cause eczema.

TREATMENT: For weeping eczema one should avoid applying powders or pastes. The best treatment is to apply a moist compress until the weeping and acute stage has passed. After this, ointments and oils such as the ones described below can be applied.

It is best to use a light linen, flannel, or gauze bandage which has been saturated with a warm tea of oak bark *(Quercus sp.)*, calendula flowers *(C. officinalis)*, chamomile flowers, chickweed *(Stellaria media)*, violet or pansy *(Viola tricolor)*, or walnut leaves. The compress is applied warm and renewed as soon as it begins to get dry or cool, about every ten to twenty minutes. Give this treatment three times daily; between treatments, tape on a bandage that has been moistened with tea.

While saturated fats can cause eczema, unsaturated fats (these are the oils and fats that stay liquid at room temperature) from good-quality vegetable oils can be used to treat it. One of the best symptomatic treatments is to make an oil by filling a widemouthed jar with finely chopped chickweed herb and calendula blossoms. Add enough olive oil to cover and let stand in a warm place for three to four days. Press-strain through a cloth and bottle for use. This oil can be freely applied for all types of eczema when it is past its weeping stage and will promote further healing.

Internally take evening primrose *(Oenothera sp.)* or borage seed oil three times daily. The seeds of these herbs are rich in an essential fatty acid called gamma-linoleic acid (GLA), which is a precursor in the body for a vital series of prostaglandins. These prostaglandins help regulate normal cellular activity. The action of these prostaglandins can be blocked by hydrogenated oils used in margarines, viral infections, alcohol, aging, zinc deficiency, and radiation. Borage seed and evening primrose are two of the highest known sources of GLA next to human breast milk. Take up to four 500 mg capsules of evening primrose capsules daily.

A good herbal tea to take is a combination of red clover blossoms, chamomile flowers, elder flowers, nettles, and violet leaves. Steep one tablespoon of the dried herbs in a cup of boiling water for ten minutes and take three cups daily before meals.

Other herbs that are good to use include burdock and yellow dock root. These can be powdered and put into 00-size gelatin capsules; take two tablets three times daily with the above tea. Finally, formulas number 99 for the skin and number 84 for the nerves are both useful to take for this condition. It is also good to consider taking triphala to promote internal cleansing and regularity.

Vitamin and mineral supplements that are sometimes effective in the treatment of eczema include vitamin A, 25,000 units taken once daily; vitamin B-complex, 100 units, and vitamin C, 1,000 mg three times daily.

Diet should be wholesome, soothing, and nonirritating. Avoid all dairy products, spices, and citrus fruits.

EPILEPSY

DESCRIPTION AND SYMPTOMS: Epilepsy is a disease characterized by uncontrolled excessive activity of part or all of the central nervous system. A person may experience an epileptic attack when the base level of excitability reaches a certain threshold. There are three primary types: grand mal, petit mal, and focal epilepsy.

Grand mal epilepsy is characterized by extreme neuronal discharges in all areas of the brain. Seizures include tonic convulsions of the entire body with a tendency to bite or swallow the tongue, difficulty breathing, and spontaneous urination and defecation. Grand mal seizures can last from a few seconds up to four minutes and are followed by postseizure depression of the nervous system.

Petit mal epilepsy is characterized by three to thirty seconds of unconsciousness with accompanying twitches and spasms of the muscles, especially of the head and eyes. This is followed by a resumption of previous activities. One may have an attack once in many months or several times in rapid succession. Petit mal usually begins in late childhood and disappears around the age of thirty. On occasion, a petit mal attack can initiate a grand mal seizure.

Focal epilepsy can involve any part of the brain. It usually results from some form of organic lesion (an accident with brain injury) or inherited or acquired functional abnormality. There are different subtypes of focal epilepsy, which include psychomotor seizure, which can cause periods of amnesia, an attack of rage, anxiety, discomfort, paranoia, incoherent speech, mumbling of some trite phrase, or an irresistible urge to hit someone. Such an individual may even be conscious of what is occurring during the seizure but is unable to control it. Focal epilepsy can also precipitate a grand mal seizure.

CAUSES: Grand mal epilepsy usually has a hereditary predisposition which occurs in one out of every fifty individuals. Attacks are precipitated by any abnormal stress. This might include emotional stress, alkalosis caused by overbreathing, drugs, fever, loud noises, or bright lights.

TREATMENT: Herbs and treatments for epilepsy include the combination of gotu kola, skullcap, peony root, and calamus root powders in equal amounts taken in two 00-size gelatin capsules three or four times a day. Another is eating three cloves of garlic daily or making a garlic and honey syrup by blending several mashed cloves in honey. This is stored in a widemouthed jar in the refrigerator, and a tablespoon or two is taken three times daily.

In East Indian Ayurvedic medicine, ghee (clarified butter made from raw, unsalted butter) is considered especially strengthening to the brain and nervous system. A few drops of ghee, aged at least five years, can be instilled into the nose each day. In addition, a teaspoon to a tablespoonful should be taken in warm milk once daily.

A combination of a few drops of garlic–olive oil and B and B tincture can be placed into the ears each night with a wad of cotton. The tincture consists of four nervine herbs that favorably strengthen and maintain the nerves. Garlic-olive oil has further healing properties and helps carry the properties of the herbs into the brain.

B and B tincture is made by powdering one ounce each of black and blue cohosh, skullcap, and vervaine. Place in a widemouthed jar covered with a pint of vodka. Let stand for two weeks, then strain and bottle for use.

Garlic-olive oil is made by blending peeled cloves of fresh garlic with enough oil to cover. Macerate in a warm place using a widemouthed jar for three or four days and then squeeze through a piece of linen or cheesecloth. The oil is then ready to bottle for use.

Supplements that have been found beneficial for epilepsy include a combination of vitamin B_6 and magnesium. Even children suffering from epilepsy have been benefited with regular daily doses of vitamin B_6 and magnesium. A conservative dosage is about 100 mg of B_6 for children under thirty-five pounds. Adults can take two or three times this amount three times daily.

Brewer's yeast is high in all the nine vitamins and three to five tablespoons can be taken on a daily basis for epilepsy and parkinsonism. Infants with epilepsy either stop having seizures or a lessening of the frequency and severity when fed approximately two tablespoons of brewer's yeast mixed into their bottle once or twice daily.

(*See also* PARKINSON'S DISEASE.)

ERYSIPELAS

DESCRIPTION: Also called St. Anthony's Fire, erysipelas is characterized by diffuse inflammation of the skin, or of the subcutaneous cellular tissue, usually with accompanying fever.

SYMPTOMS: Redness of the skin in a local area; in more advanced conditions the redness will be more pervasive and cover a wider area of the skin. Since erysipelas is generally an inflammatory condition, there may be accompanying fever and a feeling of general sickness, drowsiness, and languor. If the inflammation is not controlled in time, it can spread to the throat, glottis, and brain and have fatal results.

TREATMENT: During the acute phase, take only warm vegetable broth and thin, whole-grain porridge. Take a tea of yellow dock root, burdock root, and dandelion root in decoction, one cup three or four times daily along with echinacea tablets or extract every two hours, tapering off gradually as symptoms subside.

Topically, one can apply a number of remedies: barley flour mixed with honey and ghee, a combination of sandalwood oil and lemon juice, aloe vera juice, crushed cabbage leaves, fresh crushed and pulped comfrey or coltsfoot leaves, goldenseal tea. Bed rest is recommended.

Homeopathic remedies to consider are belladonna if the condition is of recent and rapid onset, hepar sulph 6th to 30th if the condition is associated with pus and suppuration, and silicea 6th if it seems slow to heal. Mercurius is used if the pus has formed but is slow to come to a head. Other remedies that are possible include arsenicum and lachesis. CAUTION: If symptoms do not subside after a day or two, consult a physician.

EYE INFLAMMATION AND IRRITATION

OTHER NAMES: Inflammations: blepharitis, conjunctivitis, iritis, pinkeye, scleritis, sty, uveitis. Irritations: bloodshot eye, chalazion, puffy eyes, red eye.

DESCRIPTION: The eye, like any other organ in the body, can become inflamed, infected, or irritated. Blepharitis is inflammation of the edges of the eyelids; conjunctivitis is inflammation of the membrane that lines the eyelids and connects to the eyeball; iritis is inflammation of the iris; scleritis is inflammation of the white part of the eyeball, uveitis is inflammation of the pigmented inner parts of the eye; a sty is an inflammation of an oil-secreting gland on or near the edge of an eyelid; a chalazion is a small, hard tumor that forms on the edge of an eyelid.

SYMPTOMS: Eye problems other than simple physical irritation usually involve some combination of redness, tenderness, pain, swelling, itching, tearing, crusting, oozing of pus, photophobia (sensitivity to light), and enlargement of lymph nodes.

CAUSES: Eye inflammations and irritations can result from specific causes, such as bacterial or viral infection, allergies, foreign bodies in the eye, trauma, or excessive rubbing; they can also result from general glandular congestion or a toxic system. Puffy eyes are a sign of water retention or general toxicity.

TREATMENT: Acute eye problems can be very dangerous; consult your doctor if there is any doubt about the cause or the required treatment.

If the eye is inflamed or irritated because a foreign object, like a dust particle or an insect, has gotten caught in it, do not rub the eye to try to remove the irritant. First see if the object is visible on the eye by spreading apart the upper and lower eyelids. If it is accessible, remove it with the tip of a clean handkerchief. (Cotton balls or swabs are not recommended because fuzz can stick to the eyeball.) If the object is stuck on the underside of the upper eyelid, pull the lid down over the lower lid and let it slide slowly back into position. Usually, the friction from the lower lid will remove the object. If the object is stuck under the lower lid, pull the lower lid down and remove the irritant with a clean handkerchief. If it is not possible to remove the object directly, try flushing it out by holding the eye under cool running water. Thorough irrigation with running water is also a critical first-aid measure if the eye has been exposed to irritating chemicals; then see a physician as soon as possible.

If a relatively large object is stuck in the eye, do not remove it. Cover the eye and the object with a clean paper cup or a similar item and use a bandage or cloth to keep it in place. Get to a doctor or hospital immediately.

According to Traditional Chinese Medicine, the eyes are ruled by the liver. Congestion of the liver and hypertension can also cause eye inflammation sometimes known as "pinkeye" or conjunctivitis. It is treated internally with a tea of Oregon grape root, one ounce simmered in two cups of boiling water for twenty minutes; take three cups daily along with one or two 00-size capsules of goldeneal powder. One can also use Bupleurum Liver Cleanse (formula number 13) three times daily.

A simple eyewash can be made using horsetail tea or a tea of triphala combination. Triphala is also very beneficial to take internally each evening. The diet should be corrected; strong heating, spicy, and stimulating foods including sugar should be avoided.

Triphala (formula number 89) is a very highly effective herbal combination for all eye problems, including cataracts, glaucoma, eyestrain, and itchy, scratchy eyes. Dissolve four tablets of triphala in a cup of boiling water and allow to cool. Carefully strain off the clear tea, leaving the solid residue at the bottom of the cup to be discarded. Store in a small, airtight jar. Using an eyeglass, rinse each eye with a solution of the triphala tea for approximately twenty to thirty seconds, rolling the eyeball around in the tea. Repeat this two or three times daily.

Both triphala and Planetary formula number 8 (Bilberry Eye Complex) can be taken daily for cleansing and strengthening the eyes.

Homeopathic remedies to consider include belladonna 6th to 30th at the earliest stage of inflammation; euphrasia (eyebright) 6th to 40th when there is copious flow of tears but perhaps a feeling of grittiness and dryness; and apis 6th to 30th if there is great redness of the conjunctiva with sensitivity to heat.

Sties are treated internally with River of Life and triphala formulas. Externally, one would use triphala as an eyewash.

Homeopathic remedies to consider for sties include pulsatilla, if it is on the upper eyelid and there is a discharge of yellow to green pus; hepar sulph if the eye is swollen, sensitive to touch, and relieved with warmth; apis when the eyes burn and sting. These are all in the 6th to 30th potencies.

EYESTRAIN

OTHER NAMES: Asthenopia, tired eyes.

DESCRIPTION: Eyestrain is a general term for tiredness or weakness of the eyes. It is a secondary condition associated with vision disorders, use of the eyes in dim lighting, stress, and infections in other parts of the head. The sensation of "strain" is a manifestation of fatigue in the internal and external muscles of the eyes, which are overworked or weakened by the underlying condition.

SYMPTOMS: The symptoms often associated with eyestrain include blurred or otherwise imperfect vision, headaches, a feeling of pressure behind the eyes, squinting, difficulty in keeping the eyes open, dizziness, and constant rubbing of the eyes.

CAUSES: As already suggested, eyestrain can have a variety of causes. What they have in common is their detrimental effects on the muscles of the eye. Infections in other parts of the head and use of the eyes in poor lighting place a direct physical stress on the eye muscles, a temporary effect that usually disappears when the cause is removed. More complex is the problem of chronic eyestrain associated with vision disorders and psychological or emotional stress.

TREATMENT: The following techniques are helpful for relaxing the eyes:

1. *Blinking:* Frequent binking will help relieve eyestrain. When you are reading, blink between lines.

2. *Palming:* Sit at a table and place the palms of your hands over your eyes. Relax with your elbows on the table and exclude all light from your eyes, being careful not to put any pressure on the eyeballs. At first, you will see many colors and lights; your goal is to see a field of black. Imagining the inside of a black box lined with black velvet (or imagining any other totally black item) is useful. When you achieve this goal, your eyes will be totally relaxed. You can't overdo palming; the more time you take, the better.

Palming is one of the finest aids in helping to restore normal vision.

3. *Swinging:* While standing, swing your arms and body from side to side in a twisting pattern. Relax your eyes as you do this, allow them to see what they will. This is a great relaxer.

4. *Sunning:* Lie or sit facing the sun with your eyes closed. Turn your head from side to side so that all parts of your eyelids are bathed in sunlight. Keep it up as long as you like (but not long enough to get sunburned). After a week or two of sunning with the eyes closed, change to blinking at the sun, or rather "reverse blinking," because you open the eyes momentarily from a closed position. Start slowly and gradually pick up the pace, but always stay at a rate that feels comfortable. (CAUTION: Do not stare at the sun under any circumstances!) Sunning is an excellent way to apply the long-known healing power of sunlight to eyestrain and other eye problems.

5. *Eyebaths:* Cold-water eye baths taken for one to two minutes in the morning and evening are very therapeutic. Use only distilled or pure spring water. (See Part Three.)

6. *Nose writing:* To relieve general muscle tension in the neck and face, try using your nose as if it were a pen. Keep your neck loose and relaxed and your eyes unfocused.

7. *Massage:* Massage the muscles around your eyes, being very careful not to put any pressure on the eyeballs.

8. *Clamping:* Clamp your eyelids together as tightly as you can and then open them wide. Repeat half a dozen times.

9. *Herbal applications:* Sliced cucumbers placed over tired eyes are very soothing. A compress of chamomile, goldenseal, or borage tea will also relax and soothe tired eyes.

Eyestrain can be relieved by regularly rinsing the eyes with triphala tea, horsetail, or eyebright herb. See CATARACT for the recommended eyewash. Chrysanthemum and lycii berry tea is a good herbal combination for strengthening and benefiting the eyes.

FATIGUE

Includes all diseases associated with chronic fatigue, including Epstein-Barr, mononucleosis, adrenal fatigue, anemia, and many others.

OTHER NAMES: Chronic fatigue syndrome, exhaustion, tiredness, weakness, weariness.

DESCRIPTION: Fatigue is a state of extreme physical depletion in which the individual is unable to exert physical effort or respond normally to any stimuli because the body's vital powers are sapped. Acute fatigue has a well-defined beginning and is relieved by resting; chronic fatigue is continuous.

SYMPTOMS: Fatigue includes lack of energy, tiredness, weakness, apathy, drowsiness, prostration, and depression. People have been known to sleep up to three to four days when extremely exhausted. There are many accompanying symptoms including joint pains, digestive weakness, nervousness, and lowered resistance to disease.

CAUSES: Normal fatigue may result from acute or prolonged physical or emotional stress. Examples of physical stress are overexertion, heat exposure, illness, fever, malnutrition, allergies, and exposure to drugs, chemicals, and environmental pollutants. Emotional stress generally has its origin in major life changes, in socioeconomic conditions, and in the quality of relationships with others at home, at work, and in society in general.

TREATMENT: Where appropriate, treat the cause of the underlying stress. For acute fatigue, pay attention to your body and it will tell you how much rest it needs to recover. For chronic fatigue, the conditions that promote the rejuvenation of vitality are rest, good nourishment, appropriate physical exercise, a clean environment, and avoidance of physical and emotional stress.

Wholesome foods described in the macrodiet are combined with various tonic herbs according to the condition. These include ginseng *(Panax ginseng)*, astragalus *(A. membranicus)*, and suma *(Pfaffia paniculata)*, taken to tonify energy; dong quai *(Angelica sinensis)* and yellow dock root *(Rumex crispus)*, taken to tonify blood; rehmannia root *(Rehmannia glutinosa)*, American ginseng *(P. quinquefolia)*, ophiopogon *(O. japonicus)* and lycii berries *(Lycium chinensis)*, Iceland moss *(Cetraria islandica)*, taken to tonify body essence. These can be combined and taken as a tea, porridge or soup. The ginseng formula number 40 can be simmered into a stock in which some organic meat or rice porridge is cooked. For vegetarians, these herbs can be taken as a powder, tablet, or extract along with a glass of boiled warm milk in which is added a few slices of fresh ginger and a teaspoon of honey. Such an herb food is taken once or twice daily.

There are many Planetary formulas that are useful for fatigue. But first, trying to determine the cause of the fatigue and rectifying it is of primary importance. Next, one can select formula number 38 (Ginseng Classic), based on the Four Noble Herbs of Chinese medicine, to tonify qi (vital energy) and improve digestion. Ginseng Elixir is particularly useful for prolapsed conditions associated with fatigue. It is a primary formula to be used for Epstein-Barr virus and chronic fatigue syndrome. Ginseng Revitalizer combines five different types of ginseng with dong quai and other herbs to raise vitality. If one is burned out from overwork, formula number 67 (Rehmannia Endurance) is the one to use.

Cordycep mushroom *(Cordyceps sinensis)* is sometimes called "winter worm" because it is a small fungus that resembles a worm. The naturally occurring growth of this mushroom on pristine mountain peaks in the Himalayas is remarkable. A small caterpillar becomes host to a fungus, which in turn devours the insect and then grows from the animal's carcass, retaining the exact shape of the caterpillar even though at this stage it is truly a fungus. This remarkable mushroom tonifies the kidneys and lungs and is used for a variety of debilitating conditions such as lower back pain; chronic, consumptive coughing; and general lack of energy and stamina. It can be combined or alternated with ginseng with good effect.

For debility, Ayurvedic medicine prescribes a tonic called chyavanprash, named after an ancient sage who was able to regain vigor and potency despite his advanced years. This mixture is available from Indian import houses and other suppliers. It should be taken by stirring 1 or 2 tablespoons of the herbal jam into a glass of scalded warm milk. Michael prefers fresh goat's milk because it is better absorbed by humans. Chyavanprash is made with 50 percent amla *(Emblica myrobalans)* fruit, which is the highest known source of assimilable vitamin C. This remarkable fruit is one of the three ingredients of triphala. Despite its preparation in long-sustained heat, the vitamin C in amla is bound with certain tannins that keep it intact and bioavailable. The remaining 50 percent of the formula of chyavanprash consists of approximately fifty herbs, each in small amounts that serve to amplify the bioavailability of the entire formula.

Another Planetary formula that is specific for adrenal exhaustion is number 73 (Schizandra Adrenal Complex), which tonifies kidney yang (sympathetic nervous system) and yin (parasympathetic nervous system) equally. If there are symptoms of coldness, low libido, and lack of motivation with aching joints, one would use formula number 68, which is a kidney yang tonic. If there are symptoms of wasting, low-level inflammations, and diseases associated with exhaustion, one would use formula number 67 (Rehmannia Endurance). Often there is a combination of both yin and yang deficiency so that an appropriate combination of the vitalizing and the endurance-promoting formulas are taken together, such as two tablets of Rehmannia Endurance with one tablet of Rehmannia Vitalizer.

To avoid congestion, one should consider using triphala or guggul once or twice daily to promote balanced elimination and circulation.

Diet is of great importance. One must be careful to get a regular source of easily assimilable protein as well as vitamin B_{12}.

FEVER

OTHER NAMES: High temperature, hyperpyrexia, hyperthermia.

DESCRIPTION: Fever is the elevation of body temperature above the normal level, which ranges from 96°F to

100°F for different individuals. True fever, as distinguished from an environmentally induced rise in body temperature (such as occurs in a sauna), is a physiological reaction to invasion of the body by many types of foreign organisms or substances. Fever is the predominant symptom in a number of diseases, including malaria, scarlet fever, and typhoid fever.

Fevers can be roughly classified as mild (up to 101°), moderate (101° to 104°), and high (over 104°). Fever higher than about 107° can cause death.

SYMPTOMS: During its rising and stable stages, fever is accompanied by hot, dry skin; rapid pulse; chills; and body aches. These are associated with the body's technique of raising its internal temperature by reducing perspiration and increasing metabolic and muscle activity, such as shivering. Thirst occurs during a fever because the body continues to lose water by transpiration (the emission of water as a vapor through the pores), which does not have the cooling effect that perspiration does. This dehydration also reduces the flow of urine, which becomes darker and more concentrated. High fever can cause delirium and convulsions, especially if the temperature rise is rapid. In the declining stage of a fever, perspiration increases as the body uses its natural cooling mechanism to restore is normal temperature.

CAUSES: The body responds to invasion by many sorts of foreign matter, particularly invasion in the form of bacterial and viral infections. Fever appears to be triggered by the activity of white blood cells when they attack foreign substances in the blood. This is why fever is generally associated with specific ailments or injuries, or with reactions to drug treatments for them.

TREATMENT: In one sense, fever is not an ailment to be treated at all: It is one of the ways in which the body attempts to heal itself. In fact, "fever therapy" has been used successfully against certain bacteria and viruses that do not tolerate high temperatures well. In most cases, then, it is probably best to put up with some discomfort and let fever run its course. Appropriate treatment of the underlying cause, of course, will also "treat" the fever by eliminating the need for it.

A high fever, however, must be carefully watched. If the temperature rises very rapidly or goes much beyond 105° (less for older people and those with heart conditions), steps should be taken to control the fever directly. Effective methods include partial or full body wraps, using a cloth dampened with water or with a mixture of water and vinegar (see Part Three), cool sponge baths, and lukewarm to cold immersion baths (may include lemon juice, vinegar, or sage tea in the water.) Sweating should be induced only when the fever is in the safe range and it is desired to bring it down even more.

Choose herbal remedies which are suitable to the cause underlying the fever. Preparations of willow bark act directly (like aspirin) to reduce fever. Quinine (from cinchona bark) is a specific remedy against malarial infection and fever. Lemon juice and fruit juices are good for relieving thirst and nourishing the body without putting heavy digestive demands on it. Vitamin and mineral supplements can be helpful, except for iron, which many infectious bacteria and fungi need to survive.

Many herbal teas are excellent for treating fevers: These include sweet basil tea, a combination of yarrow, mint, and elder flowers, red clover tea, gotu kola tea and one of the most effective, boneset tea (Eupatorium perfuliatum). For babies and small infants, herbal baths in a decoction of willow leaves or willow bark, white poplar bark, or oak bark tea will be just as effective as giving them teas internally. Diet should be very light, consisting of warm vegetable broths, or thin porridge.

A Planetary formula to use with fevers is formula 110 (Yin Chia Echinacea Complex). Fevers can be dangerous; be sure to obtain appropriate medical assistance as necessary.

Homeopathic remedies for fevers, especially during the first stages with sudden onset, are aconite 6th to 30th if the condition has been triggered by exposure to cold and extreme stress. Belladonna 6th to 30th is used if there is a flushed face, hot skin, redness and flushing, and in extreme conditions of delirium. Belladonna is most commonly given for simple fevers in children. Ferrum phos 6th is also a useful remedy for fevers and most acute diseases.

FIBROID TUMORS

OTHER NAMES: Fibroids, fibromata, uterine fibromyomas.

DESCRIPTION: Fibroids are benign (noncancerous) tumors that form on or in the wall of the uterus. They are hardened nodules consisting mostly of muscular tissue encapsulated in connective tissue, and range from the size of a pea to that of a grapefruit or, in rare cases, even larger. Although they may occur singly, they generally form as multiple tumors. Fibroids most commonly appear in women between thirty and forty-five years old, and black women are more likely than other women to get them. New tumors rarely form—and existing ones tend to shrink—after menopause.

SYMPTOMS: Small fibroids may be present without any symptoms at all, although a uterus with fibroids tends to become enlarged. Larger tumors may cause a variety of symptoms, particularly menstrual disturbances. Usually, menstrual flow increases (menorrhagia), but sometimes it decreases (dysmenorrhea); a whitish discharge (leukorrhea) may also occur. In addition, there may be either irregular or light but continuous bleeding between menstrual periods. As tumors grow, a sensation of pressure or weight may develop in the pelvic area, accompanied by constipation and by painful urination and defecation. Well-developed tumors may cause intermittent backache and pain in the lower abdomen and the thighs, particularly when the person is standing and during the menstrual period. Eventually, a lump may appear that can be felt with the hand.

CAUSES: There is no general agreement on what actually causes fibroids to form; the female sex hormone estrogen is suspected of playing a role. However, because fibroids afflict only some women—and those differently at different stages of life and according to ethnicity—it seems safe to say that susceptibility is a key causal element, one that is apparently in part genetic and in part environmental. If so, then keeping the body healthy is the main way to prevent the formation of fibroids and to control them if they do form. Whatever impairs the health of the body—such as poor dietary habits, drug or alcohol abuse, psychological stress, and a sedentary life-style—can be considered a cause of fibroids (and many other ailments as well).

TREATMENT: Fibroids can be diagnosed through a pelvic examination and, if necessary, by X rays or other imaging techniques. When they are diagnosed, nine times out of ten (or more often) there is no need for immediate drastic action—that is, for surgery. Generally, there is time to undertake a much safer natural course of treatment while keeping the tumors under close observation. If the tumors do not respond to the treatment, an operation can still be performed. But give the body a fighting chance first.

Except in immediately critical cases, in fact, the body may be its own best weapon against fibroids. Through a process called autolysis, the body has the ability to break down and absorb its own tissue. The normal functioning of this process can be seen in the absorption of scar tissue and in the breaking down of stored body fat and other tissue to replace food when a person is dieting or fasting. Since the body breaks down the least essential tissues to nourish the rest, its autolytic capability can often be turned effectively against fibroids. This is done through supervised, controlled fasting and dieting.

A typical ten-day program might start with three days of taking nothing but citrus fruit juices; it is best to make this a period of complete rest. Then for three days add raw fruit to the citrus juices, and drink sixteen ounces of vegetable juices a day. The most helpful juices are those made from carrots, beets, celery, parsley, cucumbers, spinach, and watercress. These can be taken in combinations (usually including carrot juice, which tastes the best). Finally, for the last four days follow a diet something like the following:

- Breakfast: raw fruit and citrus juice.
- Lunch: a starchy food (such as bread or potato), raw salad, and raw fruit.
- Supper: a combination of steamed vegetables, cheese or milk, and fresh fruit.
- At bedtime, drink a glass of raw vegetable juice.
- For hunger between meals, drink a glass of raw vegetable juice or eat a raw fruit.

Keeping protein out of the diet promotes the absorption of such nonessential tissue as fibroids.

This ten-day program can be repeated every two months until the fibroids are eliminated or stabilized without symptoms. Between programs (and after the last one), maintain a balanced diet low in fat and moderate in animal protein content.

If constipation becomes a problem, take a mild herbal laxative until the bulk provided by the diet is adequate to stimulate normal bowel movement. Exercise and sitz baths can also contribute to relief of constipation, and even of the fibroid condition itself. Particularly appropriate are the knee-chest exercise (while lying on your back, draw the knees up to the chest and hold the position for two to three minutes), pelvic muscle exercises, and swimming, as well as cold or alternating hot and cold sitz baths. These may be done daily, to the extent that physical condition allows.

The basic reason for fibroids is similar to that of cysts and breast lumps. When the liver becomes overloaded either from environmental or dietary stress (exogenous toxins) or emotional stress (endogenous toxins), it can store toxins in the breast or uterus. Thus, treatment of fibroids should always include draining the liver with herbs such as Oregon grape root, bupleurum, dandelion root, and others such as those found in formula number 13.

In addition there are some herbs that seem to be specific for promoting pelvic circulation and helping to dissolve fibroids. A good combination can be made by combining the following liquid extracts; vitex or chaste berries *(Agnus castus)*, yarrow *(Achillea millifolium)*, motherwort *(Leonorus cardiaca)*, blue cohosh *(Caulophylum thalictroides)*, sequoia tree buds (if available), and lady's mantle *(Alchemilla vulgaris)*. Combine the extracts in equal parts and take one teaspoon two or three times daily with raspberry leaf tea.

If there is a tendency toward anxiety and emotional imbalance, include tincture of fresh valerian root to the above combination and/or formula number 8. If there is a tendency toward bleeding, double the amount of lady's mantle and consider using tincture of the extract of fresh shepherd's purse.

FIBROMYALGIA

OTHER NAMES: fibromyositis; fibrositis; myofascial pain syndrome. Sometimes this condition is understandably confused with chronic fatigue, having many similarities both in terms of cause and treatment.

DESCRIPTION AND SYMPTOMS: This is a common rheumatic condition characterized by widespread pain in fibrous tissues, muscles, tendons, and other connective tissues throughout the body. Associated symptoms are fatigue, morning stiffness, insomnia, headaches, numbness of the hands and feet, irritability, and anxiety.

There must be at least three months of widespread pain in a least eleven areas in fibrous tissues of the muscles generally found in the following:

- neck
- shoulders
- chest
- rib cage
- lower back
- knees
- arms (elbows)
- buttocks

Unlike other kinds of pains, fibromyalgic pains are more generalized and lack defined trigger points. Trigger points only hurt when pressed, and then the patient may experience traveling or spreading pains.

Fibromyalgic pains are deep aching, radiating, gnawing, shooting, or burning and range from mild to severe. Pain tends to improve during the day and increase in severity during the evening. Pain also can increase with exposure to cold, damp weather, anxiety, and stress.

Possible causes of fibromyalgia may be similar to those for chronic fatigue syndrome, including viral and dietary causes as well as physical or emotional trauma. No microbe has been definitely identified.

CAUSES, INCIDENCES, AND RISK FACTORS: The cause of this disorder is unknown. Possible causes can include physical or emotional trauma. One hypothesis suggests that the disorder may be associated with changes in craniofacial and skeletal muscle metabolism, such as decreased blood flow, which could cause chronic fatigue and weakness. Another hypothesis is that an infectious microbe, such as a virus, triggers the illness. At this point, no virus or microbe has been identified. One of the exacerbating factors for the treatment of this condition is lack of sleep.

TREATMENT: Since the customary chronic pain-relieving measures may not be effective for fibromyalgic pains, a major strategy is to promote sleep. For this one may use a number of treatments similar to those indicated for chronic fatigue with a special emphasis in therapies to improve sleep (see INSOMNIA).

In addition to the supplement approach described under CHRONIC FATIGUE, one would add 150 to 250 mg of magnesium three times daily together with St. Johns-wort, which has antiviral properties and helps to counter-act mild depression. I use Planetary formula number 82 (St. Johnswort–Kava Compound). In addition, Michael uses formula number 33 (Flexibility) and formula number 70 (Reishi Mushroom Supreme).

Many patients have found that 5-HTP (5-Hydrozytryptophan) is effective in raising serotonin levels that will counteract depression and enable sleep.

FOOT ODOR

OTHER NAME: Sweaty feet.

DESCRIPTION AND SYMPTOMS: Although perspi-ration is normal, especially in an enclosed space like a shoe, excessively heavy perspiration is generally consid-ered a health problem—or a symptom of one. What is de-fined as excessive perspiration is somewhat subjective, but chronic foot odor and formation of salt deposits on the shoes would probably be generally accepted as indicators of a problem.

CAUSES: Here one can name only possibilities; there is no single clear cause for sweaty feet. They are most likely to be symptoms of an underlying problem, such as circula-tory or digestive problems, acidosis, nervousness or stress, thyroid disturbance, or anemia. Footwear may also be at fault, particularly if shoes and socks or stockings are made of synthetic materials that prevent the passage of air through them.

TREATMENT: If an underlying cause can be found, clearly the solution is to address that problem. At the same time, though, it is worth dealing with the objectionable symptoms of sweaty feet directly. Obviously, choose footwear materials and styles that give the feet as much air as possible. Use perspiration-absorbing insoles and foot powders to help keep the feet dry. A good foot and shoe powder can be made by combining four parts talcum powder, two parts stearate of zinc, and one part boric acid. If odor is a problem, add ten grains of salicylic acid to each ounce of this powder. Powdered hemlock spruce bark has also been recommended for use as a foot and shoe powder.

Footbaths should be a regular part of foot care, even if sweaty feet are not a problem. If they are, take frequent warm or hot footbaths (but avoid very hot baths if you have high blood pressure or circulatory problems). Some bath additives to choose from are: Epsom salts, vinegar bicarbonate of soda, lavender, menthol, camphor, calendula, hay flowers, oak bark, birch leaves, and oatmeal. Or take contrast warm and cold footbaths with plain water. For example, start with three to five minutes in water heated to about 95° to 100°F, then switch to cold water at 55° to 60°F for ten to thirty seconds. Repeat two or three times, ending with the cold water. After finishing any footbath, dry your feet thoroughly and give them a rubdown with rubbing alcohol or Juniperosan.

Another method of treatment involves wrapping both feet in cloths that have been dipped in a hay flower decoction or pine needle extract. These packs soak up the foul matter, and both herbs have a strengthening and healing effect. Take five or six of these applications within ten days, then one a day for fourteen days, along with contrast warm and cold footbaths, reaching to the calves. After that, it will be enough to use a foot pack or take a footbath once a week.

An unorthodox old-time folk remedy for foot odors was promoted during World War II. Men in close quarters would complain frequently of strong foot odors and an older man told them to urinate on their feet in the shower. Michael recommends this to a number of patients with this problem and it seems to work. Soaking the feet in black or green tea is another simple treatment.

FRACTURES AND BROKEN BONES

DESCRIPTION AND CAUSES: A bone that is injured or broken, usually as a result of a fall or injury.

TREATMENT: Seek medical assistance. To promote healing, use the Chinese liniment zhen gui shui or Planetary formula number 55 (Narayana Muscle Oil). To promote healing, apply a fomentation of Dr. Christopher's Bone Flesh and Cartilage each evening as described in Chapter Two. To relieve pain, try Planetary formula number 96 (Willow Aid).

GALLBLADDER INFLAMMATION AND GALLSTONES

OTHER NAME: Cholecystitis.

DESCRIPTION: The gallbladder is a small, pear-shaped bag at the bottom of the liver. It acts as a reservoir for bile when the digestive system needs less than the liver routinely produces; it also concentrates the bile while storing it. When more bile is needed to digest fatty food in the intestine, the gallbladder contracts to discharge its concentrated bile through the cystic duct (which is both entrance and exit) into the common bile duct leading to the duodenum. The gallbladder is also the place where gallstones most commonly form.

Cholecystitis is inflammation of the gallbladder and the cystic duct. It may range in severity from a chronic, mild condition to the development of gangrene and rupture of the gallbladder. It may be a complication of gallstones or may be associated with infection in the surrounding area. It afflicts women more than men.

SYMPTOMS: The basic symptom of gallbladder inflammation is a pain centered just below the lower right rib. In chronic cases, the pain may be merely a minor discomfort that recurs a few hours after meals. But if the inflammation is caused by a large gallstone that has become impacted in the cystic duct, severe pain (biliary colic) results when the gallbladder has to force its bile past the obstruction. This pain may radiate into the right back and shoulder and is often accompanied by nausea, vomiting, and loss of appetite. If the obstruction persists, the gallbladder may become enlarged; fever and chills occur when an enlarged gallbladder becomes infected. Unlike ulcer symptoms, those of gallbladder inflammation are not relieved by eating food.

CAUSES: Inflammation of the gallbladder comes about primarily from irritation due to gallstones. It can also result from bacterial or viral infection that spreads to the gallbladder from surrounding organs. Dietary and other habits that promote the formation of gallstones are therefore likely causes of cholecystitis also.

TREATMENT: Conventional physicians have found surgical removal of the gallbladder the "easiest" solution for both cholecystitis and gallstones; the body seems to get along just as well without this organ. Although surgery may be justified in extreme cases, the risks associated with it and the fact that it does not attack the roots of the problem suggest that a less drastic approach is normally called for. However, any treatment should be based on a competent diagnosis of the condition by a skilled practitioner, since the symptoms can be confused with those of appendicitis, indigestion, other gastrointestinal problems, and even heart attack.

Treatment during and after an acute attack is essential. Herbs said to stimulate gallbladder activity include artichoke, beetroot, calamus, celandine, dandelion root, yellow gentian, yarrow, European centaury, and radish.

A specific herbal combination for the relief of both gallstones and inflammation of the gallbladder is a combination of the following: 4 parts Oregon grape root, 4 parts wild yam root, 4 parts fennel seed.

Simmer one ounce of the above for ten minutes, cool, and drink three or four cups daily. It is very beneficial to take two to four 00-size capsules of powdered turmeric root alone or with this tea as well. Turmeric is a common spice used in East Indian cuisine and is a specific for the liver and gallbladder. In addition one would definitely use Hepato-Pure formula number 13 and Stone Free formula number 85.

Homeopathic magnesium carb 6x is specific for any spasmodic or griping pains such as those associated with gallbladder problems.

GAS AND BLOAT

OTHER NAMES: Flatulence, flatus.

DESCRIPTION: The condition referred to as "gas" or "bloat" is the presence of an excessive amount of gas in the stomach and intestines, particularly gases produced during the digestion of food. Usually a mixture of gases is involved, including oxygen, hydrogen, nitrogen, methane, and hydrogen sulfide. These are odorless gases, except hydrogen sulfide, which smells like rotten eggs. The characteristic odor of intestinal flatus, like that of the feces, is due mainly to skatol, a crystalline compound produced when bacteria break down the amino acid tryptophan, which is found in proteins.

SYMPTOMS: Normal accumulations of intestinal gas are eliminated during regular bowel movements. Excessive gas makes its presence known in various ways, some of them socially embarrassing. Symptoms include frequent release of gas, either by "breaking wind" or by belching; a generally bloated feeling; gurgling, rumbling, or other unsettled noises in the lower abdominal region; and abdominal and intestinal pain, particularly if the gas is deliberately held in.

CAUSES: The simplest cause of excessive gas is the swallowing of air or carbon dioxide while eating or drinking (especially carbonated beverages). Most problems with the gas, however, are associated with the digestive system's inability to handle the load put on it. Some foods naturally tend to produce more gas than others—beans are a notorious example, of course—but in most cases people have very individual patterns of reaction to the same kinds of food. How one eats is also important; food that is not chewed thoroughly makes greater demands on the digestive system than food that is, and may generate gas by fermentation or putrefaction if it cannot be digested quickly enough. Another cause may be heavy use of laxatives or antacids, which can disrupt the normal functioning of the gastrointestinal tract. And of course any disease or infection of the digestive system (or elsewhere in the body) can have similar results.

TREATMENT: Although measures can be taken for direct relief, only treatment of the underlying cause will eliminate the problem permanently. If certain foods invariably give you gas, change your diet to avoid them, reduce the amount of them you eat, or try to prepare them in a different way (for example, try cooking a vegetable instead of eating it raw). If you tend to eat hurriedly, take time to chew food thoroughly (and try to relax your pace of life in general). If the gas is a symptom or by-product of another physiological problem (such as constipation, indigestion, or ulcers), be sure to treat that condition as well as the gas problem itself.

Various herb teas or extracts are useful for relieving gas problems, including angelica, anise, caraway, chamomile, coriander, dill, fennel, garlic, yarrow, parsley, peppermint, and savory.

Sitz baths are helpful for gas as well as for other abdominal ailments. Try a ten- to fifteen-minute hot sitz bath followed by a quick cold gush to the area that was submerged; or alternate between three-minute hot and ten-second cold sitz baths, starting with the hot bath and taking each three times.

Planetary formula number 15 (Candida Digest) is based on the Ayurvedic formula called hingashtak, the Sanskrit name of the primary herb in the formula, which is asafetida. This herb is used widely throughout India and the Middle East along with bean dishes to prevent fermentation. It is combined with several other herbs that help digestion, including cumin and caraway seeds, ginger, two kinds of black pepper, green citrus, slippery elm bark, dandelion root, atractylodes root, and rock salt. The effect of this formula is to prevent gas by relieving abdominal tension and spasm while promoting the passage of food through the GI tract.

Taking a bitters formula such as Planetary formula number 24 before and/or after meals stimulates hydrochloric and other digestive secretions which will help to prevent or lessen gas. Other alcoholic bitters such as fernet branca, anisette, Benedictine, and Chartreuse all were developed in medieval monasteries for the prevention and treatment of gas. Planetary's formula number 23 (Digestive Comfort) can be taken for all digestive problems.

A pleasant-tasting after-dinner tea to prevent gas is made by steeping a few slices of fresh ginger with a teaspoon of chamomile in a covered cup of boiling water until cool enough to drink. Fennel seed tea is still another pleasant remedy to prevent gas and bloating.

Spices such as cumin seed, coriander seed, turmeric, ginger, asafetida, and on occasion garlic, sautéed in a bit of oil and stirred into cooked beans, vegetables, soups, or grains, is another good treatment to prevent gas.

An herb that has shown outstanding results for treatment of gas is called epazote *(Chenopodium ambrosioides)*. It is native to Mexico and is commonly cooked with beans as a condiment. It also eliminates worms and is an emmenagogue, so it should be generally avoided during pregnancy. An effective way to eliminate gas is to ingest a half to one teaspoon of powdered wood charcoal. Homeopathic Carbo.Veg. is also very effective for this problem.

GASTROINTESTINAL AILMENTS

OTHER NAMES: Dyspepsia, indigestion, upset stomach; heartburn, pyrosis; gastritis; gastoenteritis; peptic ulcers.

DESCRIPTION: As is suggested by the list of names above, a variety of problems come under the general heading of "gastrointestinal ailments." Indigestion is essentially the failure of the digestive system to digest and absorb food properly; dyspepsia (gastric indigestion) is failure of the stomach to perform its part in the process. Often what people mean by "indigestion" or "acid indigestion" is pyrosis, also commonly called heartburn. The burning sensation of pyrosis usually comes from the ejection of gastric juice upward into the esophagus. Gastritis and gastroenteritis are inflammations—the first, inflammation of the stomach; the second, inflammation of both the stomach and the intestines. A peptic ulcer is an area, usually in the stomach or the duodenum, where the protective layer of mucus has broken down, exposing the tissues beneath to gastric acid. If untreated, the ulcer can eventually penetrate the wall of the stomach or intestine and cause life-threatening peritonitis.

SYMPTOMS: The common symptom of all the gastrointestinal ailments is continuous or intermittent pain in the abdominal region. Heartburn, as the name implies, produces a burning sensation in the chest; it may be accompanied by a sensation of pressure in the stomach. Gastritis and gastroenteritis often are also marked by diarrhea, nausea, belching, coated tongue, lack of appetite, and—when chronic—by weight loss. Peptic ulcers tend to produce heartburn, belching, vomiting, and constipation. With stomach (gastric) ulcers, pain generally appears within two hours of eating and may radiate from the abdominal area into the back. Duodenal ulcers produce pain a longer time after a meal (often shortly before the next meal) and when the stomach is empty. Ulcer symptoms are most severe after consumption of fried and spicy foods, alcohol, and coffee.

CAUSES: There are two principal causes of gastrointestinal ailments: diet and stress. Through the diet, one can physically assault the digestive system with substances that tax its ability to deal with them—for example, large amounts of alcohol and coffee, foods that are hard to digest, and tissue-irritating drugs such as aspirin. Smoking can also impair the body's ability to keep the contents of the digestive system in balance. Less obviously, one can introduce bacteria or viruses into the digestive system by being careless about hygiene, particularly about washing one's hands before preparing or eating food. Heartburn sometimes also results from a hiatus hernia, in which the stomach partially protrudes upward into the chest cavity where the esophagus passes through the diaphragm.

The other great villain behind gastrointestinal ailments is stress. Stress is known to cause hormonal and other changes in the body, and the results seem to show up primarily in the digestive and circulatory systems. The digestive effects may range from "nervous stomach" to full-blown ulcers (perhaps even cancer), and people under great or continuous stress seem to be particularly susceptible to the whole range of disorders. "Executive ulcers," for example, are practically taken for granted as the price of success in the highly competitive American business world.

TREATMENT: Treatments can be grouped into physical and nonphysical, to correspond with the two types of causes.

For immediate treatment of acute symptoms, see HYPERACIDITY. For long-term improvement, the first step in treating any of the gastrointestinal disorders is to fast for two to three days, taking nothing but water or a mild herbal tea, such as balm, chamomile, or peppermint. If constipation is a problem, try warm enemas or warm to hot sitz baths. Following the fast, gradually add bland, easily digested cooked foods—such as potatoes, rice and oats—at first in liquid or soupy form. Fruit juices and milk can also be added gradually. During this time the person being treated should stay in bed and be protected from any excitement or stress. (If heartburn or the flow of gastric juices up into the esophagus and mouth is a problem, raise the head end of the bed four to six inches.) A few days of this treatment, followed by a conservative diet, should relieve the gastrointestinal ailments other than the ulcers.

For ulcers, the diet must be brought gradually back to a sound and balanced nutritional fare over a period of several months. The progression generally involves going from a limited selection of bland, cooked foods through raw fruits and vegetables to the full variety of a normal diet. Eating small amounts of food every few hours is better than eating large meals spaced further apart. Of course, you must give up those eating and drinking habits that brought on the ulcers in the first place. Because each person's dietary requirements are unique, there is no point in outlining a specific program here. A therapeutic diet should be designed individually by a competent practitioner.

Nondietary aspects of physical treatment for gastrointesinal ailments include abdominal wraps, daily sitz baths or dry friction rubs, fresh air, and exercise as allowed by the physical condition.

To deal with the nonphysical side of treatment, one

must address the problem of stress. It's likely that the majority of gastrointestinal problems are, at least in part, bodily responses to emotional stress. The basic link between stress and physical illness is by now well established, and new insights are reported regularly. Learning to cope with the detrimental stresses of one's existence (assuming that one can't eliminate or avoid them) generally involves conscientious and deliberate effort; in some cases it requires significant changes in personality or behavior. Again, the uniqueness of each individual case makes it impossible to give a detailed program for relief of stress. Nonetheless, a few general guidelines will give the idea:

- Get in touch with yourself: recognize and accept your basic nature (for example, easygoing vs. hard-driving).
- Recognize and express your feelings, and be receptive to those of others.
- Develop supportive relationships with others.
- Have specific goals against which to measure progress.
- Give yourself an outlet for playful feelings and behavior.

Ultimately, each person must develop a program suitable for his or her circumstances. There are numerous publications and professional people available to help in such efforts.

There are many effective herbal treatments for gastrointestinal problems. Most traditional cultures view the stomach and digestive system as the seat of most diseases.

If there is digestive weakness and coldness, there will be gas, bloating, feelings of coldness, tiredness, lack of appetite, and pale complexion. For this type of digestive problem, which is more the "hypo" type (such as hypoglycemia), we need warming, carminative, mildly stimulating and tonic herbs and foods. Such herbs as ginger root, galingale, ginseng, fennel seed, anise seed, and angelica root are all excellent to use for gastrointestinal problems caused by coldness, including abdominal pains, indigestion, and so forth.

Planetary formulas useful for indigestion and abdominal pains are:

- formula number 23 (Digestive Comfort) for occasional pains, bloating, diarrhea, and gas
- formula number 24 (Digestive Grape Bitters), one or two tablespoonsful 10 or 5 minutes before meals to stimulate gastrointestinal secretions for better assimilation
- formula number 15 (Candida Digest) is not only good for those suffering from candidalike symptoms of gas and bloating but any abdominal pains with gas
- formula number 89 (Triphala) is fundamental for any gastrointestinal condition
- formula number 38 (Ginseng Classic) when there is low energy with digestive weakness; this should be taken with ginger tea
- formula number 25 (Three Spices Sinus Support or Trikatu), again with much broader benefit than simply to dry up mucus; this combination of herbs is taken before meals when digestion is sluggish

Herbs that specifically help to relieve the accumulation of uric acid, which is the cause of gout, include the following:

- celery seed *(Apium graveolens)*, taken as a tea or powdered in capsules. Steep a tablespoon of the tea in a cup of hot water and drink two or three cups daily
- stinging nettles *(Urtica urens)*, the herb regarded as a botanical powerhouse of important nutrients, has also been shown to increase uric acid secretion in animal studies
- horsetail *(Equesitum arvense)* has diuretic properties which will relieve arthritic and rheumatic complaints and body stiffness and increase uric acid elimination, which is beneficial for the treatment of gout
- cherries *(Prunus species)* are well known in folk literature for relieving arthritis and gout. It was reported in a letter to *Prevention* magazine by Dr. Ludwig W. Blau, Ph.D., that eating a bowl of cherries one day led to complete relief from pain. His pain had been so severe that he was confined to a wheelchair and the day after eating the cherries his pain was completely gone. He continued to eat only six cherries daily and progressed to the point where he was able to get out of his wheelchair. Since then many others suffering from gout as well as other arthritic conditions reported that cherries helped them as well. Other reports find that for some strawberries work as well. These foods are known to help the body eliminate the uric acid that accumulates in sensitive joints of the body to cause pain.

Planetary formulas useful for treating gout include formula number 42 (Guggul Cholesterol compound), formula number 66 (Red Clover Cleanser) and formula number 18 (Complete Cat's Claw).

For an overheated condition, including gastritis, ulcers, colitis and gastroenteritis, one should use soothing herbs and foods. Foods such as okra, steamed amaranth, malva and violet leaves eaten regularly are very beneficial. It may be a good idea to begin by cleansing the intestinal tract using the laxative formula once or twice a week or taking triphala complex each evening, from two to three grams at a time. Other herbs that are specifically useful for this condition include dandelion root, marshmallow root, comfrey root, slippery elm bark, licorice root, and wild yam. Combine them all in equal parts and take as a tea by simmering one ounce of the combination in a pint of boiling water for ten to twenty minutes. Three or more cups are taken daily.

GOOSE BUMPS

OTHER NAMES: Cutis anserina, gooseflesh, goose pimples.

DESCRIPTION: Goose bumps are a roughened condition of the skin that occurs when small muscles attached to hair follicles contract, causing the hairs to become erect and pulling the follicles toward the surface of the skin to produce the bumps. This condition is not an ailment in itself; it is a temporary physiological response to certain stresses or stimuli.

SYMPTOMS: The principal symptom, of course, is the appearance of the bumps themselves. They are usually accompanied by a feeling of being chilled.

CAUSES: Goose bumps arise as an autonomic (involuntary) physiological response to various forms of stress on the body, especially cold external temperature or perceived threat. The response to cold is transmitted directly through the nervous system; the response to threat also involves the activity of the hormones that are triggered by emotional reactions to challenging situations. Both responses can be traced back to early evolutionary times, when life itself may have depended on the ability to puff up a coat of hair or fur as protection against cold or as a way to warn or intimidate a potential enemy by looking bigger. Nowadays we use clothes and weapons instead, but goose bumps still survive to remind us of our primitive past.

TREATMENT: The way to get rid of goose bumps is to eliminate their cause. If it's cold, raise the temperature, wear more clothing, or warm up the body through vigorous activity. If a threat is the cause, the situation could be more complicated and goose bumps may be the least of your problems.

Specific herbal treatments for this condition include Trikatu formula, Herbal Uprising, and Herbal Warmth. Warm cinnamon, ginger, anise seed, and angelica tea, taken three times daily, would also be very beneficial.

GOUT

OTHER NAMES: Arthritis uratica, gouty arthritis, podagra.

DESCRIPTION: Gout is an arthritic disorder found mostly in middle-aged men. It occurs when crystals of excess uric acid, a metabolic waste product, are deposited in bone joints and attacked by white blood cells, producing acute, painful inflammation and swelling. The most common form of gout is podagra, in which the joint at the base of the big toe is affected. Unless the condition is controlled, flare-ups tend to occur two or three times a year and last one to two weeks. Without treatment, attacks eventually become more frequent and other joints become affected.

SYMPTOMS: The first symptom often is a sudden excruciating pain in the big toe, followed by marked redness and swelling at the joint. (The fingers, knees, and ankles are less common sites for gout.) A slight fever and sweating may also occur. The site may become so sensitive that even the weight of bed sheets on the area is unbearable. Uric acid crystals may be excreted in the urine, and uric acid stones may form in the kidnesy.

CAUSES: Gout seems to be related to both dietary and genetic factors; it can also be associated with certain drugs used to treat high blood pressure and cancer, and with some diseases that involve rapid cell turnover. Stress may trigger an attack. Disturbances in the body's metabolism and in its elimination of purines—substances that break down into uric acid—are the immediate cause of the excess of uric acid that gives rise to gout. A diet high in purine-rich foods will tend to aggravate the condition.

TREATMENT: During the acute phase, apply either ice or a hot compress to the inflamed area if the contact can be tolerated. Liniments of mullein or comfrey can be helpful. This is also an appropriate time to undertake a four- to seven-day fast with fruit juices or fruit or one with carrot, parsley, pineapple, and potato juice, or a water diet with daily enemas (see Part Three). Supplements of vitamin B-complex, vitamins C and E, and pantothenic acid will help decrease the inflammation. If a related cause of the gout can be identified, treatment of that problem should be started as well.

To reduce susceptibility to gout attacks, a low-purine diet is recommended. The foods to avoid or minimize are meats (especially organ meats), fowl, and fish, as well as legumes (peas, beans, lentils), mushrooms, asparagus, spinach, and wheat. Also eliminate alcohol, black tea, salt, sugar, chocolate, and spicy foods. Buttermilk, goat's milk, citrus fruits, strawberries, and cherries are good alkalinizers and help dissolve uric acid crystals. Finally, try to reduce sources of emotional stress or improve your ability to cope with it.

Planetary formulas useful for treating gout include numbers 42 (Guggul Cholesterol compound), 66 (Red Clover Cleanser), and 18 (Complete Cat's Claw).

GUM DISEASE

OTHER NAMES: Gingivitis, periodontal disease, periodontitis, pyorrhea.

DESCRIPTION: The most common gum affliction is gingivitis, which is inflammation of the gums resulting from bacterial infection under the gum line. This condition often leads to pyorrhea, or periodontitis, in which the bones and ligaments holding the teeth deteriorate because of chronic infection. In its advanced stages, gum disease will result in loosening and loss of teeth. Both gingivitis and periodontitis are distressingly common in the United States—so much so that many people assume it is normal to lose their teeth as they get old. In fact, it is no more normal than getting cancer or any other disease.

SYMPTOMS: Gum disease can be insidious because there is usually no pain, but there are readily observable symptoms. In gingivitis, the gums become red, swollen, and perhaps tender, and they bleed easily, especially during brushing. With periodontitis, the gums tend to recede and detach themselves slightly from the teeth; the formation of pus in the resulting infected pockets also contributes to bad breath.

CAUSES: The direct cause of the inflammation and infection is the deposit of a bacterial film called plaque in parts of the mouth that are not easily cleaned, especially between the teeth and along the edges of the gums. Plaque is normal in the mouth and is harmless if it is not allowed to accumulate in one place. When it does, the toxic products and enzymes produced by its bacteria irritate and inflame the surrounding tissues, causing gingivitis. With time, the plaque can mineralize into tartar, which becomes a hard crust that causes further irritation. Without treatment and good oral hygiene, this accumulation of plaque and tartar progresses unchecked to become advanced periodontitis.

Inadequate dental hygiene is obviously an important contributing cause of gum disease and loss of teeth. Other contributing factors include habitual clenching or grinding of the teeth, diabetes, thyroid disease, smoking, oral contraceptives and some other drugs, vitamin deficiency, and stress. Temporary gum inflammation also tends to occur during puberty and pregnancy, suggesting that hormonal changes also play a role. Finally, a very basic problem is the modern Western diet. Many people in underdeveloped countries who eat natural, unprocessed foods have no gum problems, even though they never see a dentist. But when typical Western diets with sugar and refined foods are introduced into these societies, tooth and gum diseases follow.

TREATMENT: Home treatment and oral hygiene cannot substitute for regular professional dental care; both are
essential. Depending on the condition of your teeth and
gums, you should have a professional dental checkup and
cleaning at least twice a year, or even more often for acute
problems. Try to find a dentist who is oriented toward nutritional and natural treatments.

To prevent gingivitis and periodontitis:

1. Eat a natural-food diet and rinse your mouth
   with water after every meal.
2. Brush thoroughly and use dental floss regularly;
   be sure to clean along and under the gum line.
   For brushing, try a natural toothpaste or powder
   that contains charcoal, baking soda, anise, myrrh,
   and goldenseal. An oral-irrigation device (for
   example, a Water Pik) will help remove food
   lodged between the teeth but will not remove
   plaque.
3. Use a toothpick (a piece of white-oak bark will
   do nicely) for about five minutes a day to scrape
   along the gum line and between the teeth. In
   addition to removing plaque, this helps toughen
   the gums so that they form a better barrier
   against infection.

To treat gingivitis and periodontitis:

1. Make up a tooth powder of witch hazel, white-
   oak bark, yellow dock, bayberry, goldenseal, and
   myrrh by grinding and sifting the dried herbs
   together. Brush two to three times a day and
   rinse often with water containing the mixture.

2. A solution of one teaspoon apple cider vinegar in a glass of water can be used as a mouthwash and also for brushing the teeth. It also helps to prevent and remove plaque and tartar and keep them from forming.

3. Washing the mouth with comfrey root tea four times a day will help heal the inflammation.

4. Take a therapeutic vitamin/mineral supplement daily. Minimize the intake of refined, highly processed foods, especially sugar.

5. A relatively new approach to treating gum disease is the Keyes technique, which combines nonsurgical professional treatment with home care based on simple antibacterial substances. In the home treatment, a paste made by mixing one-half capful standard 3 percent hydrogen peroxide with one tablespoon baking soda is worked into the spaces between the teeth and gums to destroy the plaque bacteria hidden there. This is followed by saltwater irrigation with a dental irrigator. Although you can't hope to treat gum disease effectively without professional help, it may be helpful to use the Keyes paste in place of regular toothpaste. For an integrated program, try to find a dentist or dental hygienist who has been trained in the Keyes technique.

Use anti-inflammatory or blood-purifying herbs such as formulas 14 and/or 15. A tincture of the following is a good alterative combination: 1 ounce echinacea, 1 ounce blue flag, 1 ounce burdock root, 1 ounce Oregon grape root, ½ ounce American mandrake root, 2 teaspoons licorice root. Dose: Take one-half to one teaspoon in hot water before meals three times daily; for children, less, according to age.

In addition, apply witch hazel extract each morning and oil of eucalyptus each evening directly to the gums.

From the Japanese tradition, the burnt calyx of the pomegranate is powdered and the ash is used to brush the teeth and gums.

GYNECOLOGICAL PROBLEMS

OTHER NAMES: Irregular menstruation, premenstrual syndrome (PMS), infertility, leucorrhea (vaginal discharge), trichomoniasis, and menopause.

IRREGULAR MENSTRUATION: There are at least three general types, including dysmenorrhea, or painful menstruation; amenorrhea, or stopped menses; and menorrhagia, or excessive bleeding or flooding during menstruation. In addition, one needs to differentiate between those conditions that are caused by excess and those that are caused by deficiency. Finally, there is the general disease called premenstrual tension (PMT or PMS), which can cause physiological symptoms along with irritability, moodiness, and other emotional imbalances.

The normal menstrual cycles should occur about every thirty days. A twenty-eight- or thirty-six-day cycle is still within the normal range, however. If the cycle is too short, it occurs in only two to three weeks; if too long, over forty days. If there is no illness or marked discomfort during either a short or long cycle, it is still regarded as normal. Irregularities are common during puberty, lactation, or menopause.

Herbal treatment for short or frequent menstruation includes the use of a teaspoon of fresh shepherd's purse extract three times daily. Other herbs that can be used effectively instead of or together with the shepherd's purse include lady's mantle *(Alchemilla vulgaris)*, oak bark *(Quercus alba)*, witch hazel bark *(Hamamelis virginiana)*, raspberry leaf tea *(Rubus idaeus)*, or wild geranium *(Geranium maculatam)*. These all possess gentle hemostatic properties. One can make a tea by combining three or four together with a small amount of ginger and cramp bark *(Viburnum opulis)* in a formula. Another way is to combine the herbs and powder them in a coffee mill and take two 00-size capsules three times daily with shepherd's tincture and raspberry leaf tea. Planetary formulas number 85 (Women's Dong Quai Treasure) or 56 (MenoChange) should be taken along with formula number 10 (Bupleurum Calmative).

Chinese tienchi ginseng *(Panax pseudoginseng)* can be taken in a dose of 3 to 6 g three times a day to regulate bleeding. Another patented Chinese formula specific for all bleeding and injuries is called yunnan baiyao; it can be used both for acute bleeding or to regulate and prevent flooding. As a tonic for anemia, take formula number 6; Chinese medicine also uses black donkey skin hide gelatin (ai yao) with dong quai. This syrup is also available from Chinese pharmacies and is called Dang Quai Gin. There are two varieties, one with a sugar-based syrup and the other without sugar.

Painful menstruation or dysmenorrhea is caused by clots or obstructed menstrual flow. It is always good to try to understand the reason why one is experiencing irregular menstruation. However, in general, one should begin treatment with herbs and less invasive methods. If the condition is not resolved, then one should seek professional assistance.

Women who are underweight, recovering from a prolonged debilitating illness, or are highly athletic may have insufficient menstrual flow, and for these one should treat the underlying cause by increasing proteinaceous food intake. In addition a soup made with one whole chicken, 6 grams of dong quai cooked with brown rice, sautéed onions, and fresh ginger should be taken daily. They should also take formula 85 or 84, (Women's Dong Quai Tonifier or Eight Precious Herbs).

For any menstrual irregularities, one should at least follow a strict herbal program for three months. When the period is more regular, the herbs should be taken one week before the period is due.

PREMENSTRUAL SYNDROME (PMS) OR PREMENSTRUAL TENSION (PMT): For this one should take a combination of vitex (Agnus cactus) alone or together with formula number 10 (Bupleurum Calmative Compound).

Vitex is one of the most important gynecological herbs. It is the fruit of a tree that is commonly found in North America and used as an ornamental. It is especially effective for relieving PMS symptoms and similar symptoms accompanying menopause. It has unique pituitary-stimulating compounds that increase progesterone and help stimulate the sloughing off of the corpus luteum associated with normal menstruation.

Planetary's formula number 10 (Bupleurum Calmative) is based on the classic Chinese formula called Xiao Yao Wan, which means the "free and easy wanderer." It contains bupleurum root, which relieves liver stagnation;

dong quai root, which promotes blood circulation; atractylodes root, which assists digestion and tonifies qi; poria mushroom, which relieves edema; licorice root, which harmonizes; and Chinese mint, which is an antidepressant. The combination is an ancient formula that is specific for symptoms of liver qi stagnation, which gives rise to symptoms of moodiness and depression. It is the most revered herbal formula known for this condition. It is specific for PMS, all kinds of irregular menstruation, and for menopause.

Short or frequent menstruation can be caused by inflammation, tipped uterus, uterine swelling, and abnormal ovarian function. It may be accompanied by hypertension, heart disease, pains in the kidneys, and constipation. Excessive bleeding as a result of short or frequent menstruation can lead to anemia and low energy. As a result, there will also be increased emotional instability.

INFERTILITY. After ruling out any mechanical physical reason(s) that may require medical intervention, many herbs and formulas are known traditionally to be effective for infertility. These include Chinese dong guai, known to increase blood circulation and treat female infertility. The Planetary formula that has been known to be effective for infertility is formula number 85 (Dong Quai Women's Treasure). Male infertility is also a factor that should be considered, such as insufficient sperm count and/or decreased sperm motility. The traditional Planetary formula specific for this condition is formula number 73 (Schizandra Adrenal Complex).

Shatavari *(Asparagus racemosus)* is not the common garden variety asparagus but is more closely related to ornamental asparagus. In Indian Ayurvedic medicine the root is highly esteemed as a female tonic. One to 12 ounces of the finely powdered herb is mixed with clarified butter, honey, and raw sugar together with an eighth of an ounce each of black pepper, ginger, and anise seed to form a paste. A tablespoon of this paste is mixed with a cup of boiled warm milk and taken twice daily. Besides its value in toning and strengthening the female reproductive system, shatavari is specific for female infertility and to increase semen count for men. Shatavari is one of the most effective herbs for women. It is available from Planetary Formulas both alone and in a special complex formulation, which is generally more effective.

LEUCORRHEA: The vagina is a naturally moist environment. Since, like the lungs and bronchioles, it is a mucous membrane, it can develop excess mucus discharge for many of the same reasons. Overeating of refined foods, white sugar, saturated fats, and dairy, as well as stress, can cause an increase in these secretions, inviting the proliferation of various purulent microorganisms. It is normal for a woman to have an increase in vaginal discharge two or three days before or after her menstrual cycle. It is also normal for a pregnant woman to have an increase in vaginal discharge so long as it is thin, white, and colorless. Vaginal discharge during menopause, however, should be evaluated medically for possible carcinoma. In leucorrhea, there is usually a milky, yellowish discharge—sometimes with blood. If it is caused by cancer or abortion it tends to be more odorous and should be diagnosed professionally.

In general, detoxifying herbs for the liver are used, such as Oregon grape, barberry root *(Berberis* species), or yellow dock root *(Rumex crispus),* which helps the liver in its process of detoxification. In addition, drying, astringent herbs such as raspberry leaves *(Rubus idaeus)*, white oak bark *(Quercus alba)*, or wild geranium *(Geranium maculatum)* should be added to the formula. A combination might be a combination of the following:

6 parts Oregon grape root
6 parts yellow dock root
3 parts oak bark
3 parts red raspberry leaves
12 parts lobelia inflata herb
12 parts ginger root

Purchase or collect these herbs fresh. Mix and combine together. Bring three cups of water to a rolling boil. Mix in about one and a half handfuls of the premixed combination. Turn the flame down and continue simmering for another twenty minutes, covered. Allow to cool and strain. Take one cup three times daily, sweetened or unsweetened as preferred. The tea should also be used as an injection once or twice a day. Purchase a bulb syringe from the pharmacy. Lay on a board or mat, head downward. Inject about one cup or so of the lukewarm tea into the vagina and retain for 10 to 20 minutes as time permits.

Planetary formula number 99 (Yellow Dock Skin Cleanse), while described as being for the skin, is very effective for all genitourinary tract infections. Two to four tablets should be taken three times daily.

Leucorrhea can be treated effectively with diet and herbs. The diet should be the balanced macrodiet. For many, following an exclusive diet of kicharee (mung beans and rice), Japanese azuki beans, or black beans and rice, or any combination of whole grains and legumes, for seven to ten days will balance the pH of the blood and lymphatic system and can clear up many forms of leucorrhea.

HEADACHE

OTHER NAMES: Cephalalgia, migraine, sinus headache, tension headache.

DESCRIPTION: Any ache or pain in the head is called a headache. Like most pain, headache itself is not the real problem; rather, it is a symptom that something else is wrong in the body. The occasional headache that almost everyone has is not a cause for alarm. The ones to worry about are those that recur frequently or last for several days, those associated with other neurological symptoms (for example, visual problems or mental confusion), those that come on very suddenly and with severe pain, and those that are associated with fever and stiffness of the neck.

A migraine is a specific type of severe headache caused by alternating dilation and constriction of the blood vessels on the surface of the brain. Another name for migraine headaches is *hemicrania,* which reflects the fact that they usually affect one side of the head. Sinus headaches are associated with infection in the sinuses found in the forehead, cheekbones, or nasal area. Tension headaches, the most common type, are due to abnormal muscle contraction in the head and neck, usually as a result of tension and stress.

SYMPTOMS: Migraine headaches usually involve a throbbing pain in one side of the head. Often they are preceded by flashes or zigzags of light in the eyes or by sensory distortions. The pain, which may last for several days, is usually severe and may be accompanied by vision problems, nausea and vomiting, sweating, chills and fever, diarrhea, dizziness, and sensitivity to light and loud noises.

Tension and sinus headaches generally are a dull, steady pain centered anywhere in the head or neck; sometimes they feel like a tight band across the forehead. Moving the head may make the pain worse or may shift its apparent location, especially in sinus headaches.

CAUSES: What actually causes the changes in the blood vessels that produce migraines is not known. In susceptible people, a wide variety of factors will trigger this psychological response, including emotional stress, hormonal changes, chemicals or additives used in foods, specific types of foods, caffeine, drugs, cigarette smoke, alcohol, strong odors, strong light, air pollution, and even sudden changes in the weather.

Tension headaches are generally associated with tightening of the head and neck muscles due to emotional stress. Physical stress, such as eyestrain, problems with the jaw or teeth, or spinal problems can have the same effect. Sinus headaches are complications of pressure due to congestion and swelling of the mucous membranes in the nasal sinuses when you have a cold or hay fever. Finally, a headache can be a symptom associated with many other ailments, ranging from constipation to brain tumors. In all cases the first priority is to treat the condition.

TREATMENT: The underlying cause of a headache should be identified and treated. Chronic headaches, especially those that don't respond to the following treatments and are getting worse or more frequent, should be evaluated by your physician. As general dietary measures, avoid the foods and substances listed above if they trigger headaches in you. Spinach and feverfew leaves have been recommended as particularly useful for chronic migraine sufferers. The formula called HeadAid, based upon a traditional Chinese formula, is useful for many types of headaches.

The following treatments are aimed at alleviating the pain of the headache itself.

Enemas or colonic irrigations will often relieve headache pain and help begin treatment of the cause at the same time.

Place cold compresses on the forehead and the nape of the neck, either alternating or at the same time. These are especially helpful for migraine. Cold clay packs can be used instead, but these should alternate. If you feel faint or light-headed when using clay packs, stop using them and cleanse the system with enemas and colonics.

Lie down and rest in a dark, quiet room where you can relax. For tension headaches, use muscle-relaxation techniques. Gentle massage of the painful areas also helps; don't forget the neck and shoulders.

Light exercise and fresh air can also help relieve tension and improve circulation.

A mustard plaster placed on the abdomen for a few minutes at the very beginning of a migraine will often stop it. A mustard footbath, a hot-water bottle on the feet, or a hot sitz bath can also be used to draw blood away from the head. Putting your hands in hot water helps, too. The key is to not wait until the symptoms are severe.

Placing oil of rosemary, sage, lavender, or thyme on the forehead can help relieve a congestion headache.

The following herbal teas have been recommended for headache: valerian, passion flower, chamomile, lemon balm, basil, ginger, sweet marjoram, parsley, willow bark, peppermint, rosemary, sage, bergamot, betony, marigold, St. Benedict thistle, and thyme. The following are specifically for migraine: balm, buck bean, meadowsweet, nettle, fragrant valerian, lavender, peppermint, primrose, speedwell, woodruff, and yerba maté.

The cervical vertebrae (those in the neck) may need to be adjusted by a trained naturopath or chiropractor.

Zone therapy. Press a spoon or your thumb against the roof of your mouth as hard as you can for three to five minutes. Try to center the pressure under the location of the headache. Pressure on more than one area may be necessary.

Acupressure. Pressure points that can be used for headache include: the center of the mound formed when the thumb is held against the index finger; the bottom of the cheekbone, directly under the midline of the eye; directly above the inner corner of the eye, against the bone that forms the top of the orbit of the eye; at the base of the head, about an inch on either side of the midline, there is a depression: Press upward. All the points along the midline of the skull and about one and a half inches to either side of it are good pressure points for headaches.

Remember: if there is no pain when you are pressing on a point, you are not pressing in the right place.

Meditation, yoga, biofeedback, and autogenic training may be useful in helping you gain control over difficult headache problems. There are numerous sources of information and professional help for these methods.

In general, avoid using aspirin, acetaminophen, ergotamine, or other over-the-counter drugs to relieve headaches. It is always best to try to understand the cause of a headache. Chronic headaches may necessitate medical evaluation to rule out any underlying serious cause.

Migraine Headaches

Migraine headaches are classified as vascular headaches because they seem to occur when the arteries in the brain constrict and then suddenly relax. Usually they are one-sided headaches, tend to last an entire day, and, depending on their severity, can be accompanied by symptoms of nausea and a characteristic vision distortion that often precedes the headache, where one may see an aura around objects, flashes of light, tunnel vision, and/or blind spots. For some unknown reason, migraines are generally at least 50 percent more prevalent in women than men.

There are a number of foods that are known to trigger migraines. These include ripened cheese (cheddar, Brie, Camembert, blue cheese, etc.), onions, pickles, cured meats, avocados, fresh bread, red wine, sour cream, nuts, chocolate, coffee, tea, cola, and alcohol. Eliminating these from the diet will lessen the recurrence and severity of migraines significantly.

An interesting and extremely simple treatment for migraine headaches is the use of dry, powdered ginger (*Zingiber officinalis*). About 500 to 600 mg of powdered ginger should be taken at the first sign of a migraine coming on. Mercifully, many sufferers have reported that pain often subsides over the next half hour. Ginger, either dry or fresh, can be taken both for the treatment of migraines as well as to help prevent them. It seems that even cooked or candied ginger is effective for preventing and treating migraines.

Because of its ability to increase blood circulation to the brain, French researchers have found that ginkgo (*Ginkgo biloba*) leaf extract is about 80 percent effective in preventing and relieving migraines, cluster headaches, and even hangovers.

It may take a little doing to put it together, but one of the best herbal treatments Michael uses for headaches is a combination of a number of herbs, most of which contain various salicylic compounds. Mix in equal parts, either a tincture or a powder, of the following dried herbs: willow bark, white poplar bark, rosemary, chamomile, angelica root, feverfew, and chrysanthemum flowers. About 6 g, or a teaspoon, of the extract should be taken every fifteen minutes, tapering off as symptoms subside.

Planetary formula number 32 (Feverfew Head Aid) contains willow bark extract, feverfew leaf extract, schizonepeta leaf and stem, notopterygium root, green tea leaf, licorice, ligusticum rhizome, angelica root, ledebouriella, cyperus, and ginger. It has proven itself to be highly effective for many who suffer from either acute or chronic headaches.

Another useful Planetary formula for various pains, including headaches, is number 96 (Willow Aid). This consists of a formula of willow bark extract, corydalis, dong quai root, valerian root, guggul, and boswellia gum resin.

HOMEOPATHIC:

- *Natrum Muriaticum*. If there is numbness and tingling in the lips and tongue before a migraine, take a dose of 6C every fifteen minutes until symptoms are relieved, or up to ten doses.
- *Pulsatilla*. Migraines are associated with mood swings, a tendency to cry easily, relief from pressure, relief from gentle exercise. Take a dose of 6C every fifteen minutes for a maximum of ten doses.
- *Sanguinaria*. If headaches began or worsen with menopause, if they are worse at midday, or worsen with head pressure or when urinating, take every fifteen minutes for a maximum of ten doses.

HEATSTROKE

OTHER NAMES: Heat hyperpyrexia, sunstroke, thermic fever.

DESCRIPTION: Heatstroke is a severe disturbance of the functioning of the body's heat-regulating mechanism and is a profound emergency. It is seen most often in alcoholic males over forty (but may occur at any age) and in debilitated or fatigued persons who have had too much exposure to the sun or too high temperatures.

SYMPTOMS: The onset of heatstroke, which may be sudden or gradual, is marked by weakness, headache, dizziness, nausea, loss of appetite, spots before the eyes, and ringing in the ears. The skin becomes hot, dry, and flushed; the body temperature may rise to 108°F or even higher. Other symptoms include listlessness, staggering, seizures, cramps, anxiety, a dry mouth, excessive thirst, fast but strong pulse, difficulty in breathing, and collapse or unconsciousness.

CAUSES: Normally, exposure to excessive heat causes the body to sweat as a way to cool itself off. If the temperature-regulating mechanism fails, the body temperature rises precipitously, reaching 108° or higher within one to ten minutes. If the increase is not reversed immediately, the body cells—especially the very vulnerable cells of the brain—begin literally to cook and irreversible damage occurs.

TREATMENT: Heatstroke is an emergency, so call for an ambulance. Until help arrives, move the person to a cool environment, remove as much clothing as possible, keep the head elevated, and *cool the person off as quickly as possible by any means available.* A cold full bath (see "The Bath" in Part Three) is excellent, or use a cold shower or a garden hose. A very effective method is to cover the person with wet sheets on which a fan blows; other techniques are continuous washing with rubbing alcohol and application of cold packs. Speed is of the essence. Vigorous efforts to cool the person down should continue until the body temperature is below 102°.

If you find yourself becoming dizzy from excessive exposure to the sun or from being in a hot room, immediately get out of the heat and cool yourself off. Don't let yourself become drowsy and think that everything will be all right if you go to sleep.

To prevent heatstroke, dress appropriately for your environment and stay in well-ventilated spaces, especially during a heat wave. If you are elderly and your home is too hot, leave and either stay with someone who has a cool environment or seek shelter from local authorities.

There are many diseases that are caused by overexposure to the sun and heat. Cooling foods such as melons and cucumbers should be eaten in moderation during the peak season. Green mung beans are also very good as they provide a complete protein as well as help remove excess acidity and cleanse the blood. Coriander and a small amount of yogurt is excellent to take during the midday heat. Coriander, specifically, is used to help digestion and yet counteract some of the strong heating effects of some foods and spices.

Specific teas effective for heatstroke include gotu kola *(Hydrocotyl asiatica)* and/or hibiscus *(Hibiscus sabdariffa)* tea. The popular hibiscus tea originates from Sudan, where it is widely used as a cooling and detoxifying blood purifier for a wide range of diseases. It has become a popular beverage in the West but unfortunately is seldom used for its medicinal properties.

Planetary formula number 23 (Digestive Comfort), popularly sold as a Chinese patent called "Pill Curing," is commonly used for a wide variety of gastrointestinal conditions as well as heatstroke. Unlike the Chinese patent, Planetary's Digestive Comfort does not contain the heavy metal mercuric oxide.

HEMORRHOIDS

OTHER NAMES: Piles, varicosities.

DESCRIPTION: Hemorrhoids are protrusions caused by distension of the veins in the anal region. They can occur both inside and outside the anal orifice.

SYMPTOMS: The main symptom is rectal bleeding varying from slight reddening on the toilet paper through blood in the stools to dripping bright red blood into the toilet after defecating. Various degrees of itching, burning, and pain may also be felt, more so with external than with internal hemorrhoids (unless the internal hemorrhoids are pushed out through the anus during defecation). There may also be a feeling of fullness in the anus. Sometimes blood clots that form in external hemorrhoids can cause pain for a few days; they are usually absorbed naturally, leaving behind skin tags or flaps.

CAUSES: The basic cause of hemorrhoids is the exertion of unusual pressure on the rectal and abdominal vein system. Chronic constipation resulting from poor dietary habits is the most common culprit; straining to defecate, overuse of laxatives, obesity, liver problems (including those due to excessive alcohol consumption), lack of exercise, pregnancy, abdominal tumors, coughing, and sneezing all cause increased pressure in these veins.

TREATMENT: The first thing to attend to is bowel regularity. Treatment of hemorrhoids should always include the use of Planetary formula 89 (Triphala) and/or number 87 (Tri-Cleanse) as a foundation.

Next, one would use formulas such as Planetary formula numbers 47 and 46 (Horsechestnut Vein Strength and Horsechestnut Cream). Horsechestnut *(Aesculus hippocastanum)* is one of the most popular and effective herbs for all types of varicosities, including hemorrhoids. It is astringent and anti-exudative, anti-edematous, anti-inflammatory, and antispasmodic and it decreases capillary permeability. One of the active constituents is aescin, which will decrease capillary permeability and stimulate the production and release of prostaglandins, which induces venous contraction. It is specific for hemorrhoids caused by portal vein obstruction accompanied by shooting pains up the back. It should not be used by pregnant women. It is safe, however, when taken for a short term or in formula with other herbs. It is also very safe and effective when applied topically in the form of a horsechestnut cream.

For direct treatment, cold sitz baths (two minutes, twice daily) or warm sitz baths using chamomile or hay flower tea also will provide much welcome relief.

HEPATITIS

DESCRIPTION: Hepatitis is an inflammation of the liver. Broadly speaking there are two types of hepatitis: infectious and serum. While there seems to be many different subtypes of the various forms of hepatitis, the ones that will be included in our present discussion include hepatitis A, which is infectious; hepatitis B, which is serum; and hepatitis C, also serum. In general, from an herbalist's perspective, all forms of hepatitis are treated similarly, with the exception that with chronic hepatitis B, C, and D, one would be sure to include a protocol for immune support along with the standard antipathogenic program.

SYMPTOMS: Infectious hepatitis A is mostly spread person-to-person by the fecal-oral route (poor hygiene and food handling) but also may occur from food and water contamination. It is most common in unhygienic environments. Prevention through careful hygienic measures under such circumstances is important.

Hepatitis B and C is transmitted by intravenous drug use, manicure tools, razors, toothbrushes, tattooing, and body piercing as well as through sex. The sexual transmission of hepatitis is at best rare and is predicated on the possibility of blood-to-blood contact. There is a gradual degeneration of liver function over many months and years. People rarely present symptoms early on, so many have no idea how they were infected. Some 85 percent are chronic and become silent carriers. Within approximately twenty years about 20 percent of the chronically infected people show symptoms of cirrhosis and liver scarring and a smaller percentage develop liver cancer. There is no vaccine for HCV. HCV complications are said to cause as many as 800 to 10,000 deaths annually.

DIAGNOSIS: Acute infectious hepatitis has an incubation period of approximately fifteen to fifty days and is diagnosed by history, clinical symptoms, and liver enzyme and other tests as necessary. Symptoms are variable but include low-grade fever, anorexia, nausea, vomiting, headache, photophobia, pharyngitis, cough, and coryza (colds), all together similar to influenza. These will last from two to fourteen days, and there will be pain over the liver side (lower right rib cage) and possibly the left spleen side as well, and jaundice, yellowing of the eyes, dark urine, and light, clay-colored stool. The convalescent period may be protracted, over a period of a few months, with a general feeling of low energy and easy fatigue. Herbs will make a tremendous difference in both the treatment and convalescent phases of recovery for this disease.

The onset of symptoms of chronic hepatitis, including HPB, HPC, and HPD, is variable and slower, ranging from a few months to years. Because the herbal treatment of all forms of hepatitis is similar, and with HCV being the most common of all the serious contagious diseases—infecting around four million Americans—we will focus our discussion on the wonderful benefits that herbs and natural healing have to offer for this condition.

Hepatitis C was first discovered in 1989 and used to be called non-A, non-B hepatitis. At present there are two primary blood tests for hepatitis C: ELISA and RIBA assays. These detect and measure the presence of antibodies to measure hepatitis C.

ELISA assays admit a percentage of false positive readings in about one-third of the cases, while RIBA more specifically measures HCV antibodies. It determines which antigens your body is reacting to. If you react only to superoxide dismutase and not against hep C antigens, you don't have hepatitis C. If you react against two or more HCV antigens, you do have hep C. If you react against only one, you may or may not have HCV.

It is important to understand that neither of the above

tests indicates active chronic hepatitis; they measure antibody response to HCV, not the virus itself. Therefore, positive tests of any of the above can mean:

1. You have an ongoing HCV infection.
2. You've only been exposed to HCV.
3. As an infant you received an antibody to HCV from your mother.

Any positive antibody test of the above should be followed with a more definitive viral load test or RNA quantitative test. Different labs have different levels of sensitivity. A viral load of one million is borderline high. These tests can be variable episodically with different readings at different times.

Following positive tests for the above, one may go for one or a number of the following tests, depending on clinical health status:

CT scan of the liver
ultrasound of the liver
liver biopsy

A liver biopsy is the most definitive test and can rule out various serious liver diseases such as cirrhosis, infections, biliary tract disorders, liver cancers, or lymphoma. It also determines the stage or degree of HCV in the body. HCV can pass from the chronic state to the active inflammatory stage to fibrosis, and later, cirrhosis. Today, liver biopsies are an outpatient procedure requiring seconds to perform and are often done in a doctor's office. They allow mapping over years to record the progression of the disease.

After the diagnosis, one assesses the condition of the liver with hepatic function tests. These measure:

1. liver enzymes
2. bilirubin
3. albumin
4. clotting factors
5. complete blood count.

Liver Enzymes

The liver produces proteins called enzymes that exist within the cells of its membranes. These have the ability to break down raw materials introduced into the body into substances the body needs. The major enzymes measured are:

ALT (SGPT)
AST (SGOT)
GGT: gamma–glutamyl transferase
Alkaline phosphatase

When the liver is functioning normally, the concentrations of these enzymes are relatively low. When liver cells are injured, destroyed, or die, the cells become leaky and the enzymes escape into the blood that's passing through the liver. Therefore, these enzymes are highly reflective of compromised liver function.

Typically, with massive liver injury there is a marked increase in ALT. This especially happens in the earlier stages of hep C before cirrhosis. After cirrhosis, ALT may not be high, so ALT no longer is a good indicator of further liver damage.

Hep C patients show increases in ALT and AST but little in GGT and alkaline phosphatase. Patients with hep C tend to focus on ALT and AST counts, but other tests can be more important in measuring a healthy liver.

Bilirubin

When red blood cells complete their life cycle they break down in the body, producing a yellow pigment that is passed to the liver and excreted into bile. Bile, in turn, plays an important role in digestion.

Hep C patients tend to have fluctuating levels of bilirubin in their blood. When the bilirubin levels remain high, it means the liver disease is severe, with possible cirrhosis. When the liver fails to eliminate bilirubin from the blood, the skin and whites of the eyes turn yellow, the urine darkens, and the color of the stools turns lighter.

Albumin

Albumin is another protein synthesized by the liver and used to maintain the volume of blood in the arteries and veins. When albumin drops to low levels, fluid leaks out of the blood vessels into surrounding tissues. This causes swelling and edema. Unlike liver enzymes, albumin doesn't drop until hep is at a more advanced stage. This is usually when one considers a liver transplant as an option. Nevertheless, a significant decrease in albumin can be indicative of poor liver function.

Clotting Factors

The liver also produces proteins that maintain normal blood clotting. Prothrombin time (PT) is the most common test for measuring the combination of blood-clotting factors. If PT increases, it means the liver is not creating enough clotting factors. Unlike albumin, clotting factors can decrease rapidly, within days or even hours as a result of a severe liver injury. In hepatitis a patient's prolonged clotting time can be an indication of compromised liver function.

Complete Blood Count

A complete blood test can be indicative of advanced liver malfunction. If there is liver scarring, the blood flowing from the spleen to the liver through the portal vein is impaired, causing portal hypertension so that the blood backs up into the spleen. When this happens the spleen enlarges and traps blood elements with a lowering of blood counts, including white and red blood cell count.

In general, individuals with chronic hepatitis (or cirrhosis) should undergo a liver enzyme and blood test every three months until the condition seems more stabilized. The more costly viral load test need only be undertaken yearly.

TREATMENT: In addition to dandelion root tea, Michael would give two tablets three times daily of formula number 11 (Bupleurum Liver Cleanse) and number 75 (Shiitake Mushroom Supreme). Michael also recommends a good general multivitamin formula such as Source Natural's or Rainbow Light's complete nutritional formula, zinc, selenium, and the antioxidants alpha lipoic acid and n-acetyl cysteine, 600 mg of each daily.

During the acute phase of infectious hepatitis, nourishing, easily assimilated chicken broths should be taken with plenty of carrots, onions, and green vegetables. For recovery from chronic hepatitis, one cannot consume too much green in the form of steamed leafy vegetables. Carrots, beets, and celery are also very good. Michael recommends one or two glasses of fresh-juiced organic carrots, beets, and celery daily. Shiitake mushrooms have been shown to have powerfully positive effects on the immune system and on the liver particularly, so that the daily intake of shiitake mushrooms as part of one's diet also would be very beneficial. Finally, the intake of supplemental milk thistle (*Silybum marianum*), which is already in both of the above-mentioned Planetary formulas, is highly beneficial for its liver-protective virtues.

Clinically, Michael and his students have reported hundreds of cases of diagnosed hepatitis C patients whose liver enzymes have stabilized to normal, and a few cases where all other liver tests indicated a complete remission of the disease. Michael's conclusion is that herbs are the most perfect medicine for all chronic liver diseases as well as most renal diseases.

HERNIA

OTHER NAMES: Femoral, inguinal, or umbilical hernia; rupture.

DESCRIPTION: Although the term *hernia* applies to any protrusion of an organ outside the cavity that normally contains it, the usual meaning is an abnormal protrusion of intestines through an opening in the abdominal cavity.* The most vulnerable points are those where natural body structures pass through an internal channel or opening: the groin (inguinal hernia), the upper thigh (femoral hernia), and the navel (umbilical hernia). Hernias can also occur where a surgical incision has been made.*

---

*Hiatus hernia, which is not considered here, is the protrusion of the stomach upward into the chest cavity where the esophagus passes through the diaphragm. It may cause no symptoms at all, or it may cause heartburn and a flow of gastric acid up the esophagus and into the mouth (*see* GASTROINTESTINAL AILMENTS).

SYMPTOMS: Hernias produce a pear-shaped swelling through the abdominal wall that increases in size when the person stands, coughs, sneezes, cries, laughs, lifts heavy objects, or strains at the stool. Regardless of the site of the protrusion, the intestines feel doughy, often produce a colicky pain, and make gurgling sounds when returned to the abdominal cavity. In advanced stages, it may not be possible to return the protruding intestine into the abdominal cavity (irreducible hernia). In the most severe case, the opening is so constricted that blood flow to the protruding tissue is cut off (strangulated hernia), resulting in inflammation and then gangrene. Because a strangulated hernia can be fatal if undiagnosed and untreated, consult your physician if you discover a swelling in your groin, upper thigh, or umbilical area.

CAUSES: In some cases, hernias are present from birth because of imperfect development of the abdominal wall. Most hernias, though, occur later in life, usually as a result of physical strain or injury. The tissues and musculature in the susceptible areas of the abdominal wall may be weakened by failure to exercise, poor eating habits, injury, or poor circulation. A hernia then may result from strain due to constipation and straining at the stool, lifting heavy weights, poor posture, pregnancy, or obesity.

TREATMENT: If the hernia has progressed to the irreducible or especially the strangulated stage, surgery will be required. For less complicated hernias the following therapeutic alternatives to surgery can be used, but they should be undertaken under competent professional supervision.

The first order of business is to have your physician manipulate the protruding abdominal contents into their proper place. Then a truss is fitted and worn to keep them there. With these measures taken care of, home therapy can include:

1. Strengthening the abdominal muscles with daily exercise.
2. Slant board exercises with deep breathing to give your body a break from the pull of gravity.
3. Losing weight, if appropriate.
4. Local hydrotherapy with sitz baths (see Part Three).
5. Spinal and foot manipulation to improve posture and spinal alignment.
6. Local applications of white oak bark tea and vinegar fomentations to increase tissue tone.
7. Developing regular, nonstrenuous bowel habits (*see* CONSTIPATION).

Along with these measures, a natural food diet supplemented with vitamins A, B-complex, and C, and with zinc, magnesium, copper, and manganese, will be helpful.

Use the comfrey combination fomentation described in Chapter Two under Poultices, Fomentations, and Plasters.

HERPES

OTHER NAMES: Herpes simplex: cold sores, fever blisters, genital herpes. Herpes zoster: chicken pox, shingles.

DESCRIPTION: Herpes is a generic name for a group of viruses that cause a variety of diseases. The ailments people generally associate with herpes are those that produce small blisters on the skin, which open and are replaced by a crust before they heal completely. Cold sores and fever blisters (herpes simplex type 1) usually occur on and around the lips and around the eyes; genital herpes (herpes simplex type 2) usually occurs around the genital region, including the buttocks and the inner sides of the thighs. (Canker sores, which are small ulcers that form inside the mouth, are not a form of herpes infection.) Chicken pox and shingles are two manifestations of a single virus (herpes varicella-zoster), the former occurring in children and the latter in older people.

Nearly everyone has been infected by herpes in some form, but symptoms appear only when the virus becomes active. Most of the time it lies dormant, probably in the skin or in nearby nerve cells. The pattern of latency and activity depends on the specific virus and on the individual. Some people carry the virus and never have any symptoms. Others suffer occasional to regular eruptions of cold sores or genital herpes. Chicken pox and shingles usually occur only once.

On the whole, these forms of herpes are not dangerous. However, babies infected during birth by their mothers' active genital herpes are very likely to die or suffer severe brain damage because they have little or no resistance to the virus. Others whose immune response is impaired (such as cancer patients or organ transplant recipients) can be very susceptible to herpes infection. Herpes also has been associated with some forms of cancer, but the relationship is not yet clear.

SYMPTOMS: An eruption begins with a tingling or itching feeling, which is followed by blisters or sores. Because herpes blisters individually are the size of a pinhead or smaller, they may not be easily visible. Generally, the affected area will be red, tender, and mildly to severely painful. Fever, headache, and general malaise may also be present. The severity of the symptoms depends on age and on the site of the infection; also, the first attack is generally the most severe. In young children, symptoms usually are mild; from adolescence on they can be quite severe. Shingles, which erupts in a line on the skin following the course of a nerve (usually on one side of the body and most often on the chest), tends to be accompanied or followed by severe pain. The common types of herpes attacks are self-limiting: within a few weeks the symptoms disappear—at least temporarily—of their own accord.

CAUSES: The herpes virus seem to be inescapable; almost everyone has been infected by one or more of them, probably in childhood. Although some forms can be transmitted through the air or by contact with articles (especially towels) used by someone with active herpes, infection usually occurs through direct physical contact. For example, if the "sexual revolution" in the United States is indeed losing steam, the near epidemic levels of genital herpes in the country probably can take more credit (or blame) than all the admonitions of preachers.

What, then, makes some people more susceptible to outbreaks than others, and what triggers an outbreak? Both physical and mental health are key parts of the answer.

The normal defense of the body against disease can control, if not eliminate, the herpes viruses. If these defenses are weakened by illness, physical injury, fatigue, or psychological stress, herpes can erupt into an active infection. Cold sores often seem to appear under stressful conditions; and as simple an act as getting sunburned or irritating susceptible areas by shaving or rubbing can trigger an attack. Other precipitating factors include acid indigestion, fever, menstruation, toxic states, physical fatigue, emotional disturbance, and a weakened immune defense response.

TREATMENT: The best "treatment" for herpes is to control it by keeping up strong physical and mental defenses. A body kept healthy by proper nutrition and exercise has the best chance of keeping the virus under control. A positive mental attitude is also important to keep the stresses of modern life from weakening the body's resistance.

In treating an active herpes outbreak, the best approach is to work for symptomatic relief with herbal applications while strengthening the body's defense mechanisms with better nutrition and physiotherapy. In general, keep infected areas clean and dry; always dry them thoroughly after bathing or any wet treatment. Dust with calendula powder or corn starch. Specifically, one who has problems with herpes attacks should avoid hot, spicy foods, stimulating drinks such as coffee, and also alcohol and drugs (including marijuana).

Be careful to avoid spreading the infection to other parts of the body (or to others); for example, use disposable paper towels and clean the hands thoroughly after contact with the affected area. It's not necessary to become celibate to avoid spreading genital herpes, but sexual contact should be avoided during the virus's active stage.

A common European home remedy is to apply the mashed inner leaves of fresh white cabbage to the herpes sores. Baking soda compresses or zinc oxide salve can also be used, and an ointment based on lithium succinate is said to be effective in relieving herpes symptoms and healing the lesions.

To alleviate pain, use the capsaicin cream discussed below. Appropriate dietary items are raw vegetables and fruits, foods high in the amino acid L-lysine (particularly dairy foods), vitamins C and D, and B-complex vitamins, and the minerals calcium and phosphorus. Like lysine, grape juice and raw grapes have shown direct antiviral activity in laboratory tests, and they may be useful against herpes.

The following nutritional supplements are specifically suggested: vitamin C (with bioflavonoids), 1,000 mg twice daily; lysine, 1,000 mg twice daily; pantothenic acid, 200 mg per day; four to six 500 mg capsules daily of evening primrose oil from England. This oil has been demonstrated to have a direct effect on regeneration of the nerve sheath that insulates the nerve fibers.

For treatment beyond the immediate relief of active symptoms, one of the first requirements is adequate rest and relaxation: first, because of the already weakened and devitalized condition of the body; second, to build up sufficient vitality for the body to react properly to the application of natural remedies. The use of stress-reduction techniques, meditation, and relaxation exercises, in particular, should help to reduce the number of outbreaks induced by stress.

To cleanse the system, a two-day fruit juice fast is in order. Take orange or grapefruit juice every three hours; even better is to eat the whole fruit, which provides more bioflavonoids (in the white pulp and sections) as well as bulk and fiber to stimulate intestinal activity. At the same time, it is important to take a mild herbal laxative "surger" (an herbal tablet whose formula is designed to work interactively on the organs of digestion and elimination).

After two days of fasting, add fresh raw vegetables to

the diet in the form of salads. Include grated carrots and as many early spring greens as possible, such as leeks, beets, chives, dandelion, chervil, and watercress. All these plants are excellent sources of beta carotene (provitamin A), vitamin C, calcium, iron sodium, potassium, phosphorus, and sulfur. Also, drink two eight-ounce glasses of fresh carrot juice a day, midmorning and midafternoon.

The regular diet after fasting must be designed to maximize the body's own immune response capability. In addition to fresh vegetables, all fresh fruits are recommended. Avoid nuts, meat, white flour, white sugar, salt, hydrogenated (saturated) fats, coffee, tea (except herb teas), and alcohol.

For herpes zoster (shingles), red pepper applied topically as an ointment or cream will relieve the pain and even prevent outbreaks effectively. The active spicy constituent, capsaicin, has been shown clinically to be very effective for this painful condition. It is available in drugstores under the brand names of Zostrix or Capsaicin-P. Be sure to wash your hands thoroughly when using it, as it can be irritating to the eyes.

For herpes simplex and cold sores, the herb lemon balm *(Melissa officinalis)* applied topically as a tea or ointment has been found to be highly effective clinically. One can also make a strong tea by steeping four teaspoons in a cup of boiling water. Cover and allow to cool to room temperature. Use a cloth and moisten the affected area several times throughout the day. To make a simple lemon balm ointment, gently heat four parts by volume of olive oil. Into this sprinkle a considerable amount of powdered dry lemon balm leaves. Allow to cool to tolerance and strain through a cloth. Gently reheat the olive oil and add one part by volume of beeswax, allowing it to melt and mix with the oil. Pour into wide-mouthed salve jars.

Lemon balm ointment is available from Planetary Formulas or other sources.

Internally, for all forms of herpes one should take St. Johnswort *(Hypericum perforatum),* either in the form of a tea, a tincture, or a capsule. Planetary formula number 48 (Echinacea–Golden Seal with Olive Leaf) also should be taken as an antiviral internally.

HICCUPS

DESCRIPTION AND SYMPTOMS: Hiccups are an involuntary spasmodic contraction of the diaphragm that results in a sound while closing off the throat.

CAUSE: Hiccups can have many causes, such as indigestion, bad eating or drinking practices, drinking carbonated beverages, rapid temperature changes, overstretching of the neck, laryngitis, surgery, bloating, infection, diabetes, or anything that has caused an injury or irritation to the phrenic or vagus nerves in the brain. Most causes are transitory, but a few can be serious, such as a brain tumor or encephalitis.

TREATMENT: In most cases hiccups will stop quickly on their own, but there are cases where they may persist for days. Home remedies that override the spasmodic nerve relay will be effective. These may include:

- holding one's breath for as long as possible
- breathing into a paper bag
- swallowing a spoonful of sugar
- bending forward from the waist and drinking water from the wrong side of a glass
- yogurt with salt

This is from herbalist K. P. Khalsa: a small bowl of yogurt, highly salted, to taste—as salty as you can stand it. Consume normally in one sitting.

HOARSENESS AND LARYNGITIS

DESCRIPTION: Hoarseness is a strained or harsh quality in the voice. It may range in severity from a nearly normal voice with a rough edge to almost complete loss of ability to vocalize sound. Hoarseness is an inevitable part of laryngitis, which is the inflammation of the mucous membrane of the larynx, or voice box.

SYMPTOMS: Hoarseness is itself a symptom rather than an ailment. Especially when associated with laryngitis, it is often accompanied by tickling in the throat, a sore throat, a cough, pain when talking or swallowing, and mucus discharge.

CAUSES: Excessive physical strain on the vocal cords (from yelling, screaming, singing, or loud and long talking) can cause temporary hoarseness. Cysts, polyps, and cancer of the vocal cords can cause hoarseness by interfering with the cords' normal movement. Suppressive treatment for other conditions, especially fever, may cause hoarseness as a side effect. Chronic or acute laryngitis can result from breathing air filled with tobacco smoke, dust, or smog; from viral or a bacterial infection; and from exposure to cold and wet air.

TREATMENT: For nonsmokers, hoarseness that persists for longer than a month should be evaluated by a doctor. The main treatment for hoarseness and laryngitis is to rest the voice for a day or two by keeping quiet or, at most, whispering. It also helps to humidify the air around you and to use steam inhalations of menthol or eucalyptus (see

Part Three). Gargle with warm water and a small amount of orange juice, or with marshmallow, chamomile, comfrey, licorice, or ginger tea with honey. Drink liquids frequently. A light diet in general speeds recovery. Drinking hot yarrow tea will promote sweating and cleansing.

Warm lemon juice with fresh ginger juice and honey added to make a syrup is an excellent treatment for laryngitis. To make ginger juice, grate fresh ginger and squeeze the juice through a clean white cloth.

Moist clay poultices to the throat are helpful for laryngitis. Cold packs and warm compresses on the throat have also been recommended, as have hot footbaths.

HYPERACIDITY

OTHER NAMES: Hyperchlorhydria, sour stomach, and including symptoms of gastroesophageal reflux (GERD).

DESCRIPTION: Hyperacidity is the presence of more acid in the stomach than is necessary for the digestion of food. Every year, Americans spend over half a billion dollars for antacid products. These are bought without a prescription to treat hyperacidity, indigestion, the effects of excessive eating and drinking, and heartburn, as well as for long-term treatment of chronic peptic ulcers. Be wary: Most of these products carry a required warning not to use them for more than two weeks.

SYMPTOMS: Hyperacidity is usually characterized by discomfort over the pit of the stomach or by a burning sensation in the abdominal area, particularly when the stomach is empty. There may be a feeling of fullness due to gas, frequent belching or flatulence, bad breath, repeated eructation, and even occasional vomiting.

CAUSES: The most common causes of hyperacidity are stress and errors in diet and life-style. When these disturb the acid/alkali balance of the body by making it more acidic than normal (a condition called acidosis), the gastric secretions will contain more than the normal amount of acid. The symptoms, then, are often triggered when overindulgence in food or alcohol overstimulates gastric activity. Susceptibility varies with the individual, but alcohol, coffee, foods that are high in saturated fats (which are hard to digest), and tobacco are the most likely to break down the digestive system's natural protection against its own gastric juices.

TREATMENT: Prolonged use of modern antacids creates serious chronic conditions while suppressing the symptoms. Antacid products may be based on single ingredients or on combinations of ingredients: *Sodium bicarbonate*—Large doses or prolonged use may lead to sodium overload or systemic alkalosis. A mixture of sodium bicarbonate and aspirin after heavy alcohol intake may lead to vomiting of blood. *Calcium carbonate*—Side effects are constipation, neurological disturbance, kidney stones and decreased kidney function, and "acid rebound." *Aluminum hydroxide*—The most obvious side effect is constipation. Intestinal obstruction may even occur. Systemic aluminum toxicity has been discovered and related to disorders of the nervous system, such as Alzheimer's disease. *Magnesium hydroxide or Trisilicate*—The major side effect is diarrhea. Prolonged use may be related to kidney disease or kidney stones.

Needless to say, antacids are not the approved form of treatment for hyperacidity. Instead, keep a fresh lemon available. When your stomach bothers you, squeeze some juice into a little water and drink it. (Paradoxically, citrus fruits have a net alkaline effect because their citric acid is quickly broken down in the body, leaving alkaline salts behind.) The juice of raw, red potatoes is also said to be effective (one to one and a half cups a day, taken one-quarter cup at a time); chamomile tea is another remedy commonly recommended. A Kneipp remedy is to drink one to two glasses of water a day, with one drop of tincture of arnica per glass.

To be effective in the long run, treatment must focus on eating appropriate foods and managing of stress. Coffee (both regular and decaffeinated), cola drinks, alcohol, and nicotine must be avoided. In place of coffee and black tea, switch to peppermint, linden, or chamomile tea. Small and frequent meals will help minimize the symptoms as long as excess acid is still being produced. A "fruit day" once a week is recommended (see Chapter 3).

The safest way to neutralize excess acidity and build up your alkaline base reserve is through a diet that promotes and supports the natural alkalinity of the body. One of the benefits of a proper acid/alkali balance is that the body's natural immune system is strengthened. Dr. Alexis Carrel (1873–1944) demonstrated at the Rockefeller Institute that cancerous growths could be accelerated or inhibited by varying the degree of alkalinity of the blood through diet. Also, since your mental attitude plays an important role in the ways your body responds to stress, it is important to cultivate a more peaceful and tolerant attitude toward life's ups and downs and toward those around you.

The normal, healthy body is slightly alkaline, and a proper diet should also contain more alkali-forming than acid-forming foods. In the treatment of acidosis, it is appropriate to make the diet four parts alkali-forming foods to one part acid-forming foods.

Raw fruit and vegetable juices are very helpful in overcoming acute or chronic acidosis:

- Carrot juice is a rich vitamin and mineral source and an alkalizer.
- Celery juice is a mineral-rich alkalizer.
- Spinach juice is a rich mineral source; spinach is richer in protein than other leafy plants.
- Beet juice is a nerve tonic and alkalizer.
- Tomato juice helps eliminate uric acid and has antibiotic properties.

It is helpful to eat an apple when taking each of these juices.

Avoid the following foods, or use them sparingly:

- All meats, oily fish, eggs, cheese and cream, boiled or pasteurized milk, and melted butter
- All refined cereals, especially in highly processed forms such as bread, cakes, doughnuts, pastries, pancakes, and other synthetic and processed foods
- All stimulating beverages and condiments: green or black tea, coffee, cocoa and chocolate, beer, alcohol, mustard, pepper, and rich sauces

Chief among the alkalin-forming foods are fresh fruits and vegetables, including tomatoes as well as potatoes eaten with the skin. Fresh green leafy vegetables are particularly good. Certified raw milk, buttermilk, and herb teas also promote alkalinity.

Herbs that effectively neutralize acids include burdock root, dandelion root and chicory root, and violet leaves. The Japanese umeboshi plum, often found in many health and natural food stores, is excellent to use for occasional symptomatic relief. Chamomile tea taken after meals is also a very effective and simple remedy. This is because of the easily assimilated calcium in chamomile, which tends to neutralize excess stomach acids. Other herbs that are useful include alfalfa leaf, licorice root, and slippery elm bark tea.

It is important to address the underlying causes, which can be poor food combinations, eating too fast, and eating while under stress. In addition, one should restrict the usage of coffee, alcohol, sugar, and tobacco. Further, most refined and processed foods tend to cause acidity and should be restricted as necessary.

Two effective remedies are:

- A half teaspoon of baking soda dissolved in a cup of water ingested two or three times daily or as needed.
- An herbal powder consisting of a pinch of several common kitchen spices such as cardamom, cumin, coriander, fenugreek, ginger, and turmeric to make a teaspoon. Swallow this mixed in honey or in water. Probably one should exclude the use of cayenne and garlic in this combination to make it less spicy and more tolerable. Planetary formula number 24 (Digestive Grape Bitters) and/or number 23 (Digestive Comfort) would be useful for these conditions.

HYPOGLYCEMIA

OTHER NAME: Low blood sugar.

DESCRIPTION, SYMPTOMS, AND CAUSES: Excess intake of refined white sugar, hereditary factors, and stress can overstimulate the adrenals. This in turn signals a reaction from the pancreas to secrete insulin, which radically burns off the available blood sugar. Another factor is a chronic lack of protein, which can cause increased vulnerability to stress and a consequent lowering of blood sugar.

Hypoglycemia will give rise to strong cravings for food, especially sugar, headaches, cold hands and feet, heart palpitations, chronic fatigue, and nervousness and irritability.

TREATMENT: Because the most common cause of this condition is insufficient protein and carbohydrate intolerance one will find great relief by following a low-carbohydrate, high-protein, and vegetable diet at every meal. One can refer to the Atkins diet or the Zone diet for guidance for this extremely common condition. All fish, organic poultry, eggs, red meat, dairy, and soy can be used. Dairy in the form of milk should be taken scalded and warm, perhaps with a bit of honey and ginger to counteract its mucus-forming tendencies. Soy milk should only be used occasionally and for variety. It has a very cold energy and actually depresses metabolism. Soy in the form of tofu or tempeh is an excellent source of protein and has many health benefits, but these should be eaten no more than two or three times a week. Cheese is best taken baked and melted. In any case, these last foods should not be used as primary protein sources. All vegetables can be eaten, preferably steamed to make the nutrients more bioavailable. For every meal one should be conscious of having a first-class protein source about the size of the palm of one's hand and at least double or more of any number of a variety of vegetables. Whole grains such as brown rice are preferable to any flour products and should also be taken in small portions at each meal.

Morning is an important time to have the most balanced and nutritious meal of the day. To help get sufficient greens and other vegetables in the diet, a large amount can be steamed in the morning. Some of this can be eaten immediately, but the rest can be kept in a covered container and served cool. One of Michael's favorite ways to have such vegetables he learned from his southern Italian ancestry. It is to add a small amount of olive oil and seasoning. (Michael uses Bragg's Amino Acid seasoning, which has a salty flavor but is salt free. Of course it has no precedent in traditional southern Italian food preparation.) One can also add garlic, lemon juice, or balsamic vinegar. Prepared in this way, vegetables are available in a simple but delicious preparation for the entire day.

Chromium is a key constituent of the glucose tolerance factor. Without it blood glucose is elevated because insulin is blocked. Many believe that a chromium deficiency is at least partially responsible for the large numbers of cases of hypoglycemia, diabetes, and obesity in America. The recommended levels of chromium are achieved easily with a good multiple vitamin and mineral supplement with about 200 to 400 mg of chromium daily being critically important.

Herbs that may be useful include herbs for the liver such as bupleurum, dandelion root *(Taraxacum officinalis)* or Oregon grape root *(Berberis aquifolium),* ginseng *(Panax ginseng)* or its milder cousin, Chinese codonopsis *(Codonopsis pilosula),* skullcap *(Scutellaria lateraflora),* and ginger *(Zingiber officinalis).* These should be combined in a tea using an eighth part ginger.

Planetary formulas numbers 10, 38, and 84 would be useful, along with Triphala formula number 89.

INFECTIONS

DESCRIPTION: An infection occurs when the body as a whole or in part is invaded by a pathogenic agent such as a bacteria, virus, parasite, fungi, or rickettsia (microorganisms originating from arthropods such as lice, fleas, mosquitoes, or ticks). There are five classical symptoms, including pain, heat, redness, swelling, and disordered function.

CAUSES: Infective agents may be local or general. Depending on their type, they may be airborne, transmitted from animals, from direct contact with another who is infected, from food or drink, from another person who may not themselves suffer from symptoms, from insects, or from soil. In addition, fetuses can contract infection from the mother.

Prevention is always recommended. This is accomplished by isolation from the infective source, avoiding direct contact with individuals or clothing worn by another individual who has been infected, through hygiene, and through maintaining a strong immune system. Airborne bacteria, for instance, must enter through the eyes, nose, or mouth, so frequent washing of one's hands with a good antibacterial soap and scrupulously avoiding touching one's face until the hands are cleaned is very effective in preventing many airborne infections. Take appropriate precautions to avoid food, drink, clothing, or bedding that may carry infective pathogens.

TREATMENT: Most infections are potentially serious, so any nonmedical treatment should be undertaken if:

1. appropriate drugs are unavailable
2. the patient is unable to tolerate conventional drug treatment

3. the patient is not responding favorably to conventional drug treatment

Whenever possible one should seek out a qualified practitioner who has experience assessing the gravity of the situation or progress.

Having said this, if treated appropriately as described below, most common infections can be overcome successfully through natural forms of therapy. Nevertheless, time is of the essence. The longer pathogens are allowed to proliferate unimpeded, the more difficult they are to overcome. If they are acute or life-threatening in any way, Michael expects to see significant signs of improvement based upon the parameters described above within three days or the treatment approach should be changed, which may involve resorting to the use of conventional drugs.

One of the primary reasons for first turning to alternative remedies for the treatment of infections is because the frequent use of antibiotics, for instance, will cause the pathogens to develop resistance to them, so that in the event they are needed, the body will not respond sufficiently to overcome the infection. Another reason is because antibiotics are generally nonselective and will wipe out the favorable bacteria in the body and actually lower one's innate immunity. Still another reason is that viruses are not affected by antibiotics. Usually many of them, such as the cold or influenza viruses, are self-limiting, meaning they will run their course without any intervention. However, this is not always true and it is possible to develop bacterial complications from a primary viral infection so that the use of certain antibiotic and antiviral herbs as described below can be very beneficial, especially since they involve little risk of side effects when used in the ways described.

While there is a difference between the treatment of bacterial and viral infections in Western medicine, natural medicine hardly distinguishes between the two. The reason is that herbs work best when working with the body's innate defense systems rather than to kill or destroy anything. So if we were to use an herb as an "anti-" anything we would have to use so much more that it could produce undesirable side effects not unlike but hardly as bad as antibiotic drugs would.

Having said that, in treating an acute condition such as an infection one would need to load initially for the first day by taking double the recommended dose and then continue with frequent smaller doses every two waking hours until the symptoms diminish. In general, young children under the age of eight should be given a half to a quarter dosage; however, taking too much of any of the herbs described below is usually not a problem. One should expect signs of less pain, swelling, redness, or oozing of pus within the first three days of treatment or the condition may require more drastic medical intervention or the guidance of an experienced clinical herbalist.

The first thing is to avoid feeding the infection. Use a bland type of diet, based on completely avoiding all sweets, flour, or foods with sugar. The diet ideally should consist primarily of beans, rice, and steamed vegetables.

There are many herbs one can use for treating infections. Following are a list of some of the more effective Michael has used in his practice.

Echinacea root *(Echinacea purpurea, E. angustifolia, et species)* has proven itself to be one of the most effective single agents. It is too bad that commercial herb companies have tried to capitalize on the use of echinacea as an immune stimulant for the common cold and flu. While it is somewhat effective for these conditions, the primary reason it is sold for this reason is because there will be a great volume of sales, because more people will use it for these reasons rather than for serious infections.

To maximize the efficacy of echinacea, one should take a full teaspoon of the 20 percent alcoholic extract at least every two hours. If the infection is local, on the skin, a cotton soaked with the tincture should be applied topically with a bandage. This protocol should be followed for three days before cutting back to a teaspoon three times daily to be continued for two weeks to be sure the body has overcome the infection fully. Michael has found that echinacea can be effectively taken in pill, tea, or powder form or in formulas with herbs such as goldenseal, andrographis, dandelion, plantain, or garlic. In this way one is not overdosing on any single herb but is taking advantage of the synergistic action of the combination.

Goldenseal *(Hydrastis canadensis)* in this day and age should only be purchased "organically grown" because it is endangered in the wild. It contains berberine, which makes it useful for a wide variety of microbes. It works well synergistically when combined with other antibacterial and antiviral herbs such as echinacea with which it is frequently paired. It is often known as the "king of the mucus membranes" because it is particularly effective for infections of the sinus, respiratory organs, and genitourinary organs. Goldenseal also is used for the treatment of cancer.

Garlic *(Allium sativum)* has a long, well-earned reputation as a fighter of infections of all kinds. It is antibacterial, antiviral, and antifungal. For best results it should be taken raw and in large quantities. It can be used both internally and externally, although for external use it should be crushed with olive oil as it can be a little harsh when used alone directly on the skin. During the plagues of Europe, the populace ate garlic freely and even wore crushed garlic externally, since the medicinal oils evaporated into the immediate area around it; it repels and kills pathogens as well. It was crushed and mixed with other herbs in the famous "four thieves' vinegar," which was taken by them when they would steal valuables from those who died of the plague. Garlic has many other uses as well, such as preventing and eliminating parasites and lowering serum cholesterol. One of the active antibiotic compounds found in garlic is sulfur. One of the best ways to take garlic is to crush several cloves in olive oil and take a teaspoonful every hour or two as needed.

Andrographis *(A. paniculata)*, called "chuan lian zi" by the Chinese, is virtually a ubiquitous weed throughout many Asian countries. It has effective antibiotic, antiviral, and anticancer properties. Its major constituents include andrographolide. It has been found to be effective for staphylococci, pneumococci, streptococci, dysentery, typhoid, tuberculosis, and most gram-positive bacteria. Besides having these potent antibacterial properties, andrographis has been found to help the body overcome antibacterial resistance so that it is a very good herb to take with any antibacterial herb or drug. It is widely used throughout Asian countries as an antibacterial and antiviral for both acute colds and flus as well as for more serious diseases, including cancer. Andrographis can be taken alone or in combination with any or all of the above-mentioned herbs.

Olive leaf *(Olea europa)* has been used for centuries for the treatment of high fevers and various infectious diseases, including malaria. In 1995 some of the biochemical components were identified, and they included elenolic acid, with its salt and calcium elenolate. Olive leaf is effective for all bacteria and viruses as well as for yeasts and fungal diseases. It is most effective when used as a concentrated extract. The effective dosage is approximately two 00-sized capsules of the powdered extract taken three times daily, making a total of six capsules a day. For serious conditions, Michael recommends beginning with four capsules and continuing with two capsules every two waking hours for three days and then tapering down as symptoms improve.

Isatis *(I. indigotica* or *I. tinctoria),* also known as da qing ye in Traditional Chinese Medicine, contains indican and isatin B among other compounds and is known to have potent antibacterial properties against staphylococci, pneumococci, and meningococci, which means that it is useful for virtually all common bacterial infections. It is also a potent antiviral and has been found to be effective for a wide range of viruses, including those causing influenza, meningitis, encephalitis, and warts. It is anti-inflammatory and increases phagocytosis (the pathogen-destroying capability of white blood cells). The effective dose is about 2 g of the powder taken four to six times daily.

Dandelion root and leaf (*Taraxacum* species) is one of the most common weeds found growing throughout the world. If people only knew its many healing virtues, it might be a more welcome guest rather than a pest in the garden. Western herbalists use it widely for its beneficial effects in treating all liver diseases, from hepatitis to cirrhosis. They also recognize that it is one of the most effective botanical diuretics (called "piss-a-bed" by the French). However, the Chinese recognize and use it as a potent antibacterial, antiviral, and anticancer agent.

The most reliable overall home treatment for all infections is to take one or two teaspoons of echinacea every hour. This should be combined with taking high doses of raw garlic. The best way to take this is to blend about twenty or more cloves in olive oil and dip whole wheat bread into it. This should be the sum total amount consumed in a single day. This should be repeated over the course of three to seven days, tapering off gradually as symptoms subside. Then one should go on a maintenance dose of sixty drops of echinacea tincture and two garlic cloves three times a day for at least seven days after all symptoms have subsided. Among the many advantages of this therapy over drugs is that it works for all infectious agents, and second, there will be no problem with the pathogens developing resistance to the treatment. Michael also recommends high amounts of probiotics in the form of acidophilus, to be taken each day.

This program should be used for all infections, with the addition of the specific herbs described under each for added benefit and to direct the effects of garlic and echinacea to the affected site.

For convenience, all of the above herbs, with the exception of garlic, are found in tablet form in Planetary formula 48 (Echinacea–Golden Seal and Olive Leaf Combination). Planetary also has high-quality echinacea liquid extract in various pleasant flavors to assist palatability. I have found that homeopathic hepar sulph 6X to 30X potency is effective for many bacterial infections. Other homeopathic remedies to consider are *Calcarea sulphurica* 6X when there is general toxicity. For pus abscesses and boils, silicea 6X is sometimes effective. Choose either calcarea sulph or silica according to symptoms. Take twice a day alternating with hepar sulph.

INFLUENZA

OTHER NAMES: Flu, grip, grippe.

DESCRIPTION: Clinically, the difference between a cold and a flu is that flu presents with fever, general achiness, malaise, and sore throat; the common cold usually only affects the nasal and upper respiratory passages. Usually, both are caused by viruses. The influenza virus, is, however, typically more serious. Natural and herbal treatment are the same for both, so they will be discussed together.

SYMPTOMS: An attack of influenza is marked by the sudden onset of fever, chills, headache, prostration, a feeling of malaise, aches and pains in the neck and back, runny nose, sore throat, congestion, and swollen lymph nodes. The symptoms that predominate will change with the progress of the disease. If symptoms are not obviously reduced after two weeks, see a physician.

CAUSES: The direct cause is direct contact with the influenza virus, of which there are many strains. Influenza virus is communicated directly through contact by mouth, eyes, or nose. Commonly people catch the flu by touching someone who has it and then touching their own eyes or face. Therefore, washing one's hands frequently, especially if there is an opportunity for a lot of direct contact with others who may be infected, is one of the best ways to avoid influenza.

Of course, not everyone who is exposed to flu viruses becomes ill. The difference lies in the adequacy of the body's immune system to deal with the invading viruses, and the health of the immune system in turn depends on the general health of the body. The "causes" of this susceptibility, then, are all the practices and habits that promote poor health: poor dietary habits, such as eating processed and synthetic foods, fatty foods, excess animal protein, mucus-forming foods, and sweets; deficiencies of vitamins, minerals, and essential fatty acids; overindulgence in alcohol, tobacco, and drugs; lack of exercise; and overwork, depression, worry, and other stresses. Recent acute or chronic disease, including allergies, will also make a person more susceptible to the flu. Finally, repeated exposure to sudden changes in external temperature or exposure to cold, wet weather without proper protective clothing puts a strain on the homeostatic mechanisms of the body and thereby also makes it more susceptible to infection.

TREATMENT: As for other viral diseases, prevention is the only effective direct treatment for the flu. This means keeping the body healthy through a natural diet rich in fruits, nuts, grains, vegetables, and seeds, as well as maintaining healthful living habits. Taking five drops of cinnamon oil in a tablespoon of water several times a day has been recommended as a preventive measure to be taken before any symptoms appear.

Once the infection has begun, the only recourse is to treat the symptoms, try to support the body's fight against the viruses, and prevent complications. Treatment of the symptoms is described under COLDS. To strengthen the body, rest in bed as much as possible, at least double your normal vitamin intake (unless you are already on a megavitamin diet), and take lots of food even if you have little appetite. Soups and juices may be more appealing than solid foods. Freshly extracted juices from citrus fruits, strawberries, and black raspberries are an excellent source of vitamin C, which is useful for both prevention and treatment. Extra amounts of vitamins A, B₁, B₂, and B₆, as well as niacin and pantothenic acid, may also be beneficial. The body's need for protein—especially for certain amino acids—is higher during illness; some good foods to fill this need are cheddar cheese, lentils, peanut butter, poultry, and salmon.

Some herbal remedies to help ease the miseries of flu include taking lemon juice in warm water, three or four drops of eucalyptus oil in a teaspoon of water twice a day, or herbal teas made from yarrow, sage, mullein, echinacea, comfrey, goldenseal, coltsfoot, lungwort, and chamomile. A tea made from equal parts of sage, wormwood, licorice root, and alpine speedwell has also been used.

Historically, American boneset *(Eupatorium perfoliatum)* has been known to be one of the most effective herbs in the treatment of influenza, acute colds, and fevers. This, combined with elder flowers, honeysuckle flowers, chrysanthemum flowers, and a half part of licorice, is a powerful antiflu viral formula. This should be taken by steeping an ounce of the combination of herbs along with two slices of fresh ginger in a pint of boiling water, covered for fifteen to twenty minutes. Three cups are taken daily.

Elderberry flowers and berries have a well-established reputation for influenza and colds. Only the black elderberries *(Sambucus nigra)* should be used. Typically, an ounce of the flowers is combined with an ounce of peppermint and infused in a covered pot of water that has been brought to a boil for twenty minutes. Strain, and when sufficiently cool to drink, the patient should have one or two cups of the tea, following which he should lie perfectly still under several thick blankets to induce sweating. Allow profuse sweating but not for so long as to create exhaustion. Then have a sheet that has been wrung out in cold water ready to quickly wrap around the patient, neck to toes. Place plastic between the patient and the bedding and have him return to bed. This procedure should be repeated every two hours during the first day, then two or three times a day for three days afterward. At the same time the tea should be taken freely throughout the day.

Research from Israel has substantiated that elderberry extract significantly shortens the length of time one may have the flu. One study found that individuals with the flu who took an elderberry extract called "sambucol" improved or resolved, with fever reduction sometimes in as shortly as two days.

Kathy Keville describes making elderberry syrup as follows:

2 cups of dried elderberries
1 quart of boiling water
¼ cup of honey
¼ cup of lemon juice

In an uncovered pot, pour boiling water over the elderberries. Cover and allow them to soak overnight. The next day, simmer them for thirty minutes. Puree the warm berries in a blender and add the remaining ingredients as you blend. Pour the syrup into a clean bottle and store in the refrigerator. If you don't have time to prepare this, Planetary Formulas also has both elderberry extract and syrup as well as formula number 94 (Well-Child Echinacea and Elderberry Syrup), which are useful for both the prevention and treatment of influenza and colds. Elderberry syrup or "sambucol" (available as a liqueur in liquor stores) can be taken freely as needed.

Other remedies for influenza include:

Planetary formula number 36 (Ginger Warming Compound), a variation of the early North American Composition Powder, is specific for the first sting of either a cold or flu. It contains cinnamon—which has known antibacterial and antiviral properties—cayenne pepper, and ginger, which act to warm and mobilize the body's defense systems quickly at the first sign of an invading pathogen. The other great influenza formula from the Chinese tradition is called "yin chiao." This is a complex Chinese formula that combines powerful antibiotic and antiviral herbs, including honeysuckle and forsythia blossoms, burdock seed, bamboo, black soy bean, schizonepeta, and licorice. This is the classic version; clinically Michael has developed his own preferred version, which adds a number of Western herbs, including elecampane, echinacea, boneset, isatis, and horehound. These are Planetary formulas number 100 and 101.

One of the most effective homeopathic remedies is gelsemium 6th, which conforms to the classic picture of most flu symptoms, including tiredness, weakness, heavy and sick feelings. There will also be associated chills, runny nose, burning sore throat, and headaches that extend from the back over the top to the forehead.

INSECT STINGS AND BITES

In general one should follow the recommendations, using high, concentrated doses of echinacea and garlic, described under INFECTIONS. However, there are many other remedies that have been known to be effective for venomous bites and stings. An all-time favorite is plantain leaf (*Plantago* species). Simply chew a wad of the fresh leaf and apply it directly to the affected area. Plantain leaf can and should also be taken internally as a tea or powder. The most effective species of plantain is broadleaf plantain *(P. major)*. One folk treatment for wasp or bee stings is to apply baking soda mixed with a little vinegar directly to the affected area; another is to apply a cut onion or slice of garlic to relieve the pain and inflammation. Dermatologists have found that simply applying hot water (from 120° to 130°F) can relieve itching for several hours. Of course, if there is any associated burn or blister, these may be too irritating and should not be used. Adolph's Meat Tenderizer is based on the enzyme papain derived from papayas, and mixing it with a little vinegar to form a paste and applying it directly to stings and bites, including jellyfish stings, can be effective and is traditionally used by the Hawaiians for treating the painful sting from the man-of-war jellyfish that often plague swimmers. As for the use of Adolph's Meat Tenderizer, simply dissolve a couple of teaspoons in a little white vinegar and dab it over the affected area(s).

INSOMNIA

DESCRIPTION AND SYMPTOMS: Inability to fall asleep, inability to remain asleep for a sufficient period, lack of restful sleep.

Sleep is defined as a state of unconsciousness from which a person can be awakened by various appropriate means. Applying this definition, the unconscious state caused by anesthesia, coma, or petit mal epileptic seizures, however much similar, would not be considered deep, restful sleep.

Thus it is important to understand that an individual suffering from a chronic sleep disorder may be experiencing quite a different problem from another with occasional insomnia. Slow wave sleep is the deep, restful sleep that most people are seeking when they wish to go to sleep. In this, the individual experiences a profound slowing of the brain waves to one to two per second. Paradoxical or rem sleep exhibits a brain wave pattern that is more similar to normal waking state. It is normal to have some rem sleep which signifies dreaming or some active mental process of discharging emotions during normal sleep. An extreme of mental activity during sleep times causes wakefulness or at least a sense of insomnia.*

What can be concluded from this is that one who experiences normal, slow wave sleep awakens refreshed and renewed with the genuine feeling of having slept. The individual who is anesthetized, awakens from a coma or petit mal seizure, or who primarily has paradoxical or rem sleep may complain of insomnia, despite their superficial appearance of having slept.

CAUSES: For occasional sleep disorders, there may be dietary and environmental imbalances, emotional and physical stress, worry, anxiety or sensitivity to moon phases (full and new moon), or other cosmic influences.

Paradoxical or rem sleep disorders can have a variety of psychophysiological causes. One is a kind of hyperactivity of the brain that is due to chronic neural, hormonal, or possibly digestive factors.

It is interesting to note that Traditional Chinese Medicine associates insomnia with disorders of the heart. Since the heart is said to rule the mind, such sleep problems are

---

*Rem sleep can be identified upon closer examination by another as being accompanied with a slight twitching of the closed eyelids, signifying rapid eye movement (rem) and an irregularity of heart rate and respiration.

treated with acupuncture points on the heart meridian called "shen men" (spirit gate) or herbs that calm and sedate the spirit (and are also classified as entering the heart meridian). What we might consider in some cases is that a sleep disorder may be indicative of a functional heart problem that may not at that stage be clinically noticeable.

TREATMENT: Some basic guidelines that will relieve 90 percent of sleep difficulties are as follows:

1. Consider any possible medical problems, such as pain, hormonal imbalance, hypoglycemia, and depression, which may cause insomnia. This should also include dependency on sleeping pills or alcohol.
2. Avoid taking any stimulants such as coffee, tea, or alcohol two hours before going to bed.
3. Avoid taking naps or going to bed early, which can result in more restlessness at night.
4. Use your bed only for sleep and possibly sex to avoid wakeful associations.
5. An ideal sleeping environment is a cool room, with good ventilation, a firm but comfortable mattress, absolute quiet, and dark.
6. If you are not able to sleep for any period of fifteen minutes, get up from bed and read or do something quiet until drowsiness sets in, then return to bed. This is considered to be the most effective method and should be repeated as needed.
7. Meditation before retiring, repeating a word such as *peace* four times while inhaling and four times while exhaling, is also very effective for many people.

Many people have what is called habit-bound insomnia. This is when the act of sleeping has become associated consciously or unconsciously with some traumatic event such as a nighttime trauma, sexual molestation, fear of death, trauma during an operation, recurring nightmares, or dreams, and even the repeated failed struggle to go to sleep.

Overcoming these causes for insomnia may necessitate professional care, but creating a peaceful environment without a lot of stimulation, such as avoiding the late-night news, listening to peaceful music, meditation, and perhaps the assistance of a mild herbal sleep aid formula described below, will eventually prove to be very helpful.

There are a number of natural sleep remedies that are very effective for occasional insomnia. One thinks about Sir Arthur Conan Doyle's Sherlock Holmes (a cocaine addict!) using his drops of valerian extract each evening before retiring.

In addition to valerian *(Valeriana officinalis)*, there is passion flower *(Passiflora incarnata)*, hops *(Humulus lupulus)*, catnip *(Nepeta cataria)*, lemon balm *(Melissa officinalis)* and skullcap *(Scutellaria lateriflora)*—all having mild but effective sedative properties. At least one advantage of herbs over Western drug sedatives is that they are nonaddictive and without side effects. Thus, herbs have always been associated with their calming and relaxing properties.

Unlike Valium, the sedative effects of valerian are due to the combined effects of a complex organic substance. Thus the body is able to utilize the benefits of the herb without the severe side effects of the sedative drug. It is one of the volatile oils (isovaleric acid) that causes the sedative effects of valerian. Dosage is important. One can begin with a dose of ten to thirty drops, but for many, a dose of a teaspoonful repeated if necessary every fifteen or twenty minutes is required. A valerian tea using one teaspoon of the dried herb steeped in a cup of boiling water is also effective.

While the majority of people experience sedative and calming effects when using valerian, some paradoxically have bouts of increased anxiety or wakefulness—precisely what they are trying to overcome. One reason offered is that only fresh valerian should be used, as one of the biochemical constituents alters chemically to cineole, to which some individuals are highly sensitive. From the Chinese medical perspective, most sedative herbs tend to be energetically cool in nature, which means they tend to lower metabolism, which is ideal for sleep. Valerian has volatile oils that have a warm, stimulating effect. For some who are predisposed, having already too much hypermetabolism or heat, the stimulating effect of valerian takes precedence and overpowers the sedating effects.*

Another sedative herb which also contains isovaleric acid is hops. The dried strobules or flowers are what is used. Hops are also an effective remedy in tinctures or teas for insomnia. Its special sphere of action is when there are associated digestive disorders. Hops are also considered a mild anaphrodisiac and thus calms sexual excitement as well. Hops are usually combined with valerian for greater effectiveness and in more or less equal amounts. Thus ten to thirty drops of the tincture of hops and valerian can be used as one dose.

---

*This may not occur with the fresh valerian because Chinese medicine classifies fresh herbs with their added fluid content as cooler. Further, herbs that are extracted in alcohol are generally said to have a warmer action because of the influence of alcohol.

Hops tea is also effective but because the hops flowers are light and bulky, the dose appears much larger than that of a condensed root such as valerian. A small pillow filled with dried hops and slept on is a well-known folk remedy in many European countries for inducing a calm, restful sleep.

Another interesting fact that was noticed by young girls and women who were hops pickers for the brewing industry was their effect on the genital organs. It seems that hops also contain estrogenic plant hormones that would cause female hops pickers to have early menstruation. This may explain their anaphrodisiac effects on men.

Passion flower is a vine originating from South America of which the whole herb has mild sedative and hypnotic properties. Its action is based upon a number of nontoxic alkaloids and is useful for the treatment of insomnia either alone or in combination with valerian, hops, and skullcap. Like these other herbs, passion flower is useful for all neurological complaints including Parkinson's, chorea, shingles, and neuralgia. It is usually taken by steeping one teaspoon of the dried plant in a cup of boiling water. It can also be taken in an alcoholic tincture or extract.

Skullcap is a member of the mint family and is considered one of the best nervine tonics because of its propensity to relieve nervous tension while, unlike valerian, for instance, it refreshes the mind. It is one of the best herbs to use for delirium tremens, hysteria, PMS, epilepsy, and seizures. One or two teaspoons of skullcap is steeped in a cup of boiling water as a single dose.

Lemon balm is another nervine that is a member of

the mint family.* It is an herb traditionally prescribed for depression and melancholy as well as indigestion, gas, and fevers. One or two teaspoons are steeped in a cup of boiling water, then covered until cool enough to drink.

Lemon balm is frequently combined with chamomile and a slice or two of fresh ginger to make a pleasant tasting tea that is generally calming and quieting to the nervous system, and a good remedy for colds, flus, fevers, digestion, and menstrual pains. Try a combination of lemon balm, skullcap, passion flower, and chamomile, made into a tea by combining a tablespoon of the combined herbs and steeping them in a cup of boiling water, to which one may add a teaspoon of honey. Planetary formula number 2 (Calm Child), containing among other herbs both chamomile and lemon balm, while intended primarily for hyperactive children, is useful for adults as well.

One of the errors in treating intransigent insomnia is to resort to the use of herbs only when immediately needed—for instance, before retiring. Insomnia is a condition that is created throughout the day and sometimes over a prolonged period. What is needed is a gradual feeding of the nervous system throughout the day. For this reason it is better to take a balanced nervine formula such as formula number 71 (Stress Free) three times throughout the day; then, in the evening before retiring, make a soothing tea such as the lemon balm, skullcap, passion flower, and chamomile described above before retiring to bed. Depending on one's tolerance, add warm milk and

---

*Generally all mints, including spearmint, peppermint, and catnip, release surface tension because the oils, excreted by the pores of the skin, induce a light perspiration that in itself is sedating.

honey to the tea as well. The calcium in the milk has a mild sedative effect and the honey helps to remedy a tendency toward hypoglycemia that may be a contributing factor to sleep troubles.

Another consideration in the treatment of insomnia is that there may be a generally toxic condition of the liver or blood, and perhaps accompanying constipation, so that along with formula number 71 one might also take formula number 11 (Bupleurum Liver Cleanse) or 10 (Bupleurum Calmative). The latter formula is especially useful if there is a tendency toward depression. Two to four tablets of formula 89 (Triphala) should be taken in the evening after food.

Diet and sleep represent the foundations of natural healing. Anxiety or a state of hyperactivity can be due to either emotional or nutritional causes and commonly a bit of both. A diet high in carbohydrates, including sugar and flour products, and lacking in sufficient protein can contribute to nutritional causes of restlessness. A simple remedy for this is to have a warm glass of cow's milk to which one has added a teaspoon of honey about twenty minutes before retiring to bed. Other Planetary formulas that have been developed especially to be taken before going to bed in the evening are formula number 35 (Kava Dreams) and formula number 36 (Valerian Easy Sleep).

Kava Dreams contains kava kava, zizyphus seed, poria, ligusticum, anemarrhena, and a small amount of ginseng. Except with the addition of the anti-anxiety herb kava, the remainder of the formula is a respected Chinese herbal combination used for centuries to calm the nervous system and treat insomnia. It may be taken throughout the day but not if one needs to be especially alert and wakeful, such as when driving a car.

Kava *(Piper methysticum)* is one of the most remarkable herbs, which in formula is very safe.* Like all good things it can be abused, but in moderate dosage it has the following properties:

1. It is a most effective anti-anxiety herb (anxiolytic).
2. In the South Seas it is regarded as an anti-hate herb and used for conflict resolution.
3. It is a near specific for gonorrhea and urinary tract infections.
4. It relaxes tension, but in moderate dosage will not cause drowsiness.
5. It contains kavalactones, considered to be important for its anti-anxiety effects.

Homeopathic treatments for some forms of insomnia can be very effective. Following the principle of like cures like, one of the most common homeopathic treatments for insomnia is coffee 10th to 30th potency. This remedy is especially indicated for insomnia or restlessness caused by exhaustion and overexcitability. It is taken about a half hour before bedtime. Belladonna 10th to 30th is useful for

---

*A few recent reported cases of liver toxicity attributed to the use of kava remain a controversial issue which is at variance with its longstanding use by traditional South Sea island people, who use it ritually in what by our standards would be considered huge amounts and very frequently. This practice has been occurring over the course of centuries with no severe or chronic adverse effects. In Michael's as well as other professional herbalists' practices, kava appears to be very effective and safe. It is conjectured that the reported adverse effects by a few individuals may be due to some other causes yet to be determined.

interrupted sleep with restlessness and sometimes a throbbing headache.

MULTIPLE SCLEROSIS

OTHER NAMES: MS

DESCRIPTION, SYMPTOMS, AND CAUSES: Multiple sclerosis (MS) is a nerve disturbance resulting from the gradual loss of the myelin sheath that surrounds the nerve cell. Since one of the major functions of the myelin sheath is to transmit nerve impulses, there is a gradual decline in nerve function. It is a progressive disease that usually begins early in adult life. The symptoms are transient motor and sensory disturbances, including blurred vision, dizziness, muscle weakness, and tingling sensations.

The cause of MS is uncertain, but many currently believe that it is first caused by a virus, with measles virus being the most suspicious. Others have tried to correlate autoimmune and dietary factors and the inability to detoxify free radicals as causes.

The major diagnoses are clinical symptoms followed by laboratory and MRI evaluation.

TREATMENT: Michael has found that a prolonged course of acupuncture and herbal and dietary intervention will significantly slow the course of the disease, lessen the symptoms, or in some cases result in complete remission.

Following is a treatment protocol for multiple sclerosis developed by AHG (American Herbalists Guild) herbalist Alan Tillotson with my own modifications:

Protocol for using Planetary formula number 58 (Myelin Sheath Support) for 130- to 160-pound person:

1. Myelin Sheath Support: 2 pills three times a day
2. alpha-lipoic acid, 600 mg, 1 pill twice a day
3. vitamin E (mixed tocopherols), 800 IUs, 1 pill twice a day
4. DHA 250 mg, 1 pill twice a day or evening primrose, 500 mg (hexane-free with 135 mg gamma linoleic acid [GLA]), 2 pills twice a day
5. blueberries, ½ cup a day or one frozen bag a week

Estimated Length of Therapy

At least three months are needed to assess the usefulness of the therapy. There is an initial increase in energy, followed by a much slower gradual return of function. Michael estimates that in six to nine months, major benefits will begin to level out and hold steady, though some patients continue to improve very slowly over the next several years. Severely damaged nerves cannot be restored, so advanced cases improve, but not completely. Fatigue returns whenever patients discontinue the therapy for more than a week or so.

DIETARY INSTRUCTIONS: In general, base your diet on organic and naturally raised foods, cooked vegetables (because they are easier to digest), sea vegetables (because of the abundance of minerals they contain), animal protein (mostly fish, other seafood, and fowl), dairy (should be lightly scalded goat's milk, plain or with honey and ginger added), goat cheese, whole fruits in season, beans (especially mung beans), tempeh made from soy, almonds, walnuts, whole grains (especially rice, preferably brown rice if one can digest it), oils and fats such as ghee (clarified butter), olive oil, and sesame oil; sweeteners used in moderation (because these are inflammatory in nature), moderate use of maple syrup, blackstrap molasses (mineral rich), sucanat (whole, unprocessed sugar), or fruit juice used for sweetening special desserts; and moderate use of spices.

Because food allergies are often suspected as a cause of MS, one should avoid other grains, pastas, and sweeteners, and limit fatty red meats, artificial anything and everything, peanuts, coffee, alcohol, drugs—recreational or otherwise unless prescribed by your doctor and you are convinced you need them—and hydrogenated fats, including margarine. Also avoid too many raw vegetables, as these can be difficult to assimilate (though a small salad once a day with olive oil and lemon dressing would be fine).

Highly nutritive and easy-to-digest foods (both, not one) are key to healing the nervous system. Favor soups and warm foods and drinks. Drink spring water, especially with meals. All foods should be fresh, and organic if possible. Try to maintain regular mealtimes and adequate sleep. Use both a multivitamin and multimineral.

- Grains. Wheat, rice, corn, or oatmeal (unless you are allergic). Favor well-cooked whole grains with spices or warm cereals.
- Dairy. Avoid dairy products; however, a warm glass of goat's milk with honey and ginger daily would be useful in supplying easily assimilable vital nutrients.
- Sweeteners: sucanat (natural cane sugar), molasses, maple syrup.
- Oils. Olive, sunflower, canola, evening primrose, fish, flax, borage. Use low quantities, high quality only.

- Fruits. Sweet fruits, including berries, grapes, cherries, melons, avocado, coconut, sweet plums, pear, banana, fresh figs, mango. Eat freely.
- Vegetables. Well-cooked vegetables, asparagus, pumpkin, squash, cucumber, potato, celery, green peas, lettuce, okra, sweet potato, beans, green beans, carrots. Eat vegetables freely, especially cooked with spices.
- Spices. Pepper, cinnamon, cumin, ginger, salt, mustard, cardamom, fennel, chamomile or ginger tea.
- Proteins. Seafood is very important at least three times a week; chicken, turkey, almonds.

Avoid/Reduce:

- General. Avoid dieting and fasting, stale foods, and ice cold drinks. Also avoid canned or prepared foods, foods with chemical additives, foods with hydrogenated oils and fats, excess alcohol, candy, cake, sugary sweets, and Nutrasweet.
- Sweeteners. Avoid unhealthy sweets like cakes, pies, etc. Natural sweets, such as fruits and grains, are much better.
- Oils: Low-quality oils are very inflammatory.
- Vegetables. Reduce raw veggies (except lettuce and carrots) if hard to digest, as well as cabbage, cauliflower, zucchini, and turnips. (All should be limited, taken in small quantities, and well cooked.)
- Spices. Avoid excess amounts of hot spices, fenugreek, cayenne pepper, chili, cloves, salt, mustard.

About Fats & Oils

Fat is the most abundant substance in your body after water. More than 70 percent of your brain and nerve cells are made of fat, and the membrane of every cell in your body is 30 percent fat.

There are about two dozen fats (lipids) in the body, and two, called essential fatty acids, or EFAs, must come from your diet. The two are omega-6 and omega-3. Your cells use EFAs for energy production, your glands use EFAs to make healthy secretions, and EFAs help your immune system work. They also nourish your skin, hair, mucous membranes, and the myelin sheath surrounding your nerves.

Bad Fats

Bad fats are those that are rancid, imbalanced, overly saturated, overcooked, or modified by modern food processing:

    margarine
    shortening
    red meats: (use leaner cuts of naturally raised meat,
        but the emphasis should be on fish)
    dairy products (goat's milk is all right in moderation)
    chips
    fried foods
    pastries

Good Fats

Good fats are those that contain a healthy balance of EFAs and are fresh, unheated, and unprocessed:

    olive oil
    canola oil
    pumpkin oil

flaxseed, an important source of linoleic acid (MS patients should have a tablespoon of flaxseed oil a day.)

Supplements:

- a high-quality multivitamin supplement
- chlorella: nutrient-dense green algae that is rich in easily assimilable protein, vitamins, and minerals. Take twice daily in doses ranging from 1 to 2 teaspoons or more at a time.
- vitamin B_{12} (methylcobalamin): 2 mg per day or up to 60 mg per day for specific therapeutic use. It imparts a sense of well-being in MS patients and slows progressive demyelination.
- flaxseed oil: 1 tablespoon daily
- evening primrose: It is anti-inflammatory and beneficial for pain (1,200 mg daily).
- Take 1,000 to 1,600 mg essential fatty acids (EPA) as fish oil. The amount per capsule and gram of fish oil differs depending on the source. Check the bottle for EPA levels. Michael recommends Eskimo Oil made by Tyler Encapsulations. *Warning:* When supplementing any fat-soluble vitamin or oil, you must also take a vitamin E supplement to protect against oxidation.
- vitamin E: 800 to 1,000 IUs daily
- Wobenzyme or another good-quality enzyme supplement maintains digestion and assimilation, activates the immune system, prevents inflammatory flare-ups, and relieves pain. Dose: 2 to 4 tablets 3 to 4 times daily a half hour before meals.
- selenium to enhance the production of the antioxidant glutathione: 200 to 400 mcg per day

- lipoic acid: an important antioxidant to counteract degenerative free-radical buildup, 600 mg per day.
- N-acetyl cystein combines with selenium to synthesize glutathione (the body's inherently manufactured antioxidant); it also protects agains DNA damage. Dose: 1,500 mg daily
- a cup of fresh or frozen blueberries or raspberries daily. These are high in antocyanins, the most potent of all naturally occurring antioxidants.

Many people, especially those suffering from inflammatory diseases, need to supplement their oils. The best choices include fish oils containing DHA and EPA, evening primrose or borage oils, and flaxseed oils. It is always important to take extra vitamin E with oil supplements to help absorb them.

Adjunct Therapies

Traditional Chinese Medicine, with specific herbal, acupuncture, and moxibustion therapies indicated for each patient, includes:

hyperbaric oxygen therapy, T'ai Qi, or Qi Gong
biozyme digestive enzymes: 1 pill twice a day (if digestion is weak or compromised)
scutellaria laterifolia herbal tincture, 25 to 35 g three times a day (if there is shaking)
Pippalyadi Churnam (Planetary formula number 86), 2 g twice a day for sluggish digestion with signs of mucus

OSTEOPOROSIS

Osteoporosis is a gradual decrease in bone density that ultimately leads to a weakness of bone structure. It is a condition commonly associated with aging that is estimated to affect up to 40 percent of Caucasian women over the age of fifty and 20 percent of men. Racially it seems more commonly to affect Caucasian and Asian women, especially small-statured and thin-boned women, the latter regardless of race.

Other risk factors for osteoporosis include smoking (smokers are 40 to 50 percent more susceptible to the disease); having a mother or grandmother with osteoporosis; and taking drugs, especially glucocortisoids (cortisone) that are commonly prescribed for arthritis, asthma, and chronic inflammatory disease. Those who have had a history of malabsorptive and digestive diseases such as anorexia, bulimia, diabetes, Crohn's disease, irritable bowel disease, hyperthyroidism, hyperparathyroidism, liver disease, multiple myeloma, and kidney failure are all at greater risk for developing osteoporosis later in life.

For women, estrogen replacement therapy commonly is used to prevent and inhibit osteoporosis. Calcium supplementation also is considered to be of benefit. In this regard, the only form of calcium that is readily absorbable is calcium citrate. Premenopausal women should take about 1,000 mg a day and postmenopausal women should take up to 2,000 mg daily. These are taken in two doses, A.M. and P.M. In addition, one should take about 400 IUs of vitamin D and 400 to 800 mg of magnesium daily. The dose for the latter mineral is controversial, as some nutritionists recommend taking twice as much magnesium as calcium.

Of all the factors that may have a positive effect on

bone density, numerous studies cite physical fitness and especially weight-bearing exercise as being most beneficial. It seems that a diet high in animal protein also represents a greater risk for developing osteoporosis. This is because a diet high in phosphates increases the excretion of calcium in the urine. Another dietary risk factor is overconsumption of sugar. With the average American consuming up to 150 g of sucrose daily, together with other refined sugars and carbonated beverages loaded with phosphates, it is no wonder that osteoporosis is a major medical problem.

Green leafy vegetables like kale, collards, broccoli, amaranth, parsley and lettuce offer significant nutritional support against osteoporosis. Because soy contains the isoflavones diadzein and genistein, also known as phytoestrogens, it seems that the regular consumption of soy two or three times a week is a good idea.

One of the most valuable herbs nutritionally is stinging nettle *(Urtica dioica)*. It is a rich source of absorbable iron, calcium, phosphorus, and even protein. When cooked, the stinging compound is neutralized. One should be sure to harvest the young green leaves, of course wearing gloves to prevent being stung by the plant. It can be steamed as a potherb or made into soup. If one prefers, the powdered dried leaf can be taken in doses up to 3,000 mg or more daily. Of course, the fresh or dried leaves also can be drunk as a pleasant tea.

Other herbs that may be useful for inhibiting osteporosis include:

Horsetail *(Equisetum hyemale, E. arvense)*, which is a natural source of silica useful for strengthening bones, nails, and hair.

Red clover *(Trifolium pratense)* and alfalfa *(Medicago sativa)*, both in the Leguminaceae or Fabaceae family, are similar to soy in that they contain weak phytoestrogens. Both plants, besides having therapeutic properties, are nutritionally dense. They do contain coumarins, which may have anticoagulant properties and should be avoided when taking anticoagulant drugs. This points out one of the problems with using herbs as a regular nutritional supplement: Besides their specific nutritional value, they may have other therapeutic effects that, if not needed, can pose a problem with longtime usage. This also further underscores the value of using herbs in complex formulas rather than single entities taken over a prolonged period.

Certain Chinese herbs, including *Polygonum multiflorum* (ho shou wou), deer antler, and *Rehmannia glutinosa,* are particularly useful tonics. Two Planetary formulas that can be taken for osteoporosis include number 73 (Schizandra Adrenal Complex) and number 67 (Rehmannia Endurance).

A product Michael has known to increase bone density is OsteOrganiCal, manufactured by Natural Option Corp. It contains organic calcium oxide derived from sea algae with magnesium. Another product, called Bone-Up, by Jarrow, is a more complex formulation and is also claimed by some to be effective for bone strengthening.

PARASITES

There are many types of parasites that can proliferate both inside and outside of the body. In general, most parasites arise in hot, humid climates and/or from close contact with humans or animals. They can be very difficult to get rid of when one's health is poor. Thus, for these, one should use a tonic strengthening and building approach while applying symptomatic remedies.

Parasites are generally repelled or destroyed by herbs with strong bitter flavors. For this reason, all antiparasite herbs usually have a strong bitter or pungent taste characterized by herbs in the wormwood family *(Artemisia species)*.

INTERNAL PARASITES

Tapeworms

Male fern *(Aspidium filix-mas)* is the primary herb of choice for the treatment of tapeworms *(taenia)*. The root stock must be used fresh or freshly prepared into a liquid extract. Large doses are poisonous and can cause toxic liver damage. However, a large dose of 8 to 10 g of the extract is considered necessary to kill the tapeworm. It should be given on an empty stomach in two portions, during the morning, at fifteen-minute intervals. After two hours give two tablespoons of castor oil as a purgative to help expel the worm. Simultaneously give a tea of dandelion root or silymarin extract to help protect the liver from the effects of the male fern.

Pumpkin seeds *(Cucurbitae pepe)* are a safe and effective remedy against tapeworms, roundworms, and pinworms in both humans and animals. While not as strong as male fern, pumpkin seeds can be used for individuals with a known history of liver disease or pregnancy. Grind 200 to 400 g of unpeeled and crushed pumpkin seeds in a food mill. Combine with milk and honey to form a porridge consistency. Again, this is taken in the morning on an empty stomach in two doses. Unlike the male fern, pumpkin seeds do not kill the tapeworm but merely paralyze it, thus it is extremely important to administer a strong purgative of castor oil two or three hours after giving the pumpkin seeds.

Homeopathic medicine uses tincture of male fern, about ten to twenty drops in a little water, three times a day. Generally it is not recommended for children.

Threadworms or Pinworms

Garlic is good for all kinds of worms and most other parasites as well. Take a clove three or four times a day or blend with olive oil and take in tablespoon doses. A clove of garlic can also be coated with olive oil and inserted directly into the rectum each evening. A retention enema is made by chopping one or two cloves and steeping in a pint of water for ten minutes or until cool enough to administer.

Carrots are another effective treatment for pinworms. This is especially effective for children. The treatment is to give nothing but grated carrots and carrot juice for two days.

Wormseed (*Artemisia cina*) is very effective against worms, including pinworms, threadworms, and roundworms; less effective is wormwood or mugwort (*Artemisia species*). Take ten to thirty drops of the tincture on an empty stomach four times a day. Since this is very bitter, for children it can be taken with honey. Homeopathic cina 1x taken four times a day for four days has also been very effective against pinworms.*

Roundworms (Ascarides)

These are considered the most difficult to eliminate. They therefore require more powerful herbs, which can have possible harmful side effects. Both male fern and several cloves of garlic taken daily over several days is sometimes

---

Artemisia annum, found in Chinese pharmacies, is a recognized legal treatment to prevent malaria.

effective. The most specific treatment for roundworms, however, is chenopodium oil made from the American wormseed *(Chenopodium ambrosioides var. anthelminticum)*. The diagnosis of roundworms can only be confirmed by the presence of worm eggs in the stools.

For each year of the child's age, give one drop in the morning of pure chenopodium oil mixed with honey. Repeat the same dose an hour later. Two hours after that, give two tablespoons of castor oil. If there is no bowel movement within three hours, repeat the castor oil hourly until bowel movement has occurred.

Bed rest is important and the treatment should not be repeated until a week has elapsed. For more delicate and frail children one should wait up to four weeks before repeating the treatment. Again give dandelion root or silymarin extract to protect the liver.

Other homeopathic remedies for worms are: Mercurius 3rd to 10th potency for various types of worms associated with itching rectum, weakness, great hunger, offensive breath. One dose is taken every three hours for four days. Santonin 3rd to 10th potency for worms accompanied with itching of the nose, twitching muscles, restless sleep. It is not effective for tapeworms.

ANTIPARASITE PROGRAM

While there are a number of specific herbs for internal worms and parasites, there are also some very effective general remedies that can be used in the event that one is unsure of the type of parasite. One should not use antiparasite herbs during pregnancy unless under the guidance of a professional herbalist.

Wormseed *(Chenopodium ambrosiodes)* is, according to

Jim Duke,★ widely used in the tropics as a dewormer. It is easy to grow and is commonly eaten with beans by traditional Mexicans both because of its flavor but also because it relieves gas and both prevents and eliminates worms from the intestinal tract. *Caution: Never take internally the essential oil of wormseed.*

Ginger *(Zingiber officinale)* is, according to Paul Shulick,† effective against many of the world's most dangerous parasites. Sushi lovers may appreciate knowing that ginger either raw or pickled commonly is eaten to prevent and treat the anisakis larvae that infect raw fish. According to Jim Duke,† ginger "will immobilize 90 percent of anisakis larvae within 4 hours and destroyed them in 16 hours."

Black Walnut hulls derived from the fresh, green, immature husk is one of the most effective herbs for parasites. It contains antiparasite and antifungal agents along with trace amounts of iodine. Generally, of the 1:1 extract, one should only take one to ten drops one to three times daily with the following tea:

½ tsp. of chamomile flowers
1 tsp. of chenopodium
fresh ginger slices
½ tsp. of rosemary leaves
½ tsp. of thyme.

In addition, I would suggest that one eat several cloves of garlic each day and an ounce of pumpkin seeds.

★*The Green Pharmacy,* (Rodale, 1997).
†*Ginger: Common Spice and Wonder Drug,* 1994.

This treatment is effective for all intestinal parasites and should be followed for approximately a month. Avoid sugar and fruit juices, which are things that parasites love.

Giardia

This program is also effective for treating giardias, which are amoebas in the intestines usually contracted from polluted drinking water. For giardias Michael has had success prescribing a very bland diet of rice, steamed vegetables, and beans for a week while taking two 00-size capsules of goldenseal powder every two hours. In addition, one should consume the equivalent of a clove of garlic every hour. A great way to take garlic is by macerating the entire clove of garlic in olive oil each morning. Then, freely dip whole wheat bread into the oil and eat at least every hour.

Triphala (formula number 89) should be taken three times daily, along with Planetary's antiparasite formula, which contains a number of the herbs discussed in this section.

EXTERNAL PARASITES

Ringworm

This is a fungoid growth which is cured by sealing it off from the air. First paint the area with undiluted lemon juice, the white of an egg, or nail varnish. Renew this treatment every few hours until the ringworm is destroyed. Take garlic internally.

Head Lice and Crabs

Crabs specifically affect the pubic hairs while head lice are specific to the head hair. Both can be treated in the same manner. First cleanse the area with soap or shampoo. Comb the hair with a fine-toothed comb or use a razor to cut off all the hairs to which the crabs and lice have attached their eggs. The eggs hatch out every two weeks, so the eggs should be cut out and the treatment must be repeated twice at two-week intervals.

Various herbal treatments are effective. A strong tea of garlic can be washed over the affected areas and left on to dry. Other herbs that are effective to use in this way include wormwood or mugwort *(Artemisia species)*, calamus *(Calamus draco)*, or rue *(Ruta graveolens)*.

The following, called Juliete's Insect Repellent Oil, is based on the recipe of Juliete de Bairacli Levy. Combine equal parts rosemary *(Rosemarinus off.)*, sweet basil *(Ocimu hasilicum)*, rue *(Ruta graveolens)*, wormwood or mugwort *(Artemisia absinthe* or *A. vulgaris)*. Infuse in one cupful of salad oil and one teaspoon of vinegar in strong sunlight for five days, shaking the jar daily. After the sun infusion, squeeze the herb oil through a cloth and add a further quantity of the powdered herbs, following the same procedure as before. Repeat once again to make a total of three. Keep the jar tightly covered to prevent the escape of essential oils.

This oil can be rubbed into the scalp or pubic area each night for the treatment of crabs and lice. When applying to the head, cover with a scarf and hair net to keep the cloth covering on the head through the night. The next morning, wash the oil out of the hair with soap and rinse with mugwort or wormwood and rosemary tea, allowing the tea to dry on the hair. Repeat for five days, after which the treatment should be successful.

It is important to carefully wash and change bedding and clothes each day to prevent reinfestation. Since the condition is very contagious, contact with others should be restricted so as to prevent reinfestation or communication of the disease.

Mosquitoes

Many herbs with strong-smelling volatile oils are useful to repel mosquitoes. The above-mentioned oil can be used but most commonly oil of citronella or pennyroyal oil *(Mentha pulegium)* is externally applied, for this purpose. Neem oil, externally applied provides hours of protection against mosquitoes and even black flies. An excellent neem mosquito and black-fly repellent is made by Neem Tree Farms.*

Scabies

This is a rash formed by the presence of a microscopic mite that burrows under the skin. It prefers tender, moist areas, the insides of the arms, neck, genitals, breasts, elbows, buttocks, and under the arms. Fortunately it is seldom, if ever, found in the hair. It is highly contagious and scratching, which is unavoidable, causes mites and eggs to collect under the fingernails so that they are spread to other parts of the body.

The traditional treatment for scabies is to apply an ointment made of a six-part solution of sulfur, camphor, and alum directly over the affected areas once or twice daily. Western medical treatment is more toxic and consists of the topical application of gamma benzene hexachloride or crotamiton cream.

To administer the above treatment, begin by bathing

---

*Neem Tree Farms, 601 Southwood Cove, Brandon, FL 33511, (813) 661-8873, NeemTreeFarms.com.

thoroughly and then applying the ointment from the neck down, covering the entire body. Wait fifteen minutes before dressing. Carefully wash all clothes and toys used prior to, or during, the treatment. Furniture and floors do not have to be cleaned with any special care. Leave the medicine on the skin for two hours before bathing. Repeat the treatment, if needed, in one week.

In general, prevention is always better than a cure. Prevention consists of avoiding contact with infected persons, living in clean, sanitary places, maintaining personal cleanliness, bathing at least two or three times a week, washing the hands before eating, and laundering clothes often.

Scabies, ringworm, and lice are among the most difficult conditions to treat naturally. Nevertheless, since these have continuously plagued the human race since the dawn of time, it is reasonable to assume that people have found effective and safe treatments for them.

The Wonders of the Indian Neem Tree

Neem *(Azadiracta indica)* is a dense, shady tree some thirty to thirty-six feet tall. All parts of the tree, including the green leaves, flowers, twigs, unripe and ripe fruits, and bark, are used as medicine. It has a nauseatingly bitter taste, but the ripe fruit is slightly sweet.

It has an incredibly wide range of uses, being easily digested, cooling, and detoxifying, with bitter and pungent flavors. It is astringent, so that it will treat diarrhea; it destroys parasites and worms of all kinds, and will relieve vomiting and ulcers in children. It acts as a bitter to increase appetite; relieves abdominal bloating, biliousness, and gas; treats infections and inflammations of all kinds, thirst, coughs, fevers, blood impurities, eye, ear, and nose diseases, and diseases of the genito-urinary tract in both men and women. Besides its use on humans and livestock, for which the powdered bark and leaves and/or an infusion can be applied, it is safe and nontoxic to humans and animals as an insecticidal garden agent.

The primary use for which neem is known, however, is for skin diseases. As such it is one of the most effective remedies for a wide variety of skin conditions. The oil expressed from the kernels of the dried neem fruits is the most useful form derived from the tree. For a variety of skin conditions, including boils, ulcers, syphilis, highly resistant ulcers, as well as funguses, ringworm, lice, scabies, and other itches, neem oil can be rubbed externally over affected areas of the skin. If for any reason this proves irritating, the oil can be diluted with olive or sesame oil.

Another medicated oil that is similarly effective when applied topically includes fresh garlic in olive oil. The essential oils derived from clove *(Szygium aromaticum)*, tea tree oil *(Maleleuca alternifolia)*, or rosemary *(Rosemarinus officinalis)* can all be mixed with olive oil for topical application for funguses (tineas), lice, scabies, ticks, and other parasites. Essential oils can be irritating to the skin, so it is important to dilute them, mixing about 1 teaspoon of the essential oil to a cup of olive oil. After washing the affected areas thoroughly, rub a generous amount of the oil onto the skin twice a day.

Tansy *(Tanacetum vulgare)* is another herb with antiparasite and antifungal properties. *The oil should never be taken internally and has been known to cause death.* However, externally it is quite safe, especially when mixed with olive oil as described above. A strong tea of the aerial portion of the plant can be used as a topical wash applied head-to-toe for skin parasites.

Ticks

Ticks are contracted while walking and brushing up against plants in wild or unsettled areas. Usually they occur most in spring and fall, so that during these times of year, it is a good idea to check oneself after returning from an outdoor trek in the woods. They can crawl up the pant leg and around the body until finding a suitable place in which to burrow. Ticks are occasionally cited as a source for the introduction of serious diseases such as Lyme's disease and Rocky Mountain spotted fever, which are diseases similar to mononucleosis, causing severely lowered resistance to disease and chronic fatigue.

Ticks need to be removed in such a way that no part remains embedded in the flesh. Mountain folk grab them firmly and twist them off counterclockwise. Another method is to first kill them by coating their body with fingernail polish and allowing it to dry before removing them. It is a good idea to take echinacea *(Echinacea species)* about four times a day for three or four days after removing a parasite such as a tick.

PARKINSON'S DISEASE

OTHER NAMES: paralysis agitans, shaking palsy.

DESCRIPTION AND SYMPTOMS: Parkinson's is a degenerative condition of the brain caused by damaged nerves that control muscle tension and movement. Onset begins with a slight tremor of one hand, arm, or leg. Characteristically, the tremor, at least during the onset, is worse when the limbs are at rest. Eventually patients manually try to hold the affected limb to stop the tremors. A characteristic of the tremors is called "pill rolling," where the patients move their fingers as if they were rolling pills. With progression, patients increasingly lose all ability to control their tremors, and the condition sadly becomes much worse.

CAUSE: Parkinson's is a disease that affects approximately 1 in 200, with men over sixty being the most susceptible. It is a serious disease that requires professional medical management: Any suggestions offered in this book should be considered as part of a more comprehensive integrated program.

TREATMENT: Michael has treated Parkinson's with acupuncture, and if the condition is treated early enough its progression can be slowed significantly and perhaps halted. Unfortunately most patients expect immediate results and are unwilling to commit to a protracted program of dietary and herbal treatment over the course of a couple of years.

Studies conducted in 1979 on twenty-one patients with early Parkinson's disease over the course of seven years found significant benefit compared to a similar comparable control group. The patients were further divided into younger and older onset groups. They were both given 3,000 mg of vitamin C and 3,200 mg of vitamin E daily. Patients with younger onset Parkinson's were able to delay the need for drug therapy for 65.3 months, while those in the older onset group were drug-free on average for 59.2 months. In contrast, the group that was not given the antioxidants required medication in 24 and 40 months, respectively. All patients eventually required conventional drug therapy (Sinemet or Deprenyl).

A further study measuring only survival rate was published in *The New England Journal of Medicine* in 1997. The survival rate of 341 patients with moderately severe Parkinson's who were given the drug selegiline together with 2,000 IUs of vitamin E daily survived 230 days, compared to only 145 days' survival for patients who took only the drug plus placebo. That's a significant one-third longer survival rate, which is considered statistically very significant.

Of course, the above studies reflect only a mild nutritional supplement program. Consider the possible benefit if one were to follow a more comprehensive nutritional program such as the one suggested at the end of this section that combines nutritional supplements with herbs to both prevent or treat Parkinson's disease.

Herbs

Herbs will make a major difference also. Certainly one herb that every Parkinson's patient should be taking is approximately 120 mg of ginkgo biloba extract daily. Other herbs that traditionally have been known to benefit brain function are gota kola *(Hydrocotyl asiatica)* and bacopa *(B. monnieri)*.

Interestingly, both herbs are called "brahmi" in Sanskrit, but while gota kola is the more famous brahmi, bacopa is considered the more efficacious for the brain. Gota kola has a cooling effect on the brain, and by eliminating the heated mental chatter it helps to improve concentration and memory. Bacopa is regarded in Ayurveda as a cure for mental retardation leading to psychosis. For over three thousand years it has been regarded as efficacious in relieving anxiety and in treating loss of intellect and memory. It has been found that the bacosides in bacopa increase protein synthesis, which helps to regnerate brain cells, making it useful for all degenerative brain disease, including Alzheimer's and Parkinson's.

Fava Beans

Dr. Jim Duke describes fava beans *(Vicia faba)* as one of nature's best sources for the compound called L-dopa, which is the precursor of dopamine in the brain. Dopamine is used in the brain to restore the normal balance between excitation and inhibition of nerve impulses. Parkinson's represents an imbalance between acetylcholine, which plays a vital role in the transmission of nerve impulses between the synapses and myoneural junctions, and dopamine. Dopamine produced in the brain serves as the controlling factor in the transmission process; if it is deficient, the result is uncontrolled movement or rigidity of various parts of the body.

Dopamine is not administered because it has a chemical structure that will not allow it to pass through the blood–brain barrier. L–dopa, administered either as a drug or through diet from regular consumption of fava beans or the lesser-known velvet bean *(Macuna* species), which has about fifty thousand parts per million of L-dopa, will convert in the brain to dopamine. Furthermore, it has been found that sprouted fava beans have ten times the L-dopa as the unsprouted.

According to Jim, one would have to consume about two pounds of unsprouted fava beans to receive a significant therapeutic dose; however, one only needs to consume two ounces of the sprouted beans daily.

The pharmaceutical L–dopa is very expensive, while a sixteen-ounce can of fava beans is a mere fraction of the cost. Of course, eating these beans, if you are not used to them, will result in gas, so one may want to invest in the over-the-counter medication Beano, which is an enzyme that helps to prevent gas.

Michael plants fava beans in his garden as a cover crop so that when spring comes there is an abundance. Some are eaten in a favorite pasta fasole dish consisting simply of pasta and cooked fava beans with olive oil and garlic. The majority is dried for future use and plantings the following late fall. The beans help fix nitrogen; after plowing, the stalks rapidly decompose, making the nitrogen available for new crops.

Other herbs that would be useful for treating and managing Parkinson's disease include skullcap *(Scutellaria lateraflora)* and the Indian herbs ashwagandha *(Withania somnifera)* and guggul.

Any serious treatment of a serious brain condition such as Parkinson's or Alzheimer's should begin with good nutrition. Besides developing a good nutritional supplement program based on that described above, it is first important to limit those foods that are known to rob the body of nutrients, including all refined foods, such as white sugar, alcohol, and coffee.

Comprehensive Supplement and Herbal Program Against Parkinson's Disease:

- high-potency multivitamin such as Rainbow Light's Complete Nutritional Program or Source Natural's Ultra Multiple
- thiamin: 3 to 8 g daily (Studies have found that geriatric patients often are deficient in one or more B vitamins, and since thiamin mimics acetylcholine, which is an important neurotransmitter, this should be added to one's daily supplement program.)
- methylcobalamin (B_{12}): 1,000 mcg twice daily
- L-acetylcarnitine: 500 mg three times daily (LAC, which converts to carnitine, is important for stimu-

lating the production of cellular mitochondria. There have been numerous studies relating to the use of LAC in treating age-related conditions related to brain function.)

- tyrosine: 1,000 mg morning or afternoon (Tyrosine is an essential nutrient for the manufacture of neurotrophin proteins, including nerve growth factor (NGF), brain-derived nerve factor (BDNF), and neurotrophins (NT-3, NT-4/5, and NT-6). Therefore, it is an important adjuvant for the treatment of Parkinson's disease.)
- A good antioxidant supplement with approximately 600 mg each of N-acetyl cysteine (NAC) and alpha lipoic acid

Herbs:

- Planetary formula number 7 (Bacopa Mind Strength)
- Planetary formula number 18 (Guggul-Cholesterol) for circulation
- Planetary's Ashwagandha liquid extract antiaging tonic (take at least thirty drops twice daily)

PHANTOM LIMB PAIN

DESCRIPTION: After the loss of a limb there is residual pain, as if the limb were still present.

TREATMENT: Massage with ginger and cayenne oil or ointment. To a pint of olive or sesame oil, add a tablespoon each of freshly ground cayenne pepper and ginger powders. Keep warm for a few days. Strain and use this oil to massage the end of the affected limb. Another remedy is made by squeezing the juice of freshly grated ginger through a cloth into sesame oil. This will have to be shaken each time before rubbing on the affected area as before. Finally, capsaicin is a topical ointment made from cayenne pepper that is available in many pharmacies and can be used similarly.

In addition, onion essence rubbed on the area of amputation also is considered beneficial. This is easily made by filling a bottle with fresh chopped onions and then covering them with 40 percent vodka and allowing it to stand in a warm place for two weeks. The liquid is then strained and bottled for use.

PNEUMONIA

DESCRIPTION AND SYMPTOMS: This is a disease of inflammation of the lungs that in Western allopathic medicine is caused by pneumococcus bacteria or a virus. The incubation period is considered to be two to six days and the attack usually begins with chills. (In children, a sudden attack may begin with convulsions). The temperature rises to 101° and higher, the pulse is rapid, and breathing is shallow and difficult. White phlegm, sometimes flecked with blood, is coughed up.

The temperature continues at around 104° for as much as a week, which signals the period in which the body is actively fighting the disease. If the disease continues after this time, there may be severe weakness and prostration accompanied by a sudden fall in temperature and copious perspiration; aches and pains that were formerly present during the acute stage may at this point diminish or cease. The disease is called double pneumonia when both lungs are affected.

Walking pneumonia may occur with no severe acute symptoms except a cough. The disease can lead to pleurisy, or accumulation of fluid in the pleural cavity of the lungs, which can be very serious.

TREATMENT: Patients should be kept warm, confined to bed, and given a light diet of warm vegetable broth, chicken broth, soupy porridge, and light dahl soup. They should be given the treatment indicated under FEVER and INFLUENZA. In addition they might be given the following tea (which is also suitable for the treatment of pleurisy): one ounce pleurisy root, one ounce eucalyptus leaves, one-quarter ounce licorice root, and six fresh slices or one dried tablespoon of ginger root. Simmer the pleurisy root and licorice in one quart of boiling water in a covered pot for twenty minutes, after which steep the eucalyptus leaves and ginger in the liquid. An infusion of either eucalyptus or thyme leaf tea is a helpful treatment against pneumonia. In addition, oil of garlic should be taken. It is made by macerating several fresh cloves of crushed garlic in olive oil: Take one teaspoon every hour or two. Otherwise purchase garlic pills and take 1,500 mg every two or three hours.

The cold wet sheet treatment given for fevers should shorten the course of the disease. In between, rub camphorated oil, eucalyptus oil, or balm on the affected side of the chest or back.

A poultice over the chest or back of six finely chopped fresh onions lightly steamed and wrapped in a white muslin or linen bag and applied as hot as possible is a very effective treatment against pneumonia. Cover the poultice or keep it warm, and as it cools, replace it with another. This should be repeated at least four times in succession.

During the sickness, frequent drinks of lemon and honey tea are most appreciated.

During convalescence, the patient should be cautioned against overexertion and going out too soon, so as to prevent a relapse. American ginseng, together with a few slices of fresh ginger, brewed into a tea, can be taken three times a day to help regain strength. Tincture of goldenseal or the bitters described previously can be taken before meals to stimulate digestion and assimilation.

In addition or instead of the above, take Planetary formula number 101 (Yin Chiao–Echinacea Complex) with number 29 (Echinacea–Golden Seal with Olive Leaf). Pneumonia can be a serious disease, and one should seek professional assistance.

POISONING

DESCRIPTION AND CAUSES: Poisoning can be caused by spoiled or contaminated food and drink, by poisonous plants, mushrooms, and other natural toxins, and by exposure to or ingestion of caustic substances such as poisonous chemicals.

TREATMENTS: Treatments vary, depending on the specific cause.

Food Poisoning

Begin by inducing vomiting. Make the patient drink copious amounts of warm water, noting exactly the amount given. If mustard is available, add a tablespoon of powdered mustard or even a couple of tablespoons of prepared mustard to the water in order to make an emetic. Otherwise, syrup of Ipecac, available from a drugstore, can be used. If vomiting does not soon begin automatically, tickle the vomit reflex at the back of the throat with a feather or finger until at least the same amount of water that was taken in has been vomited up. Repeat this process a second time if the poisonous substance has not been completely expelled.

Professional medical assistance should be obtained as soon as possible.

A strong tea of cinnamon is effective against simple poisoning caused by spoiled food. Using a heaping teaspoon steeped in a cup of boiling water. The tea can be sweetened to taste with honey and one or two cups taken over the course of a couple of hours.

Licorice tea is also a good treatment against most kinds of poisoning, and if taken strong enough and in sufficient amount will serve as a good emetic.

For amanita mushroom poisoning or poisons that can severely damage the liver, use silybum extract or the powder or extract of milk thistle seeds. To help rebuild the liver, about one teaspoon of the powdered seeds should be taken every hour and a half for the first four days and then only three times a day. Dandelion root is also very effective in reducing the impact of substances that are damaging to the liver.

Caustic or Chemical Poisoning

Never induce vomiting: A chemical poison can cause permanent damage to the esophagus when it comes back up. Instead, immediately flood the stomach with a mucilaginous substance such as milk, slippery elm, marshmallow root, or mild licorice tea; oatmeal is also good. Use anything that will protect the stomach lining and dilute the substance.

Professional medical assistance should be obtained at once, if at all possible.

Drug Poisoning

Begin by inducing vomiting if at all appropriate. If the drug is a type that is a sedative, then a stimulant such as coffee or hot pepper should be given. The patient should be given a cold shower and otherwise not be allowed to fall into a coma.

For amphetamine or stimulant type of poisoning, give a warm bath and strong sedative nervines such as valerian and skullcap tea or tincture. A hot footbath is also helpful. Get professional medical assistance if possible.

Alcohol Poisoning (Drunkenness or Hangover)

This is a condition in which one can feel better by either stimulation or sedation therapy. A simple tea made with warm ginger and lemon juice can be very helpful, as can skullcap tea, made by steeping a teaspoon in a cup of boiling water. Skullcap is also effective in withdrawal from either alcohol or drugs. A half cup of the tea, sweetened with honey to taste, should be taken every hour or two, tapering off as the acute stages of withdrawal subside.

Kudzu root or kudzu flower is a near specific against hangover and can be brewed into a tea with a couple of slices of fresh ginger root per cup of boiling water.

Homeopathically one should use nux vomica 6th to 30th potency.

PREGNANCY AND CHILDBIRTH

Pregnancy is not a disease. However, there are many symptoms accompanying this condition for which various natural remedies have been recognized by women throughout the world as most helpful.

Red raspberry leaf *(Rubus idaeus)* is one of the most

common herbs safe to take throughout pregnancy. It contains fragarine, which is a uterine relaxant and tonic. Being a very mild and gentle herb, there is no danger from its use and it should be taken throughout but especially during the last three months. Red raspberry is good to aid in female fertility by helping the egg implant into the uterus and preventing miscarriage, for morning sickness, to prepare the uterus for delivery, and finally to aid in stopping bleeding and restoring the uterus after delivery to normalcy. Make the tea using one ounce of the dried leaves steeped in a pint of boiling water. If preferred, raspberry leaf can be purchased as a powder in tablets or gelatin capsules.

Many herbs with emmenagogue properties (promoting menstruation) are contraindicated during pregnancy. This includes the regular use of spicy, acrid-tasting herbs that contain volatile oils as well as strong purging or laxative herbs. Thus, overuse of herbs such as ginger root, garlic, parsley, mints, pennyroyal, and angelica, for instance, on a regular basis is not recommended.

As stated in other sections, some recent research indicates possible dangers, especially to the fetus, from the regular use of herbs containing pyrolizidine alkaloids. Because of this it may be a good idea to avoid using herbs such as comfrey, borage, senecio, coltsfoot, boneset, and petasites during pregnancy and for infants and young children.

Infertility: There can be many causes for infertility both in terms of the man as well as the woman.

Male Infertility: To increase sperm count in men use, Planetary formula number 73 (Schizandra Adrenal complex). Ashwagandha *(Withania somnifera)* from the Ayurvedic tradition is one of the most effective reproductive tonics for both men and women. One should take thirty drops of the liquid extract three times daily. Other herbs that are good for men to use to increase their potency include garlic, saw palmetto *(Serranoa serrulata)*, and ginseng.

Female Infertility: Use herbs such as dong quai *(Angelica sinensis)*, false unicorn root *(Chaemalirium luteum)*, chaste berries *(Agnus castus)*, and saw palmetto. Chinese dong quai seems to contain important saponins which act as hormone precursors that will regulate menstruation and fertility and the general health of the female. It is taken as a tea or cooked with organic chicken or lamb with ginger. This can increase sexual responsiveness and fertility, treat anemia, regulate menses, and relieve cramps.

Anther important herb from the Native American tradition is false unicorn root, also called helonias *(Chaemalirium luteum)*. It is used for all gynecological problems and is specifically a tonic for female infertility. It is also taken together with cramp bark or black haw bark for menstrual irregularities and pains and to prevent miscarriage.

Both dong quai and false unicorn are in Planetary formula number 98 (Dong Quai Treasure). Many women who were unable to become pregnant have reported doing so after taking this formula regularly three times a day for approximately three months. It should not be taken during menstruation or pregnancy unless specifically recommended by an herbalist.

To Prevent Miscarriage: Most commonly, herbalists use a combination of tincture of true unicorn *(Aletris farinosa)* and either black haw or cramp bark to prevent miscarriage. It is taken three times a day as a preventative or frequently for threatened miscarriage. The woman should confine herself to bed at the first sign of miscarriage. This combination has a wide application of usage as a normalizer for all menstrual irregularities including cramps, pains, and PMS.

Morning Sickness: A pinch of cloves, cinnamon, or ginger taken in hot chamomile and red raspberry leaf tea can be most helpful. Both wild yam *(Dioscorea villosa)* and peach leaves seem to be effective for many women with this problem. They can be combined with raspberry and peppermint or spearmint leaves in a tea for morning sickness *(see* HYPERACIDITY).

Homeopathic nux vomica 30x and/or Planetary formula number 23 (Digestive Discomfort) is often very effective to relieve morning sickness.

To Calm a Restless Fetus: Skullcap herb tea or tincture can be taken for this problem.

Anemia: Many women experience mineral deficiencies during pregnancy. Most common is a lack of iron and calcium. For increased iron, eat more beets, nettle and yellow dock root tea, and blackstrap molasses; cook foods in iron pots and skillets. To increase calcium and other minerals, take seaweed and sesame seeds. Some women may do well to take a glass of scalded warm milk with blackstrap molasses each day.

Another remedy to counteract anemia and raise the red blood cell count is to make a syrup using yellow dock root and blackstrap molasses. One or two tablespoons of this should be taken two or three times a day. Another method is to make a tincture or extract of yellow dock root to be taken along with a tablespoon of blackstrap molasses. Other good food sources of calcium include dairy, salmon, sardines (eat the bones), almonds, tahini butter, dark leafy greens, beets, carrots, broccoli, kale, and turnip tops. A traditional method used by country folk is to make a soup stock of the bones of organically raised or wild animals. Fruits such as figs, prunes, and raisins supply both iron and calcium.

Labor and Delivery: To facilitate and hasten labor, use a tincture of black and/or blue cohosh root and spikenard. This can be taken as a tincture in the dose of five to ten drops in hot water two or three times a day, beginning about four weeks before due date. During the actual labor itself, the same dose can be taken every hour or two along with sips of raspberry leaf tea.

Many women appreciate sucking on ice cubes of raspberry leaf tea throughout pregnancy. This is good for all stages of delivery as well as helping to bring down the placenta. According to herbalist Suzun Weed, raspberry is important to use throughout pregnancy because it keeps the "uterus working strongly and smoothly." To help soften the cervix, massage oil of evening primrose directly on it.

Placenta Delivery: To facilitate delivering the placenta, use equal parts blue cohosh *(Caulophyllum thalictroides)* with spikenard *(Aralia racemosa)* tincture, fifty drops every half hour if necessary. Another near specific for bringing down the placenta is a tea of ground ivy *(Glechoma hederacea)*. It can be combined with a smaller portion of sweet basil or lemon balm if available.

Postpartum Bleeding: If the placenta has not yet been delivered, use an extract or tea of witch hazel bark. To stop bleeding after the placenta has been delivered, use thirty drops of tincture of fresh shepherd's purse. This can be taken every thirty minutes if necessary. Other herbs that are good to use are trillium root and lady's mantle herb. A good Chinese herb to use is tienchi ginseng *(Panax pseudo-ginseng)* or the patented formula Yunnan Baiyao, which contains tienchi and is used by the Chinese for serious bleeding injuries.

Tonic and Postpartum Depression: To regain strength, give ginseng and dong quai root together either in tea or cooked in a soup or brown rice porridge. These should be taken for at least a week or two after delivery. Formulas number 6 and 25 are both excellent to take as a tonic for the mother after delivery. Cherokee Indians insist that a woman rest for twenty-six days, with a nutritionally rich diet, a lot of berries, if available, and wild American ginseng. St. Johnswort *(Hypericum perfoliatum)* can also be given in tincture or extract to treat depression.

Planetary formula number 39 (Ginseng Elixir), tonifying both energy and blood, is the ideal formula for recovery from childbirth. In fact, it is beneficial for recovering from any debilitating sickness, trauma, or surgery. Ashwagandha liquid extract is also good to take. For postpartum depression, formula number 10 (Bupleurum Calmative) is used.

Mastitis: Many women develop engorged and inflamed breasts after giving birth or while tending nursing children. Specific herbs that clear up this problem are dandelion root tea taken together with a combination of three parts echinacea root tincture and one part poke root *(Phytolacca americana)*. The dose is ten to thirty drops three or four times daily.

Breast-feeding Problems: Specifically, a tea of crushed fennel, anise, caraway, cumin, dill, or fenugreek are all excellent for increasing mother's milk. Vervain is another herb that is good for this purpose. To make the milk richer, give marshmallow root tea. For cracked or sore nipples, use an ointment of comfrey and/or calendula. Finally, to dry milk flow, give sage tea. Infuse a half teaspoon of dried sage leaf in a cup of water and have three cups daily.

In addition, nursing women require extra nutrients and should take extra vitamin E, B-complex, and lecithin. Vitamin B could be taken in the form of two to five tablespoons of brewer's yeast daily.

PSORIASIS

DESCRIPTION AND SYMPTOMS: A chronic skin disease with associated scaly, red patches.

CAUSES: Psoriasis can have hereditary factors, also aggravated by acid caused by foods and drink, and emotional stress.

TREATMENT: Eliminate overly stimulating and refined foods, including strong spices, coffee, alcohol, MSG, and sugar in all forms. Try to follow the balanced diet suggestions in Chapter Three. Internally, take Planetary formula number 99 (Yellow Dock Skin Cleanse). Topically, dab garlic and olive oil over the affected areas. Make a tea with the following herbs: equal parts sarsaparilla root, burdock seed, and red clover blossoms, and add a quarter part each of ginger (a couple of slices of fresh ginger will do) and lobelia herb or seed. If you can't purchase all of these, simply use sarsaparilla root. Simmer a large handful of the herbal combination in three cups of distilled water (regular water also will work but distilled is always better for extraction) for thirty minutes. Remember, medicine teas need to be strong. You can make a half gallon at a time by increasing the percentage of herbs and water. Keep it refrigerated and periodically dab some of the tea over the affected areas. Drink a cup three times daily or a half cup four times spread out throughout the day before taking food. You will see positive effects within two weeks of following this protocol.

SCIATICA

OTHER NAMES: Lumbago, and other back pains.

DESCRIPTION AND SYMPTOMS: Pain and inflammation of the sciatic nerve which radiates down from the lower back of the leg. Sciatica is specifically a neurological pain, but many of the natural treatments for back pain work well for other types of pains, including lumbago, neuritis, and rheumatic and arthritic pains, including pains caused by slipped or ruptured disks.

CAUSES: It can be caused by a chill, exposure to damp, eating too many cold and raw foods, and poor circulation; also, highly acidic foods such as coffee, sugar, white flour, and alcohol. Any or all of these can cause nerve blockage and congestion of the blood and lymphathic system.

TREATMENT: In treating sciatica, be sure that the bowels are regular. If not, use a mild herbal laxative such as triphala each night.

A number of herbal remedies taken both internally as well as externally are effective for back pain and sciatica. One approach is to drink and bathe in stinging nettle tea (Urtica urens). If possible, pick fresh stinging nettles with gloves and use a good potful of fresh nettles per tub of water. If only the dry is available, use two to four ounces per tub of water and, if available, add several slices of fresh ginger root to the tea.

Another way to use nettles is to brush a fresh branch over the affected area. This is good for sciatica, lumbago, neuritis, and other arthritic pains. Brushing a branch of nettles over the skin of the affected area will bring instant relief. Similarly, another effective folk remedy is to capture a live bee in a jar and place it over the painful part, letting the bee sting the affected part. Be sure that you do not have any allergies to bee stings before doing this, however.

One favorite treatment for sciatica used by Cherokee herbalist David Winston is a combined extract of sweet melilot *(Melilotus alba)*, dodder *(Cuscuta americana)*, and sweet or black birth *(Betula lenta)*. This can be taken as a tea or extract three times daily. In addition, drink three glasses of fresh celery juice daily.

Another tea for both sciatica and arthritis can be made from dried mulberry bark *(Morus alba)*, angelica *(Angelica archangelica)*, and teasel root *(Dipsacus sylvestris)*.

An external fomentation of grated ginger *(see* "Poultices, Plasters, and Fomentations" in Chapter 2) can be applied over the affected area. This is even more effective if it is preceded by rubbing on a coat of castor oil.

A liniment of wintergreen oil rubbed over the area will offer symptomatic relief. One can also make a homemade liniment by mixing a tablespoon of cayenne pepper, myrrh, and goldenseal in rubbing alcohol or apple cider vinegar. To help extract the properties of the herbs into the vinegar, heat them for a short while in a covered pan. In this way, they will be ready to use immediately.

Internally, an analgesic powder of willow bark, rosemary herb, poplar bark, angelica, and wintergreen leaf can be combined in equal amounts. Take two 00–size gelatin capsules of this powder every two or three hours with warm water, red poplar, or chamomile tea. If all of these herbs are not available, just willow bark and rosemary alone will be sufficient.

Specifically for nerve pains such as sciatica and neuritis, a tincture of St. Johnswort, ten to twenty drops taken every two hours, is very effective. For general pains and the pain of a ruptured or slipped disk, a strong tea of chamomile made by steeping one ounce of the flowers in a pint of water until cool enough to drink will help tremendously. One should take at least three cups of this strong chamomile tea each day.

Cupping the affected areas of the back will usually bring immediate temporary and sometimes permanent relief. Cupping (*see* Chapter 4, "Acupuncture and Related Therapies") draws the congested blood up to the surface of the skin, thus allowing for renewed circulation of blood to the deeper underlying tissues.

For many cases in which cupping or other methods are not effective, indirect moxibustion (*see* Chapter 4) applied over the affected areas can produce excellent and fast results. Moxibustion should be done until the area being treated takes on a flushed, reddish appearance. Again, this signals the blood coming to the surface of the skin with the resultant ease of deeper circulation. Moxibustion is different in that the heat works to open and dilate the capillaries and veins, relieving spasm and tension and easing circulation.

Diet while treating sciatica should be light and simple. Avoid coffee, alcohol, and sugar, and try to eat more whole grains, steamed vegetables, and a small amount of legumes or beans.

While some form of external treatment is usually necessary, internally, according to Traditional Chinese Medicine, sciatica is very often a metabolic condition involving the kidneys and adrenals. Even Western drugstores used to sell kidney pills to relieve back pain. Planetary Formulas has a number of internal remedies that have proven to be very beneficial for sciatica, such as formula 52 (Lower Back Support) and formula number 41 (Glucosamine-MSM Herbal).

SEXUAL DYSFUNCTION

OTHER NAMES: Frigidity, impotence.

DESCRIPTION: Impotence is the inability of a man to perform sexual intercourse. Frigidity is sexual unresponsiveness or lack of interest in sex, usually in a woman. A related condition in women is vaginismus, which is involuntary spasm of the vagina, preventing entry of the penis.

SYMPTOMS: A man suffering from impotence is unable to have or maintain an erection, or he may not be able to ejaculate. Frigidity is characterized by the woman's inability to reach orgasm. In vaginismus, the vagina is extremely sensitive and closes spasmodically at the slightest touch.

CAUSES: There are numerous physical problems that can cause or contribute to sexual dysfunction, but usually there is also a psychological component. Physical causes include nerve paralysis, anatomic defects, side effects of certain drugs, alcohol (which reduces sexual responsiveness), injury or disease, hormonal insufficiency, general poor health, excessive sexual activity (either with a partner or by masturbation), and long periods of abstinence (particularly in older men).

Psychological factors impairing sexual functioning include lack of desire for the partner, lack of self-confidence, feelings of guilt, emotional stress, and deep-rooted negative attitudes toward sexuality and intimacy. In men there also may be a fear of failing to "perform," and in women a fear of pregnancy.

TREATMENT: Physical causes should be identified and dealt with. If appropriate, a cleansing diet should be undertaken to improve general health and physical functioning. Recommended dietary supplements include vitamin E, zinc, magnesium, carnitine, selenium, and, for men, manganese. Mexican damiana increases blood flow to the pelvic area but must be taken daily for a month or longer. Ginseng is a general stimulant and rejuvenator. Other herbs that are considered to have some aphrodisiac properties are artichoke, celery root, cloves, European vervain, fenugreek, jasmine, matico, peppermint, onion, common plantain, savory, saw palmetto berries, and water eryngo.

There are many herbs that are known to stimulate and build sexual energy. For women, one of the very best is dong quai. For men, there are many, including ginseng and ashwagandha. Ashwagandha *(Withania somnifera)* is the primary tonic herb in the Indian Ayurvedic tradition. It is beneficial for all debilitating conditions, including fatigue and reproductive weakness in both men and women. Popularly known as Indian ginseng, unlike ginseng, ashwagandha will relieve stress and promote sound, restful sleep. Michael has found that the majority of individuals who take thirty drops of ashwagandha liquid extract three times daily over the course of one or two months will experience a sense of rejuvenation in their sex life and often not realize that it is at least partially due to Ashwagandha.

One herb from the Chinese tradition is known popularly as horny goat weed *(Epimedium grandiflorum)* because it was seen how livestock that grazed near this plant had noticeable, increased sexual activity. It is considered a major libido enhancer in the Chinese herbal tradition, but how it works is not as yet fully understood. It seems to stimulate nerves throughout the body, especially in the genital area, in both men and women. The result is increased sexual desire, reduced fatigue, and enhanced erectile function. It may increase testosterone levels, having an androgen effect on the testes, prostate, and sexual muscles. However, it is not contraindicated for prostate enlargement; in fact, it will help normalize the prostate. Despite its benefits for men, it is no less beneficial for women; in fact, the herb is effective in relieving hot flashes associated with menopause. Horny goat weed and ginseng are two of the sexual rejuvenative herbs in Planetary formula number 13 (Damiana Male Potential).

Another herb, from the Peruvian Andes, is known to enhance sexual energy: maca *(Lepidium peruvianum chacon)*. It is a root vegetable that has been used by the natives since before the Incas. Perhaps some of the potency of this remarkable herb comes from the fact that it seems to thrive on the most rugged and barren mountain peaks of the Andes, where there are subfreezing temperatures each night. When the Spanish brought their sheep to this area they noticed they were reproducing poorly. The natives suggested they feed them maca, and the results were so amazing that they demanded maca as payment from the colonies. The libido- and fertility-enhancing properties of this root-herb may be due in part to its high content of bioavailable iodine—which enhances thyroid function—zinc, amino acids, and vitamin C. Maca is a nutritionally dense root high in protein and carbohydrates. It contains vitamins B_1, B_2, B_{12}, C, and E and is a source of glycoside steroids, which in other plants are known to be responsible for their tonic properties generally and sexual energy–enhancing properties especially. Maca is available in Planetary formulas, but it is most useful to purchase a large container of the powder distributed by Imperial Gold (http://ahealthya.com/maca.htm) so it can be taken freely with food, not only because it helps sexual function, but because it is a high-powered food good for maintaining a general sense of well-being. The taste is not unpleasant and is similar to a turnip, to which it is related. Interestingly, when maca is boiled in water it becomes very sweet.

There are a number of specific treatments used by acupuncturists for revivifying sexual energy. One that individuals can do on themselves is to use moxibustion, making the area directly above the pubic bone on the abdomen red (without burning). Another area to apply moxa to is directly on the spine on the small of the back between lumbar numbers two and three.

While heat is beneficial for restoring sexual energy, alternating cold and hot sitz baths also helps awaken nerve force in the pelvic area. Aerobic and stretching exercises such as yoga are also beneficial for maintaining sexual potency. Spinal manipulation of the lumbar and sacral areas may be indicated. If you have low back pain, consult your doctor.

Dealing with psychological causes is likely to require professional counseling, preferably with both partners involved. In any case, an understanding partner is essential. Men should know that occasional impotence is normal, and worrying about it only perpetuates it. For preorgasmic women, special classes are available that teach them about their bodies, explore their feelings about their own sexuality, and teach specific techniques for achieving orgasm. Once a woman is more secure in her own sexuality, she can convey this confidence to her partner and teach her partner in a nonthreatening way how to be responsive to her needs.

SINUSITUS

(*SEE* ALLERGIC RHINITIS)

SWEATING HANDS

Soaking the hands for ten to thirty minutes once or twice daily in a tannic acid brew such as oak bark tea or black tea will help to contract the skin to prevent excessive sweating. If one uses black tea, use approximately five tea bags per quart of water; alternatively one can use four or five tablespoons of oak bark to a quart of water. Musicians, especially pianists and string players, are prone to excessive hand sweating as a result of performance nervousness. This also can be an annoying symptom during performance and can give rise to skin fungus conditions of the hands. An immediate treatment is to wipe the hands with a cloth saturated with alcohol. This could be rubbing alcohol or gin or vodka.

SWOLLEN LYMPHATIC GLANDS (INCLUDING GOITER)

DESCRIPTION: A gland is an organ that manufactures and secretes a substance for use by the body. The body contains a wide variety of glands, whose secretions range from relatively simple substances (for example, sweat) to complex hormones that affect our most basic functions and emotions. Problems with swelling generally involve the lymph glands or nodes in the neck, the armpits, or the groin. The thyroid gland in the neck may also become enlarged, a condition known as goiter.

SYMPTOMS: The main symptom is the swelling itself, which can vary from slight to extreme. The swollen area may also be red, painful, and sensitive to the touch; fever may be present as well.

CAUSES: Although there are many specific glandular diseases that could result in swollen glands, most commonly the swelling is associated with the body's attempts to fight an infection or illness in a nearby organ. Since the lymph glands produce the white blood cells (leukocytes) that are the body's first line of defense against invasion by foreign organisms, they may swell in response to the heavy demand put on them when infection strikes. The swelling of goiter, on the other hand, may be due to a deficiency of iodine in the diet, to overproduction of iodine by the thyroid gland, or to an inability of the thyroid to process iodine properly.

TREATMENT: The first step in treating swollen glands is to determine the cause and treat it. In most cases, the swelling of the glands will go away when the cause that triggered it is dealt with. However, if the swelling has not gone down after about three weeks, or if other glands become swollen, consult a doctor. In the meantime, the symptoms may be eased by applying cold compresses made with vinegar or decoctions of oak bark, English walnut leaves, fenugreek seeds, burdock leaves, fennel, or thyme. Use of a mild herbal laxative that acts systemically such as cascara bark or triphala can increase the healing process in those with excess conformation. Ginseng tea is said to promote the restoration of natural balance to glandular activity.

Because a swelling of the thyroid gland at the front of the neck can have such diverse causes, it is best not to attempt to treat goiter without professional consultation. If increased iodine intake is indicated, use natural forms such as occur in seafood and edible seaweeds (dulse, laver, Irish moss, edible kelp).

One herb that is nearly specific for swollen glands is dried poke root. This should be used carefully so as to avoid any possible hypersensitive reaction to the herb. Begin by taking only one 00-size capsule three times a day with warm water. Generally it is best to combine it with other herbs so as to prevent any possible uncomfortable reactions. Thus poke root is included in the following formulation: equal parts poke root, burdock root, dandelion root, sarsaparilla root, echinacea root, chaparral leaves, Oregon grape root, licorice root, and kelp. This can be either taken in a tea or ground into a powder and taken in two to four 00-size capsules three times daily with boiled warm water or a tea of red clover blossoms.

Formulas number 12, 14 (Blood Purifier), and 15 are also beneficial to take along with two to six grams kelp, three times a day.

Homeopathic remedies include belladonna 6th to 30th if there is associated high fever; hepar sulph 6th if there is pain and suppuration; hepar sulph 6th after the pus has ceased to form. Generally swollen glands and most glandular problems are effectively treated with poke root tincture as well as with homeopathic 6th potency of phytolacca (poke root).

THROAT INFLAMMATION

(*SEE* LARYNGITIS, HOARSENESS AND INFLUENZA)

THYROID DISEASES

The thyroid gland is located at the lower front base of the neck. It is responsible for the secretion of hormones that serve to regulate metabolism throughout the body. As a result, thyroid hormones affect every cell of the body. Still another important link in this process is the role of the adrenal gland, which is also responsible for sending hormonal signals to the pituitary gland (located in the brain) to release thyroid stimulating hormone (FSH).

One's metabolism is to a considerable extent determined by genetics, stress, diet, climate, and other factors. It is estimated for instance that if anyone in one's immediate family has had low thyroid, there is at least a 50 percent chance that any of the progeny will also have or develop low thyroid. This is very important in determining the likelihood of a naturally occurring thyroid condition.

The primary thyroid diseases are hypothyroid (low thyroid) and hyperthyroid (high thyroid). There is also Grave's disease, which usually stems from overeating known goitrogenic foods, including all the cruciferous family vegetables, such as cabbage, mustard, broccoli, kale, collards, bok choy, and turnips, and also cassava root, soy, peanuts, pinenuts, and millet. Cooking usually inactivates goitrogens. One can take supplemental iodine-rich kelp or dulse daily, especially when consuming any of these foods, to further negate the adverse thyroid-depressing effects. Traditionally, mountain and inland people whose diet lacked iodine most commonly developed goiters. This has been largely remedied by the inclusion of trace amounts of iodine in salt.

Symptoms of hypothyroid correspond to what Chinese traditionally diagnosed as "deficient yang" and includes slow pulse, cold intolerance, fatigue, depression, coarse, dry skin, tingling in the extremities, dry hair (particularly the outer third of the eyebrows), elevated cholesterol, muscle cramps and spasms, heavier and more frequent menses, constipation, and digestive weakness, including bloating, heartburn, and loss of appetite. Low thyroid is often the underlying factor causing abnormal weight gain; it is also associated with chronic fatigue, fibromyalgia, candida yeast overgrowth, osteoporosis, and heart disease, to name a few chronic conditions.

Symptoms of hyperthyroid include rapid pulse (90 bpm or greater), heat sensitivity, hyperactivity, irritability, nervousness, insomnia, inability to gain weight, bulging eyeballs, and menstrual irregularity. Diet and herbs that have a cooling nature should be used before resorting to conventional treatment for hyperthyroid, which usually involves surgically removing part of the thyroid gland or giving spot radiation or a drug that will depress its function.

Graves' disease is when a goiter has formed due to a hyperthyroid condition. Hashimoto's disease is an autoimmune inflammatory reaction to one's own thyroid secretions and may necessitate the use of synthetic thyroid hormone as a replacement for one's own.

In the main we will confine ourselves to the subject of hyperthyroid and hypothyroid.

DIAGNOSING THYROID FUNCTION

There are three methods for diagnosing thyroid function. The first and undoubtedly the most important is the pronounced manifestation of a number of the above-mentioned clinical symptoms. The second is evaluating one's basal temperature, and the third is through laboratory blood analysis.

Taking Your Basal Temperature

Fortunately, evaluating one's basal metabolism is a simple procedure requiring only a thermometer that can be done at home.

PROCEDURE

1. Begin by shaking down the thermometer below 95° F and placing it on a table near your bed before retiring each night.
2. First thing upon waking, place the thermometer under your armpit for a full ten minutes. It is important to lie as still as possible, eyes closed.
3. After ten minutes, read and record the temperature and date on a pad of paper.
4. Repeat this for at least three mornings around the same time each day.

This should not be performed by women during the first day of menstruation, and ideally should be done on the second, third, and fourth days of menstruation. Men or postmenopausal women can perform this test at any time.

INTERPRETATION

One's basal body temperature should be between 97.6 and 98.2°F. Low basal body temperatures are common and can be an indication of hypothyroidism, especially if this accompanies other clinical signs and symptoms described above. High basal body temperatures, above 98.6°F, are less common and can indicate hyperthyroidism. Again, this is especially true if this is accompanied by clinical signs.

Thyroid blood tests measure the amount of TSH (thyroid stimulating hormone) that is present in the blood, thyroxin (T4), as well as its conversion into free T3. TSH is a hormone used as a signal from the pituitary gland of the secretion of thyroid hormone. Therefore, paradoxically, in this test, when TSH levels are high it means the thyroid is low.

One should also specify measuring T4 and free T3 levels. T4 is secreted by the thyroid and must be converted into T3 to regular body metabolism.

Thyroid function, whether high or low, corresponding to Chinese yin-yang conditions, can create an underlying predisposition to a wide number of chronic acute and degenerative diseases. Hypothyroidism, corresponding to Chinese-deficient yang, is estimated to affect as much as 40 percent of the population, with more conservative estimates putting it around 25 percent, with women being 20 percent and men around 5 percent. This is further reflected by the fact that the most common drugs, Synthroid and Levothyroxin, which is synthetic thyroid hormone, is the third most widely prescribed drug in the United States.

Conventional medical treatment for hypothyroid in all but its mildest forms involves the use of either animal-derived desiccated thyroid or synthetic hormone. The difference between the two is that synthetic thyroid hormone does not contain T3. It is felt that since T4 will eventually change into T3 the latter is not needed. In many cases this is true. However, there is some concern that an organic will always be superior to its synthetic counterpart. In fact, in the world of thyroid regulation this is not always true. Some individuals manifest an allergic reaction to desiccated thyroid with symptoms of skin itchiness and possible hyperactivity due to too much T3. This can and should be determined through blood analysis. In such instances synthetic thyroid is actually preferable. There are other cases where a combination of natural and synthetic work best for some individuals. This needs to be determined medically by someone who has experience in treating low thyroid. One of the best resources for hypothyroid on the Internet is http://thyroid.about.com/mbody.htm, where one can share discussion and information with other individuals with hypothyroid and learn about qualified thyroid practitioners.

TREATMENT: For hyperthyroid, one herb that is known to be effective is bugleweed *(Lycopus virginicus)*. This herb is known to interfere with iodine metabolism, which inhibits the formation of TSH and blocks the conversion of thyroxin (T4) to T3. One can make a tea by steeping a teaspoon of the dried herb in a cup of boiling water (covered) or of the 1:5 liquid extract, taking ten to thirty drops three times daily. Lemon balm *(Melissa officinalis)*, self-heal *(Prunella vulgaris)*, and blue vervaine *(Verbena hastata)* also are effective for hyperthyroid. As usual I recommend making a combination with equal parts of each of these herbs together with skullcap *(Scutellaria lateraflora)*. Foods to include would be more green leafy vegetables, soy, and millet, essentially all the foods one would limit for hypothyroid. This should be followed daily for at least three months.

Hypothyroid is more difficult to treat without taking some form of supplemental thyroid. However, there are a number of supplements and herbs that have proven themselves to be effective for hypothyroid. As stated, kelp and dulse are usually part of a hypothyroid program and as such play a greater or lesser role in the outcome. The Ayurvedic herbs coleus forsicholi *(C. forskohlii)* and the formula called guggul made from a variety of myrrh together with other herbs are used to stimulate thyroid function. Chinese medicine would prescribe deer antler and a variety of other herbs to stimulate yang energy.

Various nutritional supplements can be beneficial for normal thyroid function. These include zinc, vitamin E, vitamin A, vitamin C, and the B vitamins riboflavin (B_2), niacin (B_3), pyridoxine (B_6), and folic acid. One of the most useful supplements is the amino acid L-tyrosine, which is effective for counteracting stress and increasing energy.

TOOTHACHE

DESCRIPTION, SYMPTOMS, AND CAUSES: Pain from a decaying tooth.

TREATMENT: Symptomatic treatment is oil of cloves applied to the tooth. Rubbing a tincture of cayenne pepper and echinacea root over the affected area is also very effective. Prickly ash bark in the form of tincture or powder of prickly ash bark is a specific to relieve toothache problems.

TUBERCULOSIS

DESCRIPTION AND SYMPTOMS: Tuberculosis can affect any tissue of the body, but its most common site is the lungs. It may begin with a simple respiratory ailment, often mistaken for bronchitis. As it advances, the following symptoms arise: low fever, dry cough, shortness of breath, night and standing perspiration, extreme fatigue, weight loss, and low appetite. In an advanced state, there is coughing of blood.

CAUSE: While TB is no longer a major threat in Western countries, in countries where there is rampant malnutrition, poor hygiene, and inefficient methods of early diagnosis, it is still very much a problem. TB is spread by the tubercle bacillus, which can be contracted airborne from other infected individuals or transmitted through the unpasteurized milk of infected cows.

Once inside the body, the tubercle bacillus can remain dormant for years, gradually weakening the body's immune system, giving the bacillus a chance to multiply. When the bacilli have reached a sufficient magnitude, then the disease develops its more active phase.

TREATMENT: Success in the treatment of tuberculosis is dependent upon early detection. This is a serious disease that responds well to a combination of Western and traditional natural healing methods.

Diagnosis is through early detection through a chest X ray or a skin test. The skin test involves injecting a small among of tuberculin solution under the skin of the forearm and then checking for a reaction a few days later. A small hard patch of raised bumps develops on the arm. If the bumps remain small, the test is considered negative. If they exceed a certain size, then the test is considered positive.

If the disease is in an active stage, then the patient will probably have to undergo an extended period of hospital confinement. Modern drugs should not be ignored in the treatment of tuberculosis. These include isoniazid (or INH), PAS, streptomycin, and ethambutol. The strategy is to first make the patient noncontagious and secondly to eliminate the bacilli from the body.

Unfortunately, for certain sensitive patients, these drugs do have harmful side effects, especially upon the liver. This is where the addition of certain protective herbs and supplements can be of great help in preventing and lessening the side effects.

Each day one should make a porridge with six ounces of Chinese astragalus root and six Chinese red jujube dates. These are first made into a tea by cooking in three cups of water slowly down to two cups. The tea is strained and to it is added one-half cup of brown rice, which is cooked on a very low flame (in a slow cooker, for instance) overnight. This porridge is taken as breakfast each morning.

The Ayurvedic Chyavanprash formula should be taken, two tablespoons three times daily. American ginseng is also taken, about 500 mg three times a day. For the liver, silybum seed extract should be taken with dandelion root tea three times a day. Finally, garlic should be taken, about 1,500 mg of raw or partially deodorized garlic, three times daily.

Vitamin therapy can include:

Vitamin A (25,000 units)	1 capsule daily
Vitamin B-complex (100-mg formula)	1–3 times daily
Vitamin C (1,000 mg)	1–3 times daily
Vitamin E (400 units)	1–3 times daily
Folic acid (300 mcg)	1–3 times daily
Pangamic acid	1–3 times daily

A building diet consisting of two or three poached or boiled eggs is taken daily with whole wheat toast or served on top of a dish of brown rice and black beans. Between meals one should have a soya protein drink. Other meals should consist of whole grains, steamed vegetables, beans (especially black beans), rice, and about four to eight ounces of organic lamb, poultry, or fish each day.

ULCERS

OTHER NAMES: Duodenal ulcers, esophageal ulcers, stomach or peptic ulcers, ulcerative colitis.

DESCRIPTION: As described above, ulcers can form in different areas of the gastrointestinal tract. Essentially they are open sores, with rawness and disintegration of the surrounding tissue. In the case of ulcerative colitis, besides the severer abdominal pain, there are profuse and frequent blood stools with mucus and pus. Fever and a general feeling of discomfort are associated with possible attendant anemia.

SYMPTOMS: Ulcers, regardless of their location, are usually quite painful. The pain will be aggravated by any strong spices or foods that stimulate extreme acid reactions.

CAUSES: There are many possible causes, making it difficult to label any one cause as the primary cause for everyone. For some, stress is a prime consideration as a cause of ulcers. Others are very susceptible to certain foods such as dairy, coffee, chili, sugar, sodas, and citrus. Tobacco and alcohol are also factors to consider. Finally, one should not rule out the possibility of parasites either as a present or past cause.

In one test, it was demonstrated that there was a definite correlation with the use of dairy products and the presence of ulcers. A significant number of patients who were taken off of dairy products recovered completely over the course of a year, and when a few resumed the dairy, their ulcers returned.

Aspirin has been shown to be another possible cause of ulcers. Too-frequent use of it will stimulate acid reaction and aggravate bleeding.

Finally, another medically induced cause of ulcers is the abuse of steroid drugs to relieve pain such as the pain of arthritis. The problem with these kinds of ulcers is that they often appear without the usual associated pains and bleeding. Considering that they have a high incidence of hemorrhage and perforation, these kinds of ulcers can be very dangerous.

TREATMENT: Bed rest may be necessary, at least in the initial two weeks of treatment. The diet should be well-cooked porridge and puréed vegetables, taken in small, frequent amounts. A good herbal combination is that of the powders of slippery elm and marshmallow root, three tablespoons of each, made into a gruel by adding a little water until the desired consistency is formed. A small amount of honey can be added for flavor. This should be eaten three times a day and provides a significant source of nourishment.

Alfalfa tablets or alfalfa tea is another herbal remedy that many have found to be effective for the treatment of ulcers. The tablets can be taken freely every couple of hours.

Surprisingly, strong chamomile tea is one of the best treatments for ulcers. It is specific for ulcer symptoms which include spasm, inflammation, and ulceration. Often, it not only gives symptomatic relief but actually cures the problem. Use about six to ten heaping table-spoons of dried chamomile flowers steeped for twenty minutes in three cups of boiling water, covered.

It is best taken with the "roll over" technique. Drink one cup and first lie on the back for five or ten minutes, then turn to the left, then right, and finally, on the stom-ach—each position lasting about five minutes. This is to enable the strong chamomile tea to affect all the mucosa of the GI tract uniformly. This should be done about three times a day for maximum benefit.

Certain raw vegetable juices, especially fresh cabbage juice, has proven to be a very effective treatment for ul-cers. This can be combined with a little celery, carrot, or pineapple juice for flavor. An eight-ounce glass of the fresh juice should be taken three times a day. If you do not have a juicer, eating small amounts of raw cabbage leaves throughout the day will also be beneficial.

VARICOSE VEINS

DESCRIPTION AND SYMPTOMS: Swollen and en-gorged veins, usually on the legs.

CAUSES: There are many theories for the cause of vari-cosities, ranging from genetic weakness of the vein walls, excessive pressure caused by the strain of standing on one's feet for long periods or heavy lifting, inflammation, and nutritional deficiencies.

TREATMENT: One should try to alleviate any percepti-ble cause. At the same time there are a number of nutri-tional and herbal remedies that are effective for this condition. Butcher's broom *(Ruscus aculeatus)* has a long history of use for leg pains caused by swollen veins. It has both anti-inflammatory properties and astringent effects that are very beneficial for the veins. It also contains bioflavonoids, which are regarded as the most important vein nutrition. We find an abundance of bioflavonoids in citrus (especially the peel) and berries, especially hawthorn berries. They are especially abundant in buckwheat *(Fagopyrum esculentum)*. Studies substantiate that patients with varicose veins taking buckwheat or buckwheat tea daily over the course of a few weeks have significant improvement in capillary strength.

Another useful supplement for the treatment of varicose veins is bromelain. The antifibrinolytic activity of bromelain from pineapple breaks down any clots or other material that is likely to impair circulation.

One of the most popular herbs in Europe is horsechestnut *(Aesculus hippocastanum)*. This is one of the few herbs mentioned in this book that should be used only in carefully formulated commercial preparations standardized to 20 percent aescin or by a professional herbalist who is experienced in the use of this herb. Horsechestnut actually has the ability to improve the tone and tighten the elastic fibers of the veins in their walls. This remarkable herb is effective both externally and internally. Planetary formula number 47 (Vein Strength) is for internal use. It contains both butcher's broom and horsechestnut along with various highly potent herbs from the Chinese herbal tradition, such as tienchi ginseng and salvia root, that help circulation and the veins. Formula number 20 (Horsechestnut Cream) combines horsechestnut with butcher's broom, witch hazel bark extract, white oak bark extract, myrrh gum, and rosemary extract to form a cream effective for all varicosities, including varicose veins and hemorrhoids.

Vitamin E, along with a good fish oil supplement, should be taken daily for preventing and treating all varicosities.

WARTS

OTHER NAMES: Dermatomyositis, hyperkeratosis, plantar warts, venereal warts, verrucae.

DESCRIPTION AND SYMPTOMS: Warts are small growths that can occur and grow on various parts of the body. Plantar warts occur on the soles of the feet, while venereal warts occur on the reproductive organs.

CAUSES: Warts seem to be caused by a general weakening of the immune system and specifically by a virus. Venereal warts are regarded as a contagious disease.

TREATMENT: Warts on various parts of the body should be treated with a good blood-purifying or alternative tea such as formulas number 12, 13, and/or 14.

The following tea can also be taken: 4 parts yellow dock root, 4 parts sarsaparilla root, 1 part poke root, 4 parts echinacea root, 4 parts Oregon grape root, 3 parts chaparral leaf, 2 parts buckthorne bark, 4 parts sassafras bark, 1 part licorice root. Combine the herbs and use one or two teaspoons simmered for twenty minutes in a cup of boiling water (three or four cups can be made ahead of time); the dose is one cup three times daily.

Another remedy is to use St. Mary's thistle (Silybum marianum), which is good for the liver. This can be taken as a tincture, five to twenty drops in a cup of hot water to evaporate the alcohol, or as a tea.

External remedies will also hasten the removal of warts. There are a number of effective external remedies: taping a slice of fresh garlic over the wart each evening, rubbing on some fresh juice of the greater celandine herb, spurge, or the latex of dandelion.

The topical application of castor oil with crushed garlic is a very effective local treatment for plantar's warts. Another is to massage vitamin E in the form of an oil or cream directly on the wart, morning and evening.

One of the most specific remedies for warts is the tincture of the yellow cedar *(Thuja occidentalis),* topically applied morning and evening.

For venereal warts, medical doctors use extract of podophyllum, which is from the mandrake root. This is applied externally and will usually cause their removal. Applying the less irritating herbal remedies described above, such as castor oil or fresh dandelion juice, should also prove effective. Neem oil is also very effective.

However, it seems that if one does not combine the use of herbs internally, venereal warts at least seem to reoccur in many individuals. Systemically, one should take the tea and/or one of the liver-cleansing formulas mentioned above along with 25,000 units of vitamin A daily for one week to six months.

Finally, homeopathic thuja (yellow cedar) 6th to 30th potency taken three times a day for a week to one month is one of the most effective remedies for warts. Interestingly enough, it is also a useful antidote to the negative effects of vaccines, which may suggest that there is a relationship between the presence of warts, the suppression of the immune system, and the use of certain vaccines.

PART THREE

HYDROTHERAPY

Whoever understands the effects
of herbs and water
and how to use them
possesses the key
to nature's healing power.

INTRODUCTION TO METHODS
OF APPLICATION

Human beings have always instinctively used water and herbs to treat ailments, to relieve aches and pains, and to revitalize the body. But we no longer have to go on instinct in using these remedies: Scientifically designed methods of modern hydrotherapy have been developed and are universally applied at European regeneration spas.

The modern form of hydrotherapy developed gradually from the rigorous "water cure" made famous by Sebastian Kneipp in the nineteenth century. Critics often derided it as a "horse cure" because it consisted mainly of shocking cold-water treatments that only sturdy patients could tolerate. But the treatments worked.

Recognizing the value of hydrotherapy, European medical schools and universities started in about 1950 to devise a regimen that could be used by people of all ages and physical conditions. In doing so, they "gentled" the original methods so that the stimulus that produces the desired physiological reaction is moderated according to the patient's tolerance. As a result, we now have scientifically established methods of applying water and herbs in various forms that are prescribed just like any other remedy to provide specific healing effects.

All water treatments exert a *stimulus* on the body, which in turn produces a physiological *reaction* within the body. This process improves the circulation of blood to the surface tissues as well as to the deep-lying internal organs. The strength of the reaction depends on both the intensity of the stimulus and the vitality of the patient's own response. The strength of the stimulus varies with the size of the application (a footbath is a milder stimulant than a half bath, which in turn is milder than a full bath), the temperature of the water (the greater the difference between the water temperature and the body's normal temperature of 98.6°F, the stronger the stimulus is), the duration of the application (the longer an application lasts, the stronger the stimulus is), herbal or mineral additives used (the larger the quantity or the more potent the additives are, the stronger the stimulus is).

In general, the physiological reaction response to the stimulus can be recognized by the following signs:

Cold at first brings on an active constriction of the blood vessels in the part being treated and produces paleness, goose bumps, and a cold sensation. This is followed by an active dilation of the blood vessels, producing a rosy flush on the skin and a feeling of warmth and well-being—which is the essential physiological reaction.

Warm causes a passive dilation of the blood vessels, producing a rosy flush and a feeling of warmth and well-being. It is usually combined with a short, cold application to close the pores and produce a subsequent active dilation as the blood returns to the part of the body being treated.

In the following pages, we will describe the main modern forms and methods of hydrotherapy.

THE BATH

The most commonly used forms of baths are the full bath, the half bath, the sitz bath, the arm bath, the footbath, the face bath, the eye bath, and the steam bath.

Water temperature may range from cold to hot. With every cold application, certain rules apply.

Before taking a cold bath, you must be warm. The temperature in the bathroom must be at least 70°F. The patient should not undress before the bath is ready for use. If it is an early-morning bath, preparations can be made the night before. Without fail, after every cold application the patient must be rewarmed. This can be done most effectively by stimulating the body to generate its own internal warming response, as follows. After the bath, dry *only* the patient's head and hands. Then have the patient dress quickly in dry clothing. Make sure that all parts of the body except the head and hands are covered. Finally, have the patient exercise lightly by walking for as long as needed to dry the body and achieve normal warmth. If exercise is not possible, substitute dry and warm. Don't let the patient get warm to the point of sweating, however, because a cold would be sure to follow.

Where durations are given in the following descriptions, they refer to the actual immersion times. The activities preceding and following the baths should be done as quickly as possible.

THE FULL BATH

The full bath consists of immersion up to the neck in a tub of water.

THE COLD FULL BATH

TEMPERATURE: 64°F or, in most parts of the country, just as it flows from the cold-water tap.

DURATION: 6–10 seconds fully immersed. There is a range because the time depends on each patient's reaction response.

Cold full baths benefit the circulation, improve the metabolic process, and strengthen the nervous system. Initially, the cold bath puts the entire circulatory system under tension, and the heart will have to work harder at first. Therefore, cold baths are not suitable for some people who suffer from certain heart ailments. If there is any doubt, it is wise to check with your physician first.

Enter the bath slowly. First step in; then with rapid strokes wet your breast, back, and forehead. Lie back gradually. After the bath, get out quickly and follow the rewarming procedure described earlier.

If you are perspiring before taking the bath, sit down in the tub so that you are covered only to the stomach and wash the upper part of your body rapidly and vigorously. Then immerse yourself up to the neck for 2 to 3 seconds. Get out of the water at once and proceed as above.

The best time to take a cold bath is when you get up from bed in the morning. Otherwise, it should be taken 1 to 2 hours before a meal or no sooner than 2 hours after a meal.

THE WARM FULL BATH

TEMPERATURE: 98°–101°F.

DURATION: 10–20 minutes.

The warm full bath is used as an herbal bath (for a list of additives and their effects, *see* Herbal Bath Additives, pages 460–467). The warm bath can also be used for warming up before a cold-water application.

As a rule, the warm bath should not be taken more than two or three times a week; excessive use can be enervating.

Immediately after a warm full bath, a cold wash or cold gush is normally required, followed by a half hour to an hour of bed rest. If this bath is taken at night before going to bed, omit the cold application; instead, go right to bed after drying off. The warm full bath can lead to sleeplessness if a stimulating herbal additive has been used. To avoid difficulties with sleeping, use soothing, relaxing herbs such as valerian, hops, or balm.

Warm baths are particularly designed to improve the circulation of the blood so that the entire body gets better equipped to resist harmful organisms and diseases. Inhalation of herbal additives has an internal effect through the bronchial system and the lungs, promoting the evacuation of toxins that have accumulated in the blood. By adding the proper herb or herbs to the bath, you can create a soothing effect on any kind of inflammation or irritation. The glandular activity of the skin will generally be quite stimulated. Improved circulation of the blood helps the cleansing, regenerative, and eliminative processes necessary for cases of skin disease and skin infections that tend to heal very slowly.

The relaxing effect of warm baths on the vascular system brings about a corresponding relief from stress. Therefore, they are advisable in cases of muscular tension brought on by inflammation, by paralysis (stroke), and by stiffness of the joints. Exercises that are prescribed for such ailments are easier to perform in a warm bath and they cause less pain when done underwater.

Warm baths are often used to loosen up stiff joints, as in cases of arthritis and chronic rheumatism. They also usually have a very soothing effect on the nervous system. Depending on which herbal additives are used, they can be helpful for both high and low blood pressure. (*See* Herbal Bath Additives, pages 460–467, to select the herb with the desired properties.)

THE HOT FULL BATH

TEMPERATURE: 102°–112°F.

DURATION: 10–12 minutes. (As a rule, the higher the temperature, the shorter the duration.)

The hot full bath is a very strong treatment and is therefore not to be taken without trained supervision.

The procedure after the hot bath is the same as that for the warm full bath.

Any increase in the temperature of the bath also increases the activity of the heart: The heart will beat significantly faster to rush enough blood to the submerged skin areas. Therefore, people who suffer from heart ailments are less well equipped than others to tolerate the strain of hot full baths, and caution is advised. After a hot bath, a full cold wash— about three seconds—is recommended, followed by bed rest.

If a wrapper (*see* Wet Wrappers, pages 481–496) is applied instead of a cold wash right after the hot full bath, it will bring on profuse sweating. Such treatments are of great benefit, especially in cases of rheumatic diseases, some kinds of infections (such as catarrhal inflammation of the lungs), inflammation of the kidneys, and uremia. A hot full bath followed by a wrapper and bed rest for 1 to 2 hours is also effective in treating the common cold.

A cup of hot lemonade (the juice of one lemon in a cup of boiling water, plus a tablespoon of honey) is recommended immediately after getting into bed in the wrapper. A tablespoon of brandy in the cup is optional. The hot drink helps produce the perspiration that is needed. After the outbreak of perspiration, the wrapper should stay on at the most a half hour longer.

THE HALF BATH

In the half bath the water reaches only to the navel. For comparable temperature, duration, and procedure, the effect of the half bath is not as strong as that of the full bath.

THE COLD HALF BATH

TEMPERATURE: 59°F.

DURATION: 6–10 seconds.

This is an application that is used often. It produces a medium-strong stimulus. The preparations are the same as for the cold full bath. Be sure that you are feeling warm before entering the bath. The upper part of the body can remain covered to avoid chilling. Enter the bath slowly; then take some water in your hands and stroke the heart region and the lower back; sit down. Keep your arms out of the water by resting them on the rim of the tub. Leave the tub quickly and follow the usual rewarming procedures: exercise or bed rest.

A cold half bath directs the circulation toward the inside of the body. The warming reaction occurs rather quickly. Through the entire procedure, the circulation in the lower part of the body is greatly increased. Weaknesses and disorders of the lower abdomen are favorably influenced by cold half baths, as are intestinal weakness, flatulence, and constipation.

THE WARM HALF BATH

TEMPERATURE: 98°–101°F.

DURATION: 10–15 minutes.

The warm half bath is generally used as a preliminary warming up in preparation for a cold application or, with the addition of herbs, in place of a full herb bath by those for whom the effect of the full bath is too strong.

Following the bath, a cold rinse of the lower part of the body and then bed rest for a half hour are required.

THE HOT HALF BATH

TEMPERATURE: 102°–112°F.

DURATION: Not more than 12 minutes.

Like the hot full bath, the hot half bath should be used only with trained supervision. It requires the same procedures as the hot full bath.

THE FOOTBATH

COLD FOOTBATH

TEMPERATURE: 60°F.

DURATION: 15–60 seconds, depending on how long it takes for the reaction response to occur.

Cold footbaths are frequently used. They produce a light stimulation to the entire body. In addition to their immediate local effects of stimulating the metabolism in the feet and lower legs, cold footbaths also influence the circulation in the pelvic area, promote the functioning of the urinary tract and the large intestine, and relieve congestion by drawing blood away from the head and chest. They are refreshing and invigorating, even for people in good health. Cold footbaths are particularly recommended in the summertime if there is a problem with getting to sleep.

There are footbath tubs designed especially for this purpose, but any tub in which both feet fit comfortably can be used.

Do not take a cold footbath with cold feet; warm them first. When taking the bath, immerse both legs in the water to above the calf. Afterward, stroke off the excess water with your hands and go through the usual rewarming procedure.

WARM FOOTBATH

TEMPERATURE: 100°–102°F (not more than 86°F for people with varicose veins).

DURATION: 5–10 minutes.

The warm footbath is practically always used as an herbal bath (for specific uses, *see* Herbal Bath Additives, pages 460–467). It can also be useful for warming the feet before a cold footbath.

Both feet should rest comfortably in the tub, with the water level above the calf. People with varicose veins should not immerse the legs further than just above the ankles. Immediately after the bath, dip the legs in cold water or apply a cold knee gush.

Warm footbaths are helpful to anemic, nervous persons, young and old. They have also proved very effective for circulatory disturbances, congestion, headache, and cramps. Further indications are local infections of the skin, bones, and joints; in gout and rheumatic conditions; for sweaty feet; and for muscle and tendon weakness in the feet. Their reflex action is also effective in inflammatory processes and congestion in the pelvic cavities (such as suppression of urine in cases of bladder catarrh resulting from a cold or from inflammation of the kidneys) and in the relief of congestion in the throat and voice box.

CONTRAST FOOTBATH

The contrast footbath has the same extensive effects as the warm footbath, but it provides stronger stimulus to the body.

Prepare two tubs, each with water deep enough to reach just over the calves. Appropriate herbal additives should be used in the warm tub.

For the warm tub:

TEMPERATURE: 96°–100°F.

DURATION: 5–10 minutes.

For the cold tub:

TEMPERATURE: 50°–59°F.

DURATION: 10–30 seconds.

To keep the warm tub at the proper temperature, add boiling water to it while the feet are in the cold tub.

The feet and legs are thoroughly warmed for 5 to 10 minutes, then removed from the warm tub and placed in the cold tub. Repeat the sequence two or three times, ending with the cold tub unless leg cramps occur, in which case end with the warm tub. Do not use the contrast footbath if severe varicose veins are present or there is any other danger of blood clotting. In early cases of incipient varicose veins, the contrast bath may be used with adjusted durations of 3 minutes or less for the warm tub and 10 seconds or less for the cold.

THE EYE BATH

COLD EYE BATH

The cold eye bath is used to strengthen the eyes and to restore their natural expression and sparkle. Dip your face in a basin or sink of plain cold water, blink your eyes for about 5 seconds, and then lift your face completely out of the water. Wait a few moments, and then repeat the procedure three or four times.

WARM EYE BATH

TEMPERATURE: 90°–96°F.

DURATION: 5–10 seconds, repeated three or four times.

The warm eye bath is used to treat inflammation, conjunctivitis, pinkeye (such as that associated with measles), eyestrain, puffy and itching eyes, sties, and small fatty tumors in the eyelash area.

This bath is used with herbal additives, particularly eyebright, elder leaves, chamomile, hyssop, or althea.

Whichever you choose, brew it as a weak tea to be added to the water in the basin. Add one cup (eight ounces) of the tea or more, depending on the size of the basin.

An eyecup can also be used, especially if only one eye is affected. Tinctures of the above herbs can conveniently be added to the warm water in the cup. The usual dose is fifteen to twenty drops, unless advised otherwise by a physician. Hold the cup against the eye, tilt the head back, and blink ten to fifteen times. Repeat twice.

THE FACE BATH

TEMPERATURE: Not more than 64°F.

DURATION: 1 minute.

The face bath is important to the vitality of the facial skin, glands, and muscle tone. It refreshes the skin and gently stimulates the circulation in the tiny capillaries just below the surface that nourish the tissues and control the moisture level of the skin. Daily use of the face bath is recommended as a routine health measure.

Remove tight clothing from around the neck and dip the face into a large basin or sink full of cold water. Open and close the eyes repeatedly; lift the face out of the water to take breaths as needed. Repeat two or three times.

Herbal additives can be used to enhance the effect of the face bath. The herbs to use are shave grass, fennel seed, eyebright, wormwood, or chamomile. Put two to three tablespoons of herb in a quart of boiling-hot water and let it steep until cool. If using loose materials, strain the tea through cheesecloth. Add one cup (eight ounces) of the tea to the face-bath water.

THE SITZ BATH

The sitz bath affects mainly the circulation in the lower abdominal and pelvic region. It does so without influencing the circulation in the lower limbs because the legs are not immersed. It serves mainly to disperse congestion in the abdominal and pelvic organs, a common problem for sedentary workers.

Sitz baths are not to be taken more than three times a week. Convenient plastic tubs that facilitate the use of this application are available, but you can also use an ordinary bathtub.

Fill the tub about one-third full so that the water covers the upper portion of the thighs, the seat, and the abdomen up to the navel. It is most comfortable to sit crosswise in the bathtub, with the feet resting on a small stool set on the floor. In this position, the circulation in the backs of the knees will not be restricted. With practice, you will be able to take a sitz bath without having to undress completely. To avoid a chill, the upper torso should be clothed, or a light blanket or sheet should be draped over the shoulders and chest.

COLD SITZ BATH

TEMPERATURE: As the water flows from the cold-water faucet, but not more than 60°F.

DURATION: 6–10 seconds.

The cold sitz bath is not recommended as a cure for sexual overexcitability; the reaction following a cold sitz bath brings a rush of blood to the pelvic area, thereby stimulating sexual sensations rather than weakening them.

WARM SITZ BATH

TEMPERATURE: 104°F, which can be expected to cool down to 100°F during the bath.

DURATION: 10–15 minutes.

The warm sitz bath is used only as an herbal bath (*see* Herbal Bath Additives, pages 460–467). It is not to be taken if the feet are cold; if they are, first warm them in a warm footbath.

For a warm sitz bath, you will need an assistant to wrap you in the required covers. After entering the bath, lay a stick or narrow board across the tub in front of you to keep the covers from falling into the water during the packing that follows. The covers consist of a bedsheet or a very large bath towel that covers the body from neck to toe, over which is placed a light wool blanket. The feet should be wrapped in the covers. At the throat, the sheet or towel should be folded over the blanket like a collar.

The additives most frequently used are hay flowers, shave grass, and oat straw. The oat straw sitz bath is used for most gout-like illnesses.

When there is a tendency toward painful menstruation, or when the menstrual period may be suppressed because of a chill due to exposure to cold, the warm sitz bath will be found most effective for relief. One or two baths usually bring about the desired results and facilitate a free and relatively painless menstrual period. The warm sitz bath increases the circulation in the pelvic organs and relieves spasms and cramps in those organs.

CONTRAST SITZ BATH

Two sitz bath tubs are required, one for the warm bath and one for the cold bath. If you have only one tub, use a conventional bathtub for the cold bath. Both baths are prepared according to the instructions given earlier.

For the warm sitz bath:

TEMPERATURE: 104°F, which can be expected to cool down to 100°F during the bath; use herbal additives.

DURATION: 5–10 minutes.

The warm tub should be reheated by adding hot water while you are in the cold bath.

For the cold sitz bath:

TEMPERATURE: 59°F.

DURATION: 6–10 seconds.

The sequence of warm bath to cold bath should be repeated two or three times. Following the series of baths, wipe excess water from the body with your hands before getting dressed. It is very important not to omit the rewarming period: light exercise or at least a half hour of bed rest.

The contrast sitz bath is indicated for bladder weakness, prostatitis, acute and chronic inflammation of the bladder and kidneys, weakening of the stomach and intestinal musculature, and conditions arising from general congestion in the area. For specific herbal additives to use in the warm bath, choose from those listed on pages 460–467.

THE STEAM BATH

A steam bath is an application of water in the form of steam or vapor, which warms a portion of the body. This warming causes an expansion of the blood vessels, increasing the circulation in both the skin and organs and relieving congestion in the heart and central blood vessels. Steam baths are not to be taken more than three times a week. Particular caution must be observed in cases of heart or circulatory disturbance. Use only the mildest forms of steam baths, and monitor the process carefully. During serious illness, consult a physician about their use.

Like all applications of water, steam baths are effective even in their mildest forms and can therefore be used safely by almost everyone. But a word of caution is in order. What may cure a sick person when done with care and precisely according to directions may, when done carelessly or incorrectly, make a well person sick. For example, someone who, after a steam bath, goes out into the cool air without a cooling-off period can easily become sick. The key is to follow the correct procedures.

Steam baths work on the principle of providing warmth. The body must obtain a certain amount of warmth to function successfully. The healthy body produces all the warmth it needs, but the chronically sick person often feels a loss or lack of necessary warmth, and this warmth must be replaced in some way. For some patients, wrappers and compresses are sufficient; for others, the artificial addition of heat through steam baths serves the body best.

The great advantage of steam baths lies in the fact that even partial baths, which touch only parts of the body directly, nevertheless have an effect on the body as a whole.

They make the patient feel well because of their effect of dissolving, loosening, and eliminating toxic matter. Very often, one type of steam bath—particularly the head or foot steam bath—has an especially favorable effect.

FULL STEAM BATH

Use a wooden chair with an open cane seat or remove the seat. In the latter case, put some folded towels around the edge of the open area for comfort while leaving an opening through which the steam can rise. Fill two large, covered pots with water and bring to a boil. Remove from the stove and add appropriate herbs (*see* Herbal Bath Additives, pages 460–467). Place one pot on the floor directly beneath the open seat of the chair. Place the other pot on the floor in front of the chair. Put two narrow sticks across the top of the second pot for the feet; be sure that they are secure so that the feet will not slip into the hot water.

The entire body must be unclothed. Sit on the chair with your feet resting comfortably on the sticks above the hot water. Then wrap the usual coverings around the entire body up to the neck (enclosing the pots and chair as well) in such a way that no steam escapes. It is best to have someone assist you in this phase of the application.

The full steam bath is recommended whenever an intense heating of the body with subsequent perspiration is desired. The duration is normally 20 minutes. The assistant can add hot water to the pots after about 10 minutes in order to sustain the steam. After the steam bath, a dry wrapper or a full gush is applied, followed by bed rest of at least 30 minutes.

STEAM BATHS FOR SPECIFIC PARTS OF THE BODY

Alternating with other uses of water, steam baths with herbs can be beneficial for many afflictions of the eyes, ears, mouth, fingers, hands, arms, and other parts of the body. For example: for eye steam baths, use an infusion of fennel powder, eyebright, or yarrow; for ear steam baths, use an infusion of dead nettles; for hemorrhoids, add a handful of chamomile flowers to three quarts of boiling water. (Use an arrangement similar to the abdominal steam bath described below.)

The minimum time for such treatments should be 10 minutes; they should never be longer than 20 minutes. The comfort of the bather is always the first consideration. Applications of steam must be cautiously done, since scalding is possible. Steam baths used for inhalation, for internal effect, and for the eyes and ears should never be administered harshly. If the heat is uncomfortable or the recommended duration seems too long, it should be reduced. The heat can be reduced by moving the source of the steam farther away from the part being treated.

ABDOMINAL STEAM BATH

DURATION: 15–20 minutes.

The abdominal steam bath particularly affects the body below the navel; it is used mainly against colds in the lower body organs. It produces a comfortable feeling of warmth, relieving abdominal cramps and pains. It is effective for acute and chronic bladder catarrh, prostate gland inflammation, and kidney problems. It acts as a strong sweat-inducing remedy in metabolic disorders, and is a favorite for treating an enlarged or congested liver, for chronically enlarged prostate, and for frequent urination (especially during the night). It is excellent for relieving cramps in the bladder control muscles, in the kidneys and gallbladder, and in the bowels, as well as for premenstrual cramps.

Use a wooden chair with an open cane seat or remove the seat and put some folded towels around the edge of the open area, leaving an opening for the steam. Fill a large pot with water, cover it, and bring to a boil. Remove from the stove and add appropriate herbs (see Herbal Bath Additives, pages 460–467). Place the pot on the floor directly beneath the open seat of the chair. Disrobe from the waist down and sit on the chair. Wrap two large linen or cotton sheets around the waist and chair, covering the lower body, legs, and feet. Wrap two flannel or wool blankets around in the same way. See that all wrappings are snugly sealed at the waist and carefully arranged at the floor so that there are no openings through which steam can escape.

Care must be taken in removing the cover from the pot to start and control the release of steam. It is best to safeguard against scalding by placing a towel over the pot while the cover is gradually slid off an inch or two at a time to maintain a constant supply of steam. The feet must remain warm during the bath; a warm footbath can be taken at the same time, also enclosed within the coverings.

More boiling water can be added to the pot if the steam runs out too soon. After the steam bath, it is advisable to go to bed for at least 45 minutes. If the bath is taken to produce sweating, or as a metabolic process stimulant, a cold rinse is recommended after the bed rest. If it is used to relieve cramps, no cold after-rinse is taken.

FOOT AND LEG STEAM BATH

Drape a linen cloth over the seat of a chair so that it reaches the floor and encloses the legs of the chair. Place a large pot or tub, slightly more than half filled with boiling hot water, on the floor in front of the chair. Place two narrow wooden sticks across the top of the pot to rest the feet on; be sure that they are secure so that the feet can't slip into the hot water. With the upper body clothed but the legs bare, sit on the chair and rest your feet comfortably on the sticks above the hot water. Wrap a thick blanket around the feet and legs (or around the waist if the lower body is being treated) and around the tub so that no vapor escapes. The blanket and the linen cloth should form a tube through which the heat rises. An infusion of hay flowers added to the water will increase the effectiveness of the bath.

The temperature of the water and the duration of the bath depend greatly on how great an effect is desired. Sometimes only the soles of the feet are brought to perspiration (as in the case of chronically sweaty feet); in other cases, the vapor is used to bring the effect to the entire lower body, including the abdomen. The effect is the strongest when the foot and leg steam bath is combined with the abdominal steam bath.

The mildest application lasts for 15 to 20 minutes, and no extra boiling water is added to the tub during that time. But to produce the strongest effects of a real vapor bath, the duration must be 25 to 30 minutes, with boiling water being added carefully to the tub every 10 minutes. As a rule, the foot and leg steam bath should not be taken more than twice a week.

This bath is always followed by bed rest of about 45

minutes and then by a cold rinse of the parts that were brought to perspiration. However, people susceptible to leg cramps should not take a cold rinse.

HEAD STEAM BATH

The head steam bath is effective for colds, headaches, ringing in the ears, rheumatism and painful cramps in the neck and shoulders, chest congestion, and various catarrhs. As a rule, two applications within three days will bring relief. A single head steam bath will generally help a catarrhal cold when taken at the onset of the cold.

To begin, you will need a relatively deep stock pot with a close-fitting cover, two straight chairs facing each other, two bath towels, and a large wool blanket. Fill the pot three-quarters full with actively boiling water, add herbs for increased effectiveness (*see* Herbal Bath Additives, pages 460–467), cover to keep the steam from escaping, and put the pot on one of the chairs.

Remove your clothes to the waist and place one towel around the waist to catch perspiration that runs down the body. Seat yourself and rest your hands one on each side of the pot, bending the upper part of your body over the pot. Have someone place the other bath towel and the wool blanket loosely over the upper part of your body and the pot, being sure that all sides are covered and no opening exists to let any steam escape. Gradually slide back the cover of the pot to let the steam out. To avoid being scalded, be careful not to get too close or to let out too much steam at once. The steam will rise onto the head, breast, and neck, and begin its work of loosening things up.

If you are not used to high temperatures, you may at first feel frightened, but you will soon grow accustomed to the steam. As you become more comfortable, assume the stooped-over position.

The procedure lasts about 15 minutes. For the best effect, let the steam get into your nose and open mouth for about 3 to 4 minutes. It takes about 6 or 7 minutes before draining of the mucous membranes begins. For head steam baths of longer duration (a maximum of 24 minutes), keep additional water hot on a nearby stove or hot plate to be added to the pot as the water cools.

After about 15 minutes, remove the covering and dry off. Cover your upper body and head with a linen cloth and allow a gradual cooling-off period in a warm bed. The effects of this procedure are important; they react on the entire surface of the torso, opening up the pores, and also on the internal body, dissolving congestive fluids and draining them off from the nose, bronchial tubes, lungs, and so on. After the bed rest, rinse your face or your whole upper body (see Washes, pages 467–471).

Since the head steam bath has a strong draining effect and causes copious perspiration, which could be weakening, it should not be used too frequently. As a general rule, you should not take more than two a week.

FACIAL STEAM BATH

Facial steam baths can work wonders for oily, unclean, or rough skin, and for skin with poor circulation. However, they should be used economically and carefully—that is, not more than once a week. Dry skin should receive a steam bath only as treatment for a specific ailment; even then the skin should be greased beforehand and the duration should be no more than 2 to 3 minutes. Those who tend to get dilated veins should avoid steam baths altogether and use only compresses.

The daily cleaning of the face is often not enough to remove dead cells, to cleanse the pores, and to keep the skin soft and supple. The facial steam bath helps with these processes: It softens rough, callused skin; has deep-cleansing effects; stimulates circulation in the skin; widens the pores and rinses them out; and, through herbal additives, has a healing and regenerating effect. It also makes it easier to remove blackheads and soften cysts, and it makes packs, masks, and peeling especially effective—when the skin can handle them.

In all cases, the face and neck first must be cleaned with cleansing cream or lotion. Then add a handful of lime blossoms, chamomile blossoms, or sage to one to two quarts of boiling water in a wide, shallow bowl, put a large terry cloth towel over your head so that as little steam as possible escapes, and hold your face over the steam. The duration of this steam bath (from 2 to 10 minutes) depends on your skin type and compatibility: Oily, unclear, and acne-plagued skin can steam for up to 10 minutes, normal and mixed skin about 5 minutes, and dry skin for 2 or at most 3 minutes.

Afterward, dab off well with a soft cloth, clear away blackheads, and then be sure to rinse off with cold water. If you have enough time, lay on a pack and relax for 20 minutes, or apply a good herbal cream (carrot, cucumber, or chamomile) to the skin, patting it in carefully and tenderly.

A facial steam bath can also bring relief from being chilled. For a cold, try an old home remedy: a facial steam bath with peppermint leaves or with a few drops of eucalyptus oil or pine needle extract.

HERBAL BATH ADDITIVES

Although water has therapeutic value by itself, its effects can often be enhanced by adding plant and other natural materials to the bath. With the increased interest in botanical medicine, scientific research is demonstrating that substances in water can be absorbed by the body, either directly through the skin or by way of inhalation into the respiratory tract.

Herbs contain vital elements—vitamins, minerals, and essential oils—that are deficient or lacking in the diseased body. They contain them in such a finely distributed and prepared state that these elements are readily assimilated by the system and conveyed to the blood for distribution. Adding herbs to the bathwater is an effective way of making the therapeutic elements available to the body. The most popular applications and uses of herbal bath additives are for rheumatic and arthritic diseases, for nervous-system disturbances, and for skin problems. For less serious ailments, a good selection of the herbs suitable for various effects—sedatives, stimulants, calmatives, decongestants, and others—can be kept on hand.

Most of the herbal additives described below are available in concentrated liquid extract form. These are particularly convenient for adding to a bath; directions for use are on the label. However, in the descriptions here it is assumed that dried or fresh plant materials are being used. The amounts vary with the plant and the type of bath. In preparing additives for eye baths, use as much plant material as you can hold with three fingers.

Plant materials can be, but most usually aren't, added directly to the bathwater as a decoction. To make your own bath decoctions, use an enameled or nonmetallic pot.

Add plant parts to cold water and bring to a boil, or add them to boiling water. Boil for 3 to 4 minutes in both cases. Hard materials such as needles, twigs, and roots need boiling for about 10 minutes and longer, steeping to extract their ingredients. Then let the mixture steep with a cover on the pot for 2 to 3 minutes. Strain out the plant parts when pouring the decoction into the bathwater.

BRAN

For a full bath, use three pounds of wheat bran; use correspondingly less for partial baths. Bring the bran to a boil quickly before adding it to the bath.

Bran baths have a soothing effect on inflammations since they reduce stimulation of the skin. Because they help form a protective, inflammation-resistant layer over the skin surface, they are used to treat highly inflammatory skin diseases and hypersensitive skin troubled by eczema and hives.

CHAMOMILE

Prepare the bath additive by soaking chamomile flowers in cold water and then boiling them in a closed stockpot for about 10 minutes. Use one pound for a full bath, a half pound for a half bath, a quarter pound for a sitz bath, and two ounces for a footbath.

Chamomile baths are known chiefly for their volatile-oil content. Their healing effects in cases of inflammation are traditionally well known. They are used for catarrhal conditions, as well as to cleanse wounds. They also have a soothing effect on itchy skin and on easily inflamed eczema.

HAY FLOWERS

Hay flowers are the flowers and other light residue obtained by sifting hay. To prepare the additive, place hay flowers into cold water, bring to a boil, and simmer for a half hour. Boil them in a cheesecloth bag, or strain them out before adding the liquid to the bath. Use one and a half to two pounds of hay flowers for a full bath, three quarters to one pound for a half bath, a half pound for a sitz bath, and three to four handfuls for an arm bath or footbath.

Hay flowers contain numerous volatile oils, which are their valuable asset. They stimulate the skin and the metabolism. When someone with eczema or highly sensitive skin uses them, signs of skin irritation appear almost immediately. (The same effect may be observed from pine needle extract.) The favorable effects on the metabolism, in turn, are particularly helpful in the treatment of gravel and stone complains, gout and rheumatic conditions, and stiff joints. In cases of exudation, inflammation of a tendon sheath, and formation of boils, their absorbing qualities are particularly important. They also have antispasmodic properties, which are especially useful for colics of the gallbladder, stomach, colon, and kidneys.

MUSTARD POWDER

Mustard powder is generally used only in partial baths. Use two handfuls for a footbath, less for an arm bath. Pour hot water (about 120°F) over the powder and stir until the mixture thickens; then add to the bath. Mustard powder must never be cooked, since its loses its potency. Only fresh powder should be used.

The volatile oils that become liberated in the mixture

have the strongest stimulant effect on the skin of all the additives mentioned. Therefore, this application must not last more than 5 to 10 minutes, or until the patient feels a stinging or burning sensation. After the application, rinse the area with warm water to remove any mustard powder clinging to the skin.

OAK BARK

Oak bark is dried and chopped, soaked in cool water, and then boiled for about 30 minutes. The decoction is added to the bathwater. Use one and a half to two pounds for a full bath, three quarters to one pound for a half bath, a half pound for a sitz bath, and three to four handfuls for an arm bath or a footbath. Commercially made extracts are also available.

Because of its tannic acid content, oak bark is useful for combating infections and also for helping to heal wounds. It can also be used to treat chapped skin, cold sores, and varicose veins.

OAT STRAW

For a full bath, put one and a half to two pounds (correspondingly less for partial baths) of oat straw into three quarts of cold water, bring to a boil, and continue boiling for 30 minutes. Add the decoction to the bathwater.

The uses of oat straw are the same as those for hay flowers, but oat straw is milder and is therefore recommended for use by frail and nervous persons. In Europe, oat straw is used for various baths that, when taken regularly, are helpful for a number of ailments. Warm full baths are good for rheumatic problems, lumbago, paralysis, liver ailments, gout, and kidney and gravel problems. Warm sitz baths are good for bladder and abdominal problems, hemorrhoids, intestinal colic, and bed-wetting. Warm footbaths are good for tired or chronically cold feet. Poultices are good for skin diseases, flaky skin, frostbite, chilblains, wounds, and eye problems.

PINE NEEDLE EXTRACT

For the preparation of pine needle extract, use pine needles and pine sprigs, as well as the resinous cones. For a full bath, use a strong decoction made from one pound of the fresh shoots that appear at the tips of the branches in May. Let stand in three quarts of cold water for several hours. Then bring to a boil and boil briefly. Let stand for 15 minutes, then add to the bathwater.

Additives are also available in the form of pure extracts from Swiss mountain pine cones. The advantage of ready-made extracts is that volatile oils are more likely to be preserved in them than in your own boiled decoction. For a full bath, add one half to one cup of extract. Products such as pine needle tablets, powders, and salts can also be used. The normal color of a pine needle bath is brownish; tablets, powders, and crystals having an artificial green color are not recommended.

Pine needle additives are used to stimulate the skin; but, unlike other such stimulants, they tend to have more of a tranquilizing effect on the nervous system.

SALT

Salt does not require any special preparation; just add about four pounds of salt for a full bath and correspondingly less for partial baths (about a quarter pound for foot-baths).

Salt baths stimulate the skin and increase the elimination of water and carbon dioxide through the skin. Because blood circulation is improved near the skin, disturbances of the metabolism (such as rheumatic conditions) that affect the deeper-seated organs can be treated successfully. In general, salt baths help build up the body's resistance to disease.

SHAVE GRASS

Shave grass *(Equisegum sp.)* is prepared cold and then brought to a boil for about 30 minutes before being added to the bathwater. Use one to one and a half pounds for a full bath, three quarters pound for a half bath, a half pound for a footbath. Commercially prepared extracts are also available.

Shave grass is usually used in partial baths. Its main benefit is derived from its high silicic acid content. Shave grass baths are used to alleviate spasmodic conditions in the kidneys and bladder, and in cases of weak bladder and catarrh of the bladder. Small bandages soaked in shave grass extract can help in the healing of wounds.

SWEET FLAG ROOT

To prepare sweet flag root *(Acorus calamus),* soak one pound roots and leaves in five quarts of cold water for 60 minutes; then bring to a boil and steep for about 5 minutes. Use one pound for a full bath, or two to three tablespoons of the liquid extract; use correspondingly less for the partial baths.

Sweet flag root works as a strengthener; it is a good additive for the treatment of anemia. It stimulates the metabolism and is also recommended for insomnia and tense nerves. Baths with sweet flag root extract are used in treating scabs.

THYME

Thyme *(Thymus off.)* is a good remedy for acute and chronic coughing, chronic bronchitis, and chronic emphysema. Boil a half pound of thyme in two quarts of water for 5 minutes and strain; add the decoction to a warm half bath. While in the bath, breathe slowly and deeply in order to inhale as much steam as possible. Some of the volatile oils of the thyme will be taken into the lungs through the bronchial system, and some will be absorbed through the skin.

ENGLISH WALNUT

English walnut *(Juglans regia)* leaves can be used either fresh or dried. Soak the dried leaves in cold water (one and a half quarts of water per one pound of leaves), then boil in a covered pot for 45 minutes and add the strained liquid to the bathwater. Use about one and a half pounds of leaves for a full bath, correspondingly less for partial baths.

These baths generally are helpful in treating children's complaints such as chicken pox, diarrhea, cough, croup, thrush, colic, and sleeplessness.

MIXED BATH ADDITIVES

As a general principle, additives that have conflicting qualities and those that would nullify each other's effects should never be mixed. The most frequently used mixtures are: hay flowers and oat straw in equal proportions; pine needle extract with salt (add approximately two pounds of cooking salt to a regular full bath with pine needle extract); sweet flag root and English walnut leaves in equal proportions.

WASHES

Washes are an excellent means of strengthening the body. They improve blood circulation and are relaxing. Production of warmth in the body is activated by washes, and toxic substances in the blood and deposits in the limbs—with all their disagreeable consequences—are increasingly eliminated and even prevented.

Washes, the mildest form of all the water applications, spread water uniformly over the skin by means of a washcloth. Fresh, cold water should be used for every wash. All washes are best done in the morning upon getting up, in a room with the windows closed to prevent drafts. When getting out of bed, pull the covers up to keep the warmth in until you return. Take off your nightclothes. Use a piece of porous linen folded a few times as the washcloth. The cloth should be neither dripping wet nor too well wrung out. After the wash, put your nightclothes on without drying yourself, climb back into bed, and pull the covers up snugly around your shoulders. Rest in bed for 30 to 60 minutes after the wash.

Not drying off after washing allows evaporation to take place equally over the whole body. This stimulates the blood vessels equally to active constriction and dilation, a process that is especially important to increase blood circulation in cases of infection. The process also relieves the strain on a weak heart and increases metabolism and body warmth.

The principal underlying purpose of a cold application is to constrict the blood vessels next to the surface of the skin, driving the blood into the deeper-lying internal organs. As the reaction takes place, the vessels dilate and the blood surges back to the surface of the skin. There is a stronger-than-normal increase in circulation in the area of the application, without added strain on the heart; in this way, washes improve the circulation of the blood.

Similarly, washes applied to healthy people will act to prevent illness by evacuating and strengthening the body through an increase of circulation to the skin.

THE FULL WASH FOR BEDRIDDEN PERSONS

A full wash, carefully and expeditiously done, can never do any harm, even if it is done with very cold water, which is the most desirable. Just be sure that the patient is thoroughly warmed before beginning the application. No part of the body, not even the soles of the feet, should be omitted, unless the patient has athlete's foot, in which case the feet should be excluded from the wash. Wash the entire surface of the body as evenly and as quickly as possible. Try also to keep the strength of the strokes equal so as to avoid uneven body temperature effects, which—though not necessarily harmful—would be less helpful to the patient.

Have the patient sit up in bed. If he is too weak to sit up by himself, support him in a sitting position. Wash the arms, chest, abdomen, and back as quickly as possible; then also go up and down the spine. Have the patient lie down again and wash the legs. The entire process should take only 3 to 4 minutes, and the patient will feel as though he were starting out on a new life.

The wash can also be done in two parts. First, the upper part of the body is washed while the legs remain covered. Then the upper part is covered and the legs and buttocks are done.

In treating high fever, repeated full washes play a significant role and should be taken instead of the cold full bath. The time for the repetition of the full wash is indicated by a rise in temperature and the patient's anxiety and discomfort because of it. In certain circumstances, the wash may be repeated as often as every half hour.

Water diluted with vinegar is preferable to plain water for patients who are very weak. The vinegar water washes the skin more thoroughly, opens the pores, and also has a strengthening effect.

THE FULL WASH FOR AMBULATORY AND WELL PERSONS

The full wash for people not confined to bed takes in the whole body except the head and is performed in one quick operation in a place without drafts. Always start when the body is warm. Take a coarse washcloth or rough towel, dip it into cold water, and begin by washing the arms and then the neck. With long strokes, wash the chest and abdomen, then the legs and feet, including the soles. During this process, the folded wash towel has to be turned and rewetted several times. Wash the back last by unfolding the towel and drawing it back and forth vigorously across the back several times. The whole application must be completed in 1 minute or, at the most, 2 minutes.

Without drying off, put on your clothes as quickly as possible and exercise, by either working or walking, until the skin is perfectly warm and dry again. You may also return to bed in nightclothes, bundled up completely, until a feeling of warmth comes over you.

First thing in the morning is the suitable time for the full wash. The temperature of the body is at its highest because a night in bed has raised it, and the wash serves pleasantly to cool you. It is refreshing, drives away sleepiness, and provides a good start for a lively and vigorous day's work. For people who enjoy a morning walk, a full wash is particularly appropriate before starting out. However, if you are taking full washes as a preventive health measure and are too busy in the morning, any hour of the day is good. Take just 2 or 3 minutes during the part of the day that is most convenient and proceed as described above. Some people prefer to take the full wash at night before retiring, but others find that at this time it causes too much excitement of the nervous system. Therefore, try the wash at a few different times and see which is the best time for you.

THE LOWER BODY WASH

This type of partial wash affects circulation in the legs and the abdominal organs. It will also help get rid of waste matter from the upper portion of the body and consequently is helpful for cold feet, varicose and inflamed veins, leg ulcers (although care must be taken to avoid the inflamed part of the leg), stomach and intestinal ulcers, inflammation of the tissues of the pelvic cavity, bladder disorders, congestion of the lungs, strokes, and paralysis of the lower extremities.

Remove all clothing from the lower part of the body. Wash the right leg by stroking upward from the foot to the hip along the outer side of the leg, and back along the inner side. In the same way, wash the back part of the leg and the sole of the foot. From time to time, rewet the towel or washcloth in cold water. Now cover up the right leg and repeat the wash for the left leg. The abdomen and buttocks are washed with big circular movements.

For people who are ill, these partial washes may be used to stimulate the metabolism and blood circulation, and for general skin care.

THE UPPER BODY WASH

The upper body wash is used principally to affect the circulation of the blood in the organs of the chest: the lungs, pleura, and heart. Accordingly, it has been applied successfully for colds, bronchitis, catarrh of the nose and throat, influenza, inflammation of the lungs, pleurisy, and inflammation of the heart valves.

During this procedure, the lower part of the body remains covered. Begin the wash with the back of the right hand, go up to the shoulder, then back on the inner side of the arm, and up again to the armpit. Wet the armpit. Do the chest, the abdomen, and the sides of the body, using just 4 or 5 long strokes. After the application, it is important to dress as quickly as possible (without drying yourself) and then to get warm by returning to bed or by brisk walking or other exercise.

GUSHES

THE BACK GUSH

The back gush takes in the entire back part of the body, from neck to heels. Beginning at the right foot, the jet of water is brought slowly along the outside of the body up to the hip and returned downward to the inner part of the heel. This sequence is repeated on the left side. At this point, the patient, who has held his left hand ready, takes some water and washes the area around the heart.

Crossing the buttocks, the flow of water is then transferred to the right hand. With the hose in a perpendicular position, the jet of water is carried upward along the outer side of the right arm to the right shoulder blade. There special attention is paid to the right half of the back and right arm, so that a film of water covers them evenly, like a coat. Next, the water jet is brought downward and again across the buttocks to the left hand, from where the procedure is repeated on the left side. This procedure is followed several times. The change from one side of the back to the other is always made by way of the buttocks to avoid any direct gush of water onto the spine.

Since the back gush has a powerful effect on the system, it must be applied slowly and carefully and the patient must be certain to inhale and exhale calmly and evenly. As soon as the reaction to the gushing of the upper back sets in, the jet should be brought downward along the left side to the left heel, ending the application.

The back gush is a very rigorous application; it greatly stimulates breathing and heart action. The effect on the abdominal organs is particularly noteworthy. Weak and nervous patients are not able to stand the cold back gush; for these people, a warm back gush is often more acceptable.

THE CONTRAST FULL GUSH

The contrast full gush extends over the entire body. With the patient facing away from the jet, the flow of warm

water is directed to the heel of the right foot, then carried
slowly up the outer side of the right leg to the hip and
slowly down the inner side to the heel. The left side is
treated similarly. At this point, the patient washes his chest
with his hand, using water from the hose, while the attendant washes his back with the free hand. Then the flow of
water is brought across the buttocks to the right hand and
from there upward to the shoulder, from where the water
is allowed to flow evenly over the right half of the body.
The greater part of the water should flow over the back
and only a little over the front part of the body. Now the
hose is directed down along the back, across the buttocks
to the left arm, and from there upward to the left shoulder. The previous procedure is repeated on the left side.
After the water has been allowed to flow over the left side
of the body, the stream is directed to the right and left
across the back of the neck until the reaction occurs.
When it does, the flow is directed down along the left side
of the spine, continuing down the inside of the left leg
and ending at the left heel.

For the front of the body, the gush is started at the
right heel and brought up to the hip, then down the inside of the right leg to the heel. The left side is treated
similarly. Then the flow is brought up to the tip of the left
inner thigh and across to the right hand. In contrast to the
earlier procedure, the main part of the water is allowed to
flow down the front and the smaller part down the back.
Next, the flow is directed down the torso and across the
middle of the upper thighs (not across the abdomen) to
the other side and up the left arm to the shoulder, where
the same type of gushing follows as on the right side. Finally, the flow is directed from one side to the other across
the breastbone until the reaction occurs. After the onset of

the reaction, the flow is carried down the inside of the left leg to the heel. The same procedure is followed with cold water except that, at the end, the flow is directed in a spiral fashion over the abdomen. Then the patient turns around to have the soles of the feet gushed for 2 to 3 seconds each, beginning with the right foot. During the cold application, it is necessary for the patient to practice deep breathing.

The contrast full gush brings about an intense stimulation of the entire blood circulation. It is to be clearly understood that this gush may be applied only to those in general good health; in any case, however, it must be deferred until a number of less strenuous applications have accustomed the patient to this type of treatment. The reaction to this gush brings about an increased blood supply to the skin tissues and the inner organs. The principal indications for the contrast full gush are overall metabolic disorders, such as obesity. It is also used to strengthen the constitution of those in good health. The contrast full gush can also be used in cases of localized congestion in the blood vessels; however, it is not to be used if advanced arteriosclerosis, abnormally low blood pressure, or depressive states are present.

THE EYE GUSH

The eye gush is very valuable in cases of weak eyes, vision disorders requiring glasses, and redness of the eyes caused by lengthy reading or studying. This gush can also be used for paralysis of the eye muscles. The eye gush should not be applied if glaucoma or any other diseases of the eye are present.

Use a considerably smaller flow of water than for the

larger gushes, and squeeze the opening of the hose between the thumb and index finger so that a fan-like spray results. The physical arrangement and position are the same as those for the face gush (see below).

The right eye is treated first. Begin at the right temple and direct the flow slowly around the eye in a circle. Follow the same procedure for the left eye. Direct the water carefully so that you can breathe freely while the gush is changed from the right side to the left. Gushing of each eye is not to last longer than 1 to 2 seconds at a time. It is advisable to interrupt this gush every now and then during the treatment, which is not to be done more than three times.

This gush will stimulate active blood circulation in the skin surrounding the eye, the conjunctival tissue (the mucous membrane covering the eyeball), and the interior part of the eye.

THE FACE GUSH

The face gush has a remarkably stimulating effect on the blood circulation of the facial tissues, which has contributed to its reputation as a beauty treatment. Stimulating the blood supply helps prevent premature aging of facial skin, and helps flabby, faded skin regain tautness and freshness. This gush is a refreshing application for mental and physical fatigue, especially tiredness of the eyes after much studying and reading. It is also helpful for weak nerves and migraine headaches. It should not be applied if glaucoma or any other diseases of the eye are present.

To take a face gush, bend forward slightly and support yourself by placing a hand on the edge of the sink or tub. Wrap a loosely folded towel around the neck and begin by directing a gentle flow of water to a point just below the right temple. Bring the water across the forehead and circle the face several times. Direct the flow across the forehead a number of times and then slowly gush the face with upward and downward strokes from forehead to chin. Conclude by again circling the face. After the gush, dry the face.

This gush is easy to apply to yourself. If applying it to another person, take care to allow enough opportunity to breathe.

THE KNEE GUSH

The knee gush stimulates blood circulation and lightens the work of the heart. It eliminates tiredness in the feet and legs, tones the connective tissues, and prevents varicose veins. It can be applied even in the presence of varicose veins. However, in cases of phlebitis and thrombosis, knee gushes should be applied only with a doctor's prescription. It also eliminates congestion in the head, tension headaches, migraine, and symptoms of a cold in the nose and throat. The increased circulation will help get rid of waste matter from the organs of the upper abdomen, the liver, and stomach, and also the chest, head, and neck.

For the knee gush, the legs are uncovered up to midthigh. The patient faces away from the jet with feet spread slightly apart. The jet is led from the outside of the right foot slowly up the outside of the calf, stopped just above the hollow of the knee, and is moved back and forth there, before proceeding down the inside of the calf to the right heel and then over to the outside of the left foot. The procedure is repeated for the left leg, but after the pause at the hollow of the knee, the water is led over to the hollow of the right knee, stopped, led back to the left knee, stopped, and is then moved slowly down the inside of the left calf to the left heel.

For the front of the leg, the patient faces the jet, which starts at the outside of the right foot. The procedure is the same as for the back of the leg. The gush should not be applied to the shinbone, but to the muscular sides of the leg. The soles of the feet should be gushed at the end of the treatment.

The length of a single gush to the front or back part of the lower leg varies from 3 to 10 seconds for treatment. An application consists of a series of gushes, which should be stopped as soon as a reaction is noticed in the form of reddening of the skin or a feeling of warmth.

THE LEG GUSH

The leg gush is more powerful than the knee gush, particularly in its effects on the bladder, abdominal organs, and liver, and for treating lameness or paralysis of the lower limbs, sciatica, and inflammations of the hipbone, such as chronic arthritis. In this last case, the gush must be alternated with hot hay flower wrappers (see The Hay Sack, pages 507–509) or used in connection with hot baths. For treatment of hemorrhoids, however, the knee gush is preferred.

The leg gush includes those parts covered in the knee gush, and also the upper thigh as far as the hips. The clothes below the waist are removed, keeping on the upper clothing to prevent chilling. The gush is begun from the back at the outside of the right foot. The stream is directed up the outside of the leg to the hip and then down the inner side of the leg to the heel. The left leg is done in the same way. Then the stream is brought to the right hip, directed back and forth across the buttocks, and moved down the inner side of the left leg to the heel. When the front is gushed, the vertical motions should go only as high as the groin, and the horizontal ones across the middle of the upper thigh, not directly over the bladder and abdomen.

THE LOWER GUSH

The lower gush is used especially in cases of congestion of the stomach and intestines, overacidity of the stomach, and cramps of the stomach and intestinal muscles, as well as in weakened and enervated conditions of these parts. It is a very important treatment for circulatory congestion in the portal vein system, which brings blood back from the spleen, stomach, pancreas, intestines, liver, and gallbladder. The portal system carries blood that is relatively high in soluble materials, such as simple sugars, amino acids, and digested fats, that have resulted from body metabolism and are ready to be assimilated, and some accessory veins of the system go directly to the heart, so it is most important that this circulatory process not be sluggish. Swelling of the liver, accumulation of gas, and inclination to form gravel and stones also indicate the use of the lower gush.

In the lower gush, the back of the body is first covered with the water, which starts from the foot and travels up to the hips, with special attention to the small of the back and the lumbar region. The front of the body is treated the same way, and the stream of water is directed as high as the rib cage.

The action of this treatment is more intensive than that of the leg gush and resembles the effect of the cold half bath. If the patient is not thoroughly warm before the treatment, a contrast lower gush should be applied, that is, a warm gush followed by a cold gush.

THE UPPER GUSH

The effect of the upper gush is strong, both locally and in general. It involves the large areas of skin of the upper body, the muscles of the shoulder zone, and the organs of the chest cavity—the lungs with the diaphragm and pleura, and the heart. Care must be taken when there is fluid in the lungs, a tendency to hemorrhage, or arteriosclerosis of the aorta and the pulmonary blood vessels. People suffering from heart disease should take the upper gush only after becoming adapted to repeated applications of the knee gush, arm gush, arm bath, and other partial gushes and baths. For disorders of the abdominal organs, the upper gush is applied alternately with the leg and lower gushes.

The upper gush has an evacuating effect in cases of congestion of the head and abdomen, numbness, and varicose veins. This is an excellent remedy if there is a tendency toward catarrh in the upper air passages and in cases of chronic bronchitis and bronchial asthma. It is also beneficial for an inflamed or irritated throat and larynx (the vocal chords).

The usual procedure is to start off with the contrast upper or arm gush, including gushing of the chest, before changing to the cold upper gush for the treatment. This is essential if the patient is not thoroughly warm at the start of the application.

The upper gush includes the entire body—that is, the chest, back, neck, and arms. The patient undresses to the waist, also removing any constricting garments below the waist. A small bench or footstool may be placed in the tub or bathtub to make the treatment easier. The patient bends the upper body forward over the tub, placing the hands on the stool for support. The upper body should be in such a position that the water flows off the back into the tub. The patient holds the head erect but not stiff, and rotates it slowly during the application. Doing deep breathing during the gush is also recommended.

The upper gush begins with the flow being directed up the inner side of the right arm to the shoulder and then immediately back to the hand down the outer part of the arm. It is then passed across the front to the inside of the left arm, and the stream is directed upward from the hand to the armpit. With the hose in an upright position, the breast is gushed in a figure-eight pattern. Finally, the stream of water is brought slowly up to run over the left shoulder and coat the back with an even flow. The patient must breathe deeply at all times, since often a slight interruption of breathing occurs. The stream of water should never strike the spine directly, and the points of impact should be changed by gently shifting the stream evenly to the left and right.

At the start of a cure, the upper gush may be used first as a concentrated form of arm gush. The opening of the hose is always directed toward the arm. The right arm is gushed up to the shoulder, and over the shoulder blade as far as the back; the water is allowed to flow over the right side of the back and to the shoulder, breast, and arm. The stream is then brought back to the hand. The same sequence is repeated on the left side. After the gush, the body is quickly covered, and the hands, neck, and hair are dried.

WET WRAPPERS

INTRODUCTION

A therapeutic effect is obtained by wrapping up affected body parts. Frequent application of wrappers provides a constant influence on circulatory disturbances and the metabolism.

In general, we can choose between hot and cold wrappers. The hot, moist wrapper achieves a much more intense reaction and a quicker and better healing result than other types. The effect is increased even more if the wrapper is used with certain herbal additives, such as the essential oil of hay flowers, which add their own stimulative properties.

The penetrating heat has beneficial effects on the circulation in the part of the body being treated, from the skin to the lower-lying musculature with its tendons, nerves, joints, and bones. The circulation to the inner organs is also affected. The result is a deep-seated, continuous, hours-long stimulation of the metabolism, which leads to a strengthening of weak organs and to dissolution and elimination of metabolic waste.

METHODS AND MATERIALS REQUIRED

All wrappers should be applied in a warm bed, and in a thoroughly warm room. The bladder and bowels should be emptied before an application. Do not read or engage in any other kind of activity for the duration of the treatment.

There are three layers to each wrapper, in sizes corresponding to the area involved (*see* Wrapper Dimensions, page 484): a linen or coarse-woven, porous sheet (the "wet sheet"), which is used directly against the skin; a simple porous linen or 100 percent cotton sheet (the "middle sheet"), which serves as the dry covering for the wet sheet and prevents absorption of the eliminated toxins into the outer blanket; and a lightweight wool or flannel blanket, which serves as the final "outer layer."

Before starting the application, place the outer blanket on the bed and cover it with the middle sheet, which should be the same size or a little larger than the blanket. After all the preparations have been made, dip the inner wet sheet in water and wring it out well. Wrap it around the body part to be treated so that it lies close and wrinkle-free against the skin. There must be no air space between the wrapper and the skin. The middle sheet is wrapped over the wet sheet as tightly as possible without creating a feeling of constriction or interfering with breathing. The outer blanket is then wrapped tightly around the outside. The three layers should be applied in rapid succession.

After the application has been completed, remove the entire wrapper as quickly as possible. Remain in bed for at least another half hour to bring your temperature back to normal.

COLD WET WRAPPERS

Cold wet wrappers are used primarily for three purposes.

1. To withdraw heat from local inflammation of joints from sprains, and from inflammations of the veins. The wrapper is applied for short periods; after 20 to 40 minutes a fresh wrapper should be applied.

2. To increase the metabolism in chronic disease processes with insufficient development of heat, in which cases the cold wrapper stays on for 45 to 75 minutes, allowing it to cause a heat-producing (but not sweat-producing) reaction.

3. As a sweat-producing application in the treatment of colds and infections, and for strong stimulation of the metabolism, the wrapper is allowed to remain in place until it develops enough heat to bring on perspiration, usually after 90 minutes.

The cold stimulation produced by the application of a cold wet wrapper causes, through reaction, an active dilation of the blood vessels of the skin and of the deeper areas. In this way, the flow of blood and of the lymph is greatly increased locally. The deeper-lying organs will be stimulated similarly.

Do not apply a cold wrapper if the body feels at all cold. Warm yourself first, either with a heating pad in bed or by taking a warm bath. It is most important that the feet be warm.

Cold wet wrappers are usually made with fresh cold tap water. In cases of fever, be certain the water is not colder than 68°F.

The usual duration for a cold wet wrapper is 30 minutes. Repeat with a fresh wet cloth, if necessary.

WARM WET WRAPPERS

Most wet wrappers are applied cold, since the warm wet wrappers lose their heat rapidly. By their introduction of heat, warm wet wrappers bring about an immediate dilation of the blood vessels of the skin. In addition, they have a soothing effect on conditions such as cramps and colic. The blood circulation in the deeper layers of the skin and related tissues is also greatly increased, which is especially important for its effect on inflammatory processes.

The usual duration for warm wet wrappers is 45 to 75 minutes. The initial temperature at application is 98.7°F.

WRAPPER DIMENSIONS

The following are the standard dimensions for the wet sheet in the various types of wrappers:

Foot, calf, lower leg, head wrapper	32x32 in. (80x80 cm)
Leg wrapper	32x54 in. (80x130 cm)
Lumbar, chest wrapper	32x72 in. (80x180 cm)
Short wrapper	32x75in. (80x190 cm)
Lower, full wrapper	75x90 in. (190x230 cm)
Arm wrapper	28x36 in. (70x90 cm)
Hand wrapper	26x26 in. (65x65 cm)
Neck wrapper	4x24 in. (10x60 cm)

HERBAL ADDITIVES FOR WRAPPERS

Herbal additives can increase the total effect of a wrapper or bring about specific local healing effects. Cold wet wrappers are mostly applied with vinegar water, salt water, or clay water; warm wet wrappers require herbal additives.

Hay Flowers: Hay flowers help to increase the local reaction and stimulate the metabolism. They aid in dissolving and eliminating toxic accumulations. One to three handfuls of hay flowers, loose or in a small bag, are boiled in four to five quarts of water for a half hour and the liquid is stained. The wet sheet is then rolled up, dipped in the broth, and wrung out. If the broth is being used for a cold wet wrapper, let it cool down before dipping the wet sheet into it.

Oat Straw: The quantity and preparation are the same as for hay flowers. The effect is milder, and the softening effect on the surface of the skin is greater.

Shave Grass: Shave grass has a beneficial effect on wounds that are slow to heal, on leg sores, and on running eczemas. Boil 3 handfuls of shave grass for half an hour.

Oak Bark: Oak bark is of value because of its effect in healing skin cuts, minor scratches, and bruises. A handful of oak bark is boiled for a half hour. The resulting broth is usually used cold. (Note: Oak bark broth makes stains that are hard to remove from the sheet.)

Chamomile: Two to three handfuls of chamomile flowers are boiled for 15 minutes, and the broth is used hot. It has a gentle, soothing effect on the area treated.

Vinegar Water: Vinegar speeds up reactions, and the acid in it neutralizes excess alkalinity. To make it, mix one part vinegar with two parts water. Vinegar water wrappers are applied cold.

Epsom Salts Water: This application has an irritating effect on the skin and is often used to produce a skin eruption—for example, in chicken pox and measles. A solution of 6 to 10 percent Epsom salts in water is used. Epsom salts water can also be used as a wet dressing for open wounds.

Clay Water: Clay remains cold and thus has the effect of reducing inflammation. It is a valuable agent in cases of varicose veins. A few handfuls of powdered clay are mixed with two to three quarts water to make a thick paste. Clay wrappers are always used cold. (*See also* Herbal Bath Additives, pages 460–467.)

THE HAND WRAPPER

Here the whole hand is wrapped, including the wrist. The sheet is folded to form a triangle. The hand is placed on it palm down with the fingers pointing toward the tip of the triangle, allowing enough space for the turned-back portion of the wet cloth to cover the back of the hand. The right and left points of the sheet are drawn back over the back of the hand and around the wrist, where they are tucked in. The same is done with the middle layer and the wool cover, which must overlap the wet sheet. The wrapper should be tight but not constricting.

THE ARM WRAPPER

The arm wrapper includes the hand and the arm up to the shoulder. The arm is placed diagonally across the rectangle from corner to corner. Start at the tips of the fingers and continue wrapping the whole arm, following the method for the hand wrapper. It is important that the whole hand and arm be firmly wrapped and that the wrapper be well sealed at the shoulder.

Hand and arm wrappers serve mainly as local treatments—for example, in inflammations, paralysis, congestions, and swollen glands. The reflex action is beneficial for inflamed conditions of the sheath, muscles, and valves of the heart and, in combination with other appropriate measures, for sclerosis of the aorta.

THE CALF WRAPPER

This wrapper extends from the ankle to the hollow of the knee. Usually, both calves are wrapped because a general effect is desired. The technique is so simple that a person can apply the wrapper without help. Simple hand towels and a suitable wool cover suffice; of course, the general rules of the wrapping technique must be observed. If you fold a large hand towel in half and wet only one half, it may be used as both wet sheet and middle layer.

THE CHEST WRAPPER

The chest wrapper covers the area from the armpit to the lowest rib. The sheets are placed on the bed in the proper sequence; the patient then lies down on his back. The wet sheet is pulled securely across the chest and tucked in around the back, first from one side, then from the other. The middle and outer layers are similarly wrapped around the body in turn. They must envelop the body smoothly, without any wrinkling, but should not be so tight that they interfere with breathing. For best results, the patient is asked to inhale and exhale regularly and slowly. The sheets are then pulled tight in the middle of a breath, not at the deepest inhalation or exhalation.

The chest wrapper has proved beneficial for inflammations in the region of the deeper lying respiratory organs and the heart. Congestion in the lungs and bronchial tubes, dry coughs, and expectoration are also relieved.

THE FOOT WRAPPER

This wrapper is always an auxiliary application; that is, it is used to assist and complete other applications. Both feet are wrapped to above the ankles following the same procedure as for the hand wrapper. The simplest form of foot wrapper is a pair of wet socks (cotton or preferably linen) under a pair of dry wool socks. During the time of application, which lasts from 60 to 90 minutes, the patient remains in bed. If the application is specifically being used to relieve heat—as, for example, in infections of the lungs, pleurisy, or inflammation of the abdomen—the wrapper should always be rewetted as soon as considerable heat has developed.

In cases where foot wrappers are used to get rid of toxic or waste matter through the feet, to withdraw heat from an infection, or to draw the blood from the upper part of the body downward, they provide excellent results. Those who can endure this form of water application in the evening should put on wet socks when retiring, covering them with dry socks. Used in this way, the application will induce sleep, and there is no need to observe a specific length of time for the treatment. It is only necessary to remove the wet socks promptly on rising in the morning or in waking up during the night. For many who are very tired in the evening, the wet sock wrapper often draws away their tiredness more thoroughly than a cold footbath. I suggest that those who suffer from cold feet try this night wrapper just once; they will find it effective. Those bothered with perspiring feet will also benefit, but only after repeated applications.

Although fever is a natural defense mechanism against infections, sometimes something has to be done to bring it down. Foot wrappers have proved very effective in bringing down body temperature. A large cotton cloth is dipped into 65°–68°F water to which vinegar has been added (one tablespoon of vinegar to one pint of water) and only slightly wrung out. First wrap the wet cloth around the foot, then the dry covering. The application should be renewed every 20 to 30 minutes.

THE FULL WRAPPER

The entire body is wrapped from neck to feet. The preparations are the same as those for the lower wrapper, except that the blanket used for wrapping the upper part of the body has to extend to the middle of the headrest. The blanket and the middle sheet are folded over to the outside of the wrapper to ensure a close fit around the neck. While the bed is being carefully prepared, the patient must be kept warm.

When everything is ready, the patient lies down on the wet sheet. A previously wetted towel is placed over the chest and tucked between the arms and the body on both sides to ensure that the sides of the chest area are covered. The wrapping then proceeds with a technique similar to that for the lower wrapper (see page 492). However, the wrapper starts at the neck and, to obtain a good, close fit at the neck, it has to be folded. Pull the opposite upper corner of the wrapper over the neck, chest, and shoulder toward you, tucking it in under the shoulder next to you. Similarly, pull the near corner across the chest and tuck it in under the opposite shoulder. The chest, lower body, and legs are wrapped following the technique used for the lower wrapper. The feet and legs, again as in the lower wrapper, are wrapped tightly. As for the final wrapping with the blankets, work your way up from the feet, using the lengthwise blanket, and then do the upper part of the body with the crosswise blanket. A towel is wrapped around the neck to prevent rubbing by the blanket and at the same time to ensure a good seal. Warm-water bottles or heating pads may be placed at the feet and sides of the body.

THE HEAD WRAPPER

The head wrapper, which is seldom applied, covers the entire head except for the face. A large towel or linen sheet, folded into a triangle, is used as the wet sheet. The base of the triangle goes across the forehead and around to the back of the head, where the ends are crossed and tucked in along the sides. The point of the triangular sheet lies to the rear. The middle sheet and the wool blanket are applied in the same way. Patients with long hair can eliminate the wet sheet by washing their hair and leaving it wrapped around the head, thoroughly wet but not dripping. A dry towel is wrapped securely around the entire head to keep the air from penetrating into the hair. The face, however, remains uncovered. A pillow may be used to rest the head during the application. After the application, the head is thoroughly rubbed dry.

The head wrapper is used to treat eczemas of the scalp, inflammation of the hair follicles, and rheumatic ailments in the head. Since the blood vessels of the scalp and those of the brain react simultaneously, the head wrapper is used also to stimulate circulation in the brain—as, for example, in arteriosclerosis and stroke.

THE LEG WRAPPER

The entire leg is wrapped. Leg wrappers are usually applied to both legs. To fit the contours of the leg and groin, the rectangular wet sheet must be folded at one corner so that one of the sides parallel to the leg is shorter than the other. The longer side lies along the outer part of the leg, the shorter along the inner part. First wrap the foot and calf, then the thigh. The long end at the upper part of the leg can be folded back so that a firm, practically airtight closing of the wrapper results.

Wrappers applied to the lower limbs affect local circulation and metabolism and, in a reflex way, the organs of the pelvis. They have an eliminative effect on the abdominal organs—stomach, liver, pancreas, etc.—as well as on the chest and head organs. The cold leg wrapper is used for varicose vein inflammations, slow-healing wet ulcers and chronic dry leg ulcers, acute arthritis, bone diseases, tuberculosis of the joints, eczemas, and flat feet, and also for general relief of tired feet.

Leg wrappers are generally applied cold; however, the warm leg wrapper may be beneficial for chronic rheumatism of the joints and the muscular system, a late stage of inflammation of the tendons, cramps of the blood vessels or the muscles, limping that comes on occasionally, sciatica, and lameness.

The leg wrapper is valuable in the treatment of acute and chronic catarrhs of the throat, inflammation of the throat, and inflammation of the middle ear. It is also used in the treatment of meningitis, pneumonia, pleurisy, and pericarditis. The advantage of using the leg wrapper is that it puts relatively little strain on the already weakened patient, especially in cases of cardiac insufficiency.

If the patient has cold feet or is shivering, a warm leg wrapper must be applied. Its sleep-inducing effect is comparable to that of the foot wrapper.

THE LOWER WRAPPER

The lower wrapper covers the entire body below the armpits, down to and including the feet. The shoulders and arms, although not included, must be well covered by a nightgown or other covering so that there will be no opening at that end. To apply the wrapper, take two blankets and spread one—intended for wrapping the upper part of the body—crosswise over the bed, and spread the other—for wrapping the lower part of the body—lengthwise over the bed. On top of the two blankets, put a correspondingly large dry sheet as the middle sheet, followed by the wet sheet.

Start by wrapping the upper part of the body and work your way down carefully. Both legs are wrapped at the same time, and the wet sheet is tucked between them Wrap the feet as described for the foot wrapper. The legs and feet, like the rest of the body, have to be wrapped tightly so that there is no room for air between the skin and the wet sheet.

The benefits of the lower wrapper are varied. All organs of the chest area, the abdominal cavity, and the lower limbs are affected because the wrapper regulates the circulation, thereby relieving the heart. It acts as a strong stimulator of the metabolism and therefore has a very desirable detoxifying effect. It is used in cases of rheumatism, gout, obesity, chronic catarrhs, gas, climacteric disorders, and skin and infectious diseases.

THE NECK WRAPPER

You may use a hand towel, folded over several times to about a hand's width, as the wet sheet for the neck wrapper. Wind it around the neck so that it is airtight but not constricting. The middle sheet and the wool blanket have to overlap the wet sheet. The middle sheet may be omitted if a long and narrow enough towel is available for the wet sheet. Then half its length can be dipped in water and the remaining dry half can be used for the dry middle sheet.

The patient must strictly follow a physician's advice in this application, because leaving the wrapper on too long could lead to undesirable results. If the neck wrapper is used to reduce inflammation and eliminate heat, it should be removed and renewed whenever it becomes uncomfortably warm. Care must be taken, especially in the evening, that the patient does not fall asleep in the wrapper. How long each wrapper stays on depends on the patient's signs of anxiety or discomfort, which are the best indications that it is time to change the wrapper.

Aside from its inflammation-reducing action during infective processes in the neck and throat, the neck wrapper helps to regulate the blood circulation in the mucous membranes of the throat, larynx, and nose.

THE SHAWL

The shawl is a special application for the chest and the upper part of the back. The top edge of the middle sheet and wool cover are folded under along the top edge for three to four inches and are arranged on the bed so that they will reach about halfway up the back of the patient's head. For the wet sheet, a piece of coarse linen, one or one and a half yards square, is folded once into a triangle, dipped in water, wrung out, and then placed next to the skin as an ordinary shawl or muffler would be, with the base of the triangle across the shoulders and neck.

Now the patient lies down on the middle sheet and wool cover. Next, another wet towel is spread across the chest, enclosing the arms and the sides of the upper body. The middle sheet and wool cover are then wrapped around and carefully sealed. The sealing is important; the wrapper must be firmly drawn around and carefully adjusted to the contours of the neck. The ends are then tucked under the arms, first on one side and then on the other. For those just learning to use and apply wrappers, the chest wrapper can serve as an easier-to-apply "shawl."

The duration of this application may be from 30 to 90 minutes or, in rare cases when a stronger effect is desired, up to 2 hours. In the longer applications, the shawl should be rewetted after 30 to 45 minutes, which is usually when the heat becomes great and the wrapper becomes warm or hot.

Shawls and chest wrappers are used for diseases of the lungs and pleura before there is any accumulation of fluid. As cold wrappers, they are useful in cases of acute and chronic bronchitis——in the latter, when no shivering is present. Similarly, the cold wrapper works well for inflammation of the lungs. In infectious diseases where the air passage is threatened (such as measles and scarlet fever), this wrapper can be used to advantage. Because of its reflex influence on the circulation of blood through the lungs and mucous membranes, it can influence the nourishment of the lung tissue, loosen catarrhal discharge, and promote the expulsion of mucus by coughing.

Warm shawls and chest wrappers relieve cramps. They

have always been comforting to women suffering from depression. In long-standing conditions that tend to become fixed, and in asthma, they can help relieve spasms. People suffering from heart conditions that make breathing difficult cannot tolerate this wrapper well.

THE SHORT WRAPPER

The short wrapper reaches from under the armpits down to the middle of the upper thigh; in other words, it is a combination of the abdominal and chest wrappers. To apply it, follow the general instructions at the beginning of this section. Be sure that the legs are close together so that the wrapper fits tightly. The arms are not covered.

The short wrapper affects the entire body, increasing its natural body warmth or reducing its temperature, according to the length of time it is applied. Depending on what has been prescribed, the application may last from 1 to 1½ or even 2 hours. Healthy people can prevent many diseases by using the short wrapper once every week or two.

The most striking qualities of the short wrapper are its stimulating effect on the metabolism and its influence on body warmth. The short wrapper is particularly well-liked for treatment of obesity. It is also useful for all the complaints mentioned under the abdominal and chest wrappers. Even arteriosclerosis accompanied by high blood pressure (but with otherwise good condition of the heart) can be treated in this way.

THE SPANISH MANTLE

The Spanish mantle differs from the full wrapper in that a robe-like garment made of coarse linen and open in the front is used instead of the wet sheet. It reaches from the neck to over the toes, and the sleeves extend over the fingertips. The patient is helped into the wetted mantle just before lying down on the bed, which has been previously prepared with the dry layers as for the full wrapper. The mantle is then straightened out and wrapped around the patient following the procedures for the full wrapper. For a speedy warm-up, hot-water bottles may be placed at the patient's feet and sides.

The effects of the Spanish mantle are similar to those produced by the lower wrapper. Both are used to treat obesity and to produce a change in metabolism. The dissolving and purifying effects are particularly noteworthy. The duration of the application must be determined by the strength of the patient, especially by the degree of obesity; it should range from 1 to 1½ hours for a weak person to 2 hours at most for a strong man.

COMPRESSES

Compresses are water-like applications. The purpose of the wrapper used in connection with the compress is to secure and seal the compress in place.

The principal effect of the compress is very similar to that of the wrapper, the essential difference being that the entire compress application (a wet sheet folded several times) lies only on the body part being treated rather than surrounding it. Compresses, therefore, have a more localized effect than wrappers, but that effect is not to be underestimated. The middle sheet and outer wool blanket are the same sizes as for wrappers.

The materials used for compresses are porous and soft ones, such as coarse linen and cotton terry cloth towels.

The general procedure is to dip the cloth in cold (or warm) water, wring it out lightly, fold it four to six times (according to the size needed), and place it on the body part. Over this wet cloth, place a dry middle sheet and then a wool outer cover. The middle sheet must overlap the wool cover by at least an inch in all directions. The whole compress should always project about two inches beyond the affected body part. The wrapper must be well sealed and tucked in securely to prevent any heat from escaping.

The most popular additive to water used in cold compresses is vinegar, mainly to stimulate the responsiveness of the skin. Water and vinegar are used for weak persons to achieve a rapid warming effect. Other cold-compress additives include salt and clay. The effect of a warm compress is increased with various herbal additives (hay flowers, oat straw, spruce twigs, and fenugreek, for example). Bring a quart of water to a boil, turn off the heat, add a handful of dry herbs, and steep for 10 minutes.

THE COLD COMPRESS

Compresses are used whenever localized effects are indicated. There are two types of cold compresses. One is applied cold and kept cold through frequent changes; it has an anti-inflammatory, calming effect. The other, which stimulates inflammation, is also applied cold but remains on long enough to develop an intense warmth; sometimes it is even covered with a heating pad or a hot-water bottle to enhance the warming effect. Which compress to use initially is best left up to the instincts of the patient.

The anti-inflammatory, calming compress is applied at the height of an inflammation when it appears that the defenses of the body are overreacting. This compress reduces local heat and circulation, and thereby tends to relieve pain. It has a calming effect in cases of nervous excitation.

The inflammation-stimulating compress, on the other hand, is essential at the beginning of an inflammation when the body's defenses are reacting too slowly. Once this compress brings an improvement, it is advisable to switch to the cold compress.

THE HOT COMPRESS

In cases where cool, soothing compresses are not effective, hot compresses may be used to allay pain. In this case, two porous cloths four to six folds thick should be used in succession. One of them at a time is dipped in hot water (as hot as the patient can bear), wrung out, and laid on the affected part. Hot water must be available at all times for the duration of this treatment. The compress should be changed every few minutes, and should always be covered with a dry wool cloth or covering. Continued applications for a half hour are usually enough, after which they should give way to soothing compresses; or a dry flannel covering may be laid over the affected part and allowed to remain for as long as the person feels comfortable. If the pain continues, however, the cool, soothing compresses should be applied.

THE ABDOMINAL COMPRESS

The abdominal compress affects mainly the abdominal organs, especially the digestive organs, the kidneys, and the reproductive glands. It is used as a hot or cold application. For cold compresses, add about four ounces of vinegar to the water in which the compress is dipped. Cold compresses are removed as soon as they have absorbed the body warmth, which usually occurs within 60 to 75 minutes after the initial application. Hot compresses cool off in about the same time and then have to be removed or rewetted.

To prepare the abdominal compress, take a linen cloth (or a twin-size bedsheet, preferably cotton, folded lengthwise); dip it in cold or hot water, depending on the purpose of the compress; then wring it out well and apply it on the abdomen so that it covers from the rib arch to the hip area—generally fourteen to sixteen inches wide. As usual, a dry middle sheet and an outer blanket are used to complete the compress.

The effects of the cold abdominal compress are helpful for decreased muscle tone of the intestines and complaints arising from it. It also draws blood from the head downward (in case of a stroke) and calms palpitations of the heart. The cold abdominal compress is applied an hour or more before mealtimes.

The hot abdominal compress has an antispasmodic effect on the abdominal organs and therefore is used to treat stomach ulcers and cramps of the lower abdomen (menstrual pains). It is also used in the treatment of chronic catarrh of the bladder. Application of the compress in conjunction with a hot hand or arm bath of the left arm can be very beneficial in cases of irregular heartbeat (arrhythmia). The compress is applied 30 to 60 minutes after mealtimes.

THE BACK COMPRESS

The back compress affects primarily the circulation and metabolism of the back part of the body and benefits inflammatory conditions of the spinal cord (marrow). The cold–water application can have a calming effect on nervous conditions (such as sexual neurosis and involuntary emission of semen). The warm compress helps persistent rheumatic conditions of the back muscles and also relieves cramps and spasmodic abdominal attacks. In cases of infectious diseases of the spinal cord and the spinal cord membrane, the compress should preferably be applied hot or with a mustard powder additive. Increasing stiffness of the spine, lumbago, local neuromuscular disturbances, and even whooping cough are treated in this way.

A wetted sheet covers the back part of the body from the shoulders to the middle part of the upper thigh. A dry sheet and a blanket are wrapped snugly around the body over the wet sheet.

THE BREWER'S YEAST COMPRESS

Powdered brewer's yeast contains 45 to 48 percent high-quality protein, some lecithin, and significant amounts of the B-complex vitamins. In addition, and especially important to its effectiveness as a remedy for ulcers and running sores, it is a rich source of ergosterol, which is converted by the sun's ultraviolet rays into vitamin D. Its healing action takes effect on the tiny arterioles—the hairlike arteries at the skin's surface.

Varicose vein ulcerations that refuse to heal respond very well to the combined effects of brewer's yeast. The yeast holds up to 70 percent moisture, and this compress literally provides the building blocks for regenerating healthy tissue under favorable conditions: moisture, nutrients, and warmth.

The paste form is prepared in sufficient quantities to

cover the affected area. For example, if the ulcers are localized around the ankles, stir eight ounces of powdered
brewer's yeast into enough warm water (or chamomile
tea, which will provide an extra soothing effect on the
skin) to make a soft, moist paste about the consistency of
prepared mustard. Apply finger-thick directly on the affected area or spread on a wet linen or cotton cloth to be
laid on the ulcerous area. Cover this with a dry sheet and a
blanket as usual, and leave in place until the paste begins
to dry. This compress must stay moist to be effective. After
removing it, flush the area with cold water and allow it to
dry by exposing it to air. Do not rub dry; the delicate re-
growth of healthy tissue must be protected from friction,
including that caused by bedclothes or any other clothing.

THE CLAY COMPRESS

Clay compresses provide relief for inflammation of the
veins and cause a rapid decrease of infection and swelling
in cases of insect stings (for stings, renew the compress
every hour). When applied to larger parts of the body, clay
compresses are useful for the treatment of disorders of the
metabolism and extensive congestion in the tissues and
muscles.

Clay compresses are almost always applied cold. Sterilized clay should be available at your pharmacy, health food
store, or herb store. If there are clay deposits near your
house, you can sterilize the clay yourself by heating it in
the oven for about an hour, after which it should be pulverized. To prepare a clay paste, use vinegar diluted with
either water or an herb decoction, according to the effects
desired (see the introduction in this section). This thick,
ointment-like paste is spread onto a linen or cotton cloth

the size of the part of the body to be treated, or it is applied directly to the body.

Clay can be used to treat parts of the body or the whole body. In the latter case, it is usual to cover the body completely with the clay before wrapping with a dry sheet and a blanket. The cold paste should be about finger-thick. Only sterilized clay should be used in treating open wounds. A hay sack may be used to provide warmth. In general, the clay compress remains on until it is so dry that it will crumble. Then shower to remove any clay that may still be adhering to the skin; usually, the dried clay comes off easily by itself. Since clay compresses have a tendency to dry out the skin, rub in some warm olive oil or an herbal lubricating cream after the treatment.

Clay compresses remain cold for a relatively long time and have a great capacity for absorbing heat, which is of great advantage in treating inflammations.

THE COTTAGE CHEESE COMPRESS

The effects of the cottage cheese compress are similar to those of the clay compress; cheese compresses are used mainly because of their heat-absorbing qualities. The butterfat and casein contained in the curds also have an added curative effect. These compresses are used in the treatment of all diseases accompanied by high fever, such as pleurisy; pneumonia; inflammation of the joints, veins, and eyes (pinkeye); and both dry and wet leg or ankle ulcers.

Whey or milk and a few drops of vinegar are added to the cottage cheese and stirred until the mixture thickens, when it can be spread on a linen or cotton cloth; however, the best results are obtained when the mixture is applied directly to the skin. A dry sheet and a blanket are wrapped around the compress as usual. Cottage cheese compresses usually remain on until the curd has dried and crumbles. The application should be renewed several times.

THE EYE COMPRESS

Cold eye compresses are used to reduce redness and tiredness of the eyes due to eyestrain, noninfectious pinkeye, and other eye irritations or fatigue. They can also be applied in cases of minor externally caused injuries to tissues around the eyes.

A soothing, astringent solution for the compress can be made by steeping one heaping tablespoon of fresh eyebright herb in one cup of boiling-hot water for 5 minutes, then letting the solution cool. For convenience, twenty drops of tincture of eyebright to an eyecup of water may also be used.

A witch hazel lotion that can be purchased at your local health food store can make an effective compress for puffiness and redness of the eyes caused by crying. Lie down and place large cotton balls soaked in the lotion over each eye for 10 to 15 minutes, turning them as they become warm. A washcloth may also be dipped in the lotion, left wet but not dripping, and folded to fit across both eyes. Witch hazel draws out heat and reduces swelling of surrounding tissues.

For sties, a warm compress can be applied for 15 to 20 minutes every 3 to 4 hours until the sty points, opens, and drains.

For a simple warm eye compress, tie some flaxseed up in a clean cotton handkerchief. Soak in hot water for a few minutes to activate the compress effect. Hold the handkerchief gently against the closed eye for 15 to 20 minutes, rewetting it in the same hot water as the compress cools.

Here are some additional recipes for eye compresses:

Cucumber and Sage Compress

4 slices of cucumber
1 teaspoon sage seeds or 3 sage leaves

Pound the cucumber to a pulp. Soak the sage seeds in a tablespoon of water until the mixture becomes a thick mucilage, or pound the sage leaves to a pulp. To reduce puffiness around the eyes, combine the cucumber and sage and use as an eye compress.

Calendula and Carrot Compress

1 tablespoon dried calendula flowers
2½ ounces boiling water
½ cup fresh carrot pulp

Steep the calendula flowers in boiling-hot water for 10 minutes. Strain, add the carrot to the yellow infusion, and stew gently until the mixture becomes a soft mass. Allow to cool; then use as an eye compress for irritated eyes.

Comfrey Compress

A handful of fresh comfrey leaves
4 fluid ounces milk

Wash the comfrey and shake it dry. Simmer with the milk in a covered pan for 10 minutes. Lift out the herb and crush to a pulp. When it is tepid, lie down, lay the pulp over the eyes, and relax for 10 minutes. Use as a compress for tired eyes.

The following herbs are also used as compresses or lotions for the eyes:

Eyebright—infuse the whole plant, or use fifteen
    to twenty drops of tincture of eyebright in an
    eyecup.
Fennel—infuse the leaves or seeds.
Shave grass—use as a decoction for swollen eyelids.
Lemon verbena—infuse the leaves.
Rose—infuse the rose hips or soften the rose petals
    in cold milk.

Infusions of coltsfoot, chervil, borage, chamomile, plantain, and elder flowers are also good for the eyes.

THE FRONT COMPRESS

The front compress is used specifically to eliminate gases trapped in either the stomach or the lower abdomen. It is also used to treat obesity. It can affect the entire body by increasing the natural body warmth, but it can also reduce body temperature, depending on whether it is applied for a longer or a shorter period of time.

Fold a cotton sheet until it is long enough to cover the front part of the body from the neck to about the middle of the upper thigh and wide enough to extend somewhat down the sides of the body. The back part of the body is not covered. After this sheet is wetted and applied, wrap the dry middle sheet and the outer blanket tightly around the body.

The application should last for about 45 to 75 minutes.

THE HEART COMPRESS

The cold heart compress is suitable for nervous heartbeat and nervous conditional pains in the heart region. It is also applicable to inflammatory conditions of the heart, for which the cold is always beneficial. It does not necessarily follow, though, that the cold compresses have a direct cooling effect on the heart; the healing influence on the heart comes much more through distant effects on nerves in the chest.

In general, the cold heart compress has much greater effects—in the sense of slowing and strengthening the heart action—than the cold wash. The heart contracts and expands more energetically, thereby increasing the amount of blood pumped with each beat. The compress also tends to normalize an irregular heartbeat.

Cold heart compresses should not be made too small: They should cover the entire middle and left side of the chest. A handkerchief is not large enough; use a towel instead. With those forms of heartbeat problems that involve overfunctioning of the thyroid gland, apply the compress to the back of the neck, the neck, and the chest all at the same time. Wrap the towel from behind, around the nape of the neck, crossing it in front, over the neck, and spreading the ends over both sides of the chest. As usual, cover the compress with a dry cloth and an outer covering.

THE VAPOR COMPRESS

Vapor compresses relieve pain and cramps. Since the warmth of the compress stimulates blood circulation, it has a curative effect when the body does not generate enough warmth or when a functional weakness of the organs is present. It is used for the same problems as the hay sack, which is described next.

In addition to the three sheets used to prepare wrappers and other compresses, a fourth one made of woolflannel is necessary for the vapor compress. First, prepare the bed with a blanket and a dry sheet for the wrappings. Then fold a linen cloth three to four times until it is large enough to generously cover the part of the body to be treated. Roll it up and put it into boiling water for a few minutes. The addition of herbs (see pages 484–486) makes the application more effective. Use tongs to remove the cloth from the hot water and drop it onto a dry towel. Wrap it in the towel and wring out thoroughly. Then place the hot cloth on the wool-flannel sheet and fold them so that there will be only one layer of the flannel sheet on the side that will be touching the body. The dry sheet and the blanket are then wrapped around the body. Application and wrapping have to be done very carefully because of the heat. The vapor compress should be renewed when it has become cold.

THE HAY SACK

The hay sack, like other hot applications, is above all a pain reliever; however, it has added value through the special effects that derive from hay flowers.

The size of the hay sack is determined by the width of the body part being treated; two frequently used sizes are 14 x 18 inches (35 x 45 cm) and 18 x 24 inches (45 x 60 cm). Make a sack (a pillowcase folded to the appropriate size will do) and fill it three-fourths full of hay flowers. Tie the top of the sack and place it into a pot or basin. Pour boiling water over it and cover (don't put a hay sack into cold water and bring to a boil). Remove the sack after 5 to 10 minutes and put into a press. If you don't have a press, put the sack on a small wooden rack and place a wooden cutting board on top. Press on the board a few times, turning the sack occasionally, until all the excess water is pressed out. The drier the sack is, the longer it will stay warm. Then cover the sack with a wool cloth so that it will retain the heat. It is best to have the bed ready with a dry sheet and a blanket before preparing the hay sack.

When you feel that the heat of the sack can be tolerated, apply it to the part of the body being treated. Don't wrap right away with the dry sheet and blanket; rather, cover the area only loosely and lift them up a few times for a fanning effect to make the heat more tolerable. When the heat can be tolerated without this help, complete the wrapping, making sure that it fits tightly on all sides so that no vapors escape.

The duration of this application is from 45 to 75 minutes. After removal of the hay sack, the patient should rest in bed for at least a half hour to complete the effects of the treatment. The rest period should be followed by a cool full wash.

The hay sack works primarily locally; however, larger-size sacks will affect other parts of the body as well. The main areas of application are disorders of the digestive organs. Such problems as painful cramps, sluggish liver, debility, sagging of the transverse colon, and weak functioning of the glands are treated with the hay sack. Its dissolving and curative powers are evident in chronic inflammations such as in catarrhs of the upper respiratory system (bronchitis, whooping cough). Pleurisy and inflammation of the appendix can be treated with a hay sack if applied soon enough; otherwise, a cold compress and a physician are needed without delay.

The hay sack is known to absorb toxic matter excreted through sweating. It is always beneficial in the treatment of muscular rheumatism (lumbago), chronic rheumatic complaints of the joints, sciatica, and tissue changes and deposits due to gout and rheumatism. Colics suffered because of kidney stone or gallstone ailments are treated so effectively that hay sacks are called the morphine of naturopathy.

POULTICES

Poultices are similar to vapor compresses, but they retain warmth longer. A poultice is a hot, moist mass of boiled potato, ground flaxseed, powdered fenugreek, or another substance designed to hold prolonged, moist warmth between two layers of linen or coarse cotton cloth. It is applied to the skin to relieve congestion and pain, to stimulate absorption of inflammatory products, and to hasten suppuration (the draining of pus).

Before applying a poultice, check whether it will be too hot by holding it against your cheek or by testing it on the back of your hand. After applying, cover and keep it in place with a dry sheet and a wool cloth. To prevent burns, it is advisable to wait a few minutes before doing the final wrapping so that, if the poultice should still be too hot, it can be removed quickly.

THE POTATO POULTICE

Potatoes are healing, cleansing, and nourishing for the skin. The potato poultice aids in curing eczema, bleaching sunburn, and reducing puffiness under the eyes (caused by insomnia, fatigue, or strain, for example).

Boil unpeeled potatoes. Mash them. Apply as described in the introductory paragraphs, being careful not to burn the patient. Remove the poultice when it has become cold. A cold postapplication is generally not needed.

THE FLAXSEED POULTICE

The flaxseed poultice softens the skin and aids in excretion of any obstruction in hard abscesses or inflammations (as in the formation of an ulcer or carbuncle).

Depending on the size of the body part to be treated, boil two to four handfuls of ground flaxseed in water, stirring constantly until a thick paste has formed. This is then spread onto a cotton or linen cloth. A sort of package is formed by folding the cloth over the flaxseed paste, similar to the package used for the vapor compress. The flaxseed poultice is held in place by a dry sheet and a blanket as usual.

THE FENUGREEK POULTICE

The fenugreek poultice can be used in the treatment of small external complaints—for instance, in the treatment of boils, which it brings to a head more quickly.

Two to three handfuls of fenugreek powder are used for a poultice. The paste is prepared by bringing the cold water and the fenugreek powder to a boil, stirring constantly. The paste is then spread thickly onto a cotton or linen cloth. Apply to the body part being treated and cover with the usual dry sheet and blanket.

APPENDIX 1

Planetary Herb Formulas

Following is a list of herbs and formulas, including those mentioned in the text. The Planetary Formula line formulates Western, Chinese and Ayurvedic herbs together to create the most potent and effective formulas possible. They are under strict quality control and use good manufacturing practices (GMP). As well, they include products described as "full spectrum," a process developed by Planetary Formulas that combines the whole herb along with its standardized extract so they contain guaranteed potency without leaving any part of an herb out. To obtain contact: 1–800–717–5010, or *www.planetherbs.com*

FORMULA NUMBER 1: Antler Velvet: antler velvet from deer and elk; use for low sex drive, coldness, peri/menopause disorders, fatigue, infertility, impotence, cold extremities, ringing in the ears, weak low back and knees, frequent urination.

FORMULA NUMBER 2: Ashwagandha Liquid Herbal Extract: ashwagandha root extract; use for sexual debility, nervous exhaustion, problems of old age, poor memo rheumatism, fatigue, infertility, insomnia.

FORMULA NUMBER 3: Astragalus Full Spectrum Extract: astragalus, available as a tablet or as an alcohol or glycerin extract; use for fatigue, frequent colds and flu, poor digestion, exhaustion, poor appetite, diarrhea, non-healing sores, night sweats.

FORMULA NUMBER 4: Astragalus Jade Screen (traditional Chinese formula): astragalus, white atractylodes, sileris; tonifies Qi and releases to the surface; use to strengthen protective energy and prevent frequent colds and flu.

FORMULA NUMBER 5: Avena Sativa Oat Complex for Men: oat extract, saw palmetto, damiana, nettle, epimedium, ginseng, sarsaparilla, rose hips, cinnamon bark, ginkgo; strengthens sexual energy; use for low sex drive and sexual debility.

FORMULA NUMBER 6: Avena Sativa Oat Complex for Women: oat extract, *dong quai,* white peony, ligusticum, curculigo, alfalfa, vitex, ginger, cinnamon bark, jujube; use for low sex drive and sexual debility.

FORMULA NUMBER 7: Bacopa-Ginkgo Brain Strength: bacopa extract, ginkgo leaf extract, ashwagandha, guggul, saussurea, cardamom, gotu kola, asparagus root, chebulic myrobalan, Indian valerian root; use for poor memory and concentration.

FORMULA NUMBER 8: Bilberry Eye Complex: bilberry extract, eyebright, lycii, prepared rehmannia, mum, dioscorea, white peony, tribulus, fu ling, use to strengthen and improve eyesight, eyes, improve night vision.

R 9: Bilberry Vision: full spectrum

: Black Cohosh: full spectrum

FORMULA NUMBER 11: Borage Super GLA 300: borage seed oil

FORMULA NUMBER 12: Bupleurum Calmative Compound (traditional Chinese formula: Xiao Yao Wan): bupleurum, *dong quai,* white atractylodes, white peony, ginger, *fu ling,* licorice, mint; use for PMS, irregular menstruation, irritability, anxiety, depression, headache, breast distension, poor appetite, chronic hepatitis, malaria and peri/menopausal disorders with more pronounced Heat signs.

FORMULA NUMBER 13: Bupleurum Liver Cleanse: bupleurum, wild yam, Oregon grape, lycii, milk thistle extract, cyperus, dandelion extract, *dong quai,* white peony, fennel, ginger, green citrus, dandelion root, *dong quai* extract

FORMULA NUMBER 14: Cat's Claw tablets

FORMULA NUMBER 15: Calm Child: gotu kola extract, chamomile extract, zizyphus, hawthorn berry, catnip, lemon balm, longan pepper, licorice, chamomile flower, amla, anise, magnesium taurinate, calcium carbonate, clove, cinnamon bark; use for ADD, stress, hyperactivity, insomnia (hard to fall asleep), colds and flu.

FORMULA NUMBER 16: Calm Child Herbal Syrup: zizyphus, hawthorn, catnip, lemon balm, longan pepper, licorice, chamomile, gotu kola, amla, essential oils of anise, cinnamon bark, and clove; use for ADD, stress, hyperactivity, insomnia (hard to fall asleep), colds and flu.

FORMULA NUMBER 17: Candida Digest: asafetida, caraway, cumin, ginger, longan pepper, black pepper, slippery elm, dandelion, white atractylodes, rock salt, cyperus; use for loose stools, vaginal itching, poor digestion with gas, bloatedness, abdominal distension, nausea, vomiting, Candida symptoms, all due to cold.

FORMULA NUMBER 18: CholestGar: garlic, guggul, salvia, *dong quai,* gambir, *ho shou wou,* cayenne; use to lower cholesterol.

FORMULA NUMBER 19: Comfrey Care Salve: comfrey leaf, calendula flower, plantain leaf, St. Johnswort aerial parts, yarrow aerial parts, *Echinacea angustifolia* root, barberry root, lavender herb, lavender essential oil, chamomile essential oil, gum benzoin, olive oil, beeswax; use topically on wounds, cuts, sores, insect bites, and so on.

FORMULA NUMBER 20: Complete Cat's Claw Complex: cat's claw, andrographis, echinacea, isatis, oldenlandia, astragalus, reishi, reishi extract, jujube, cardamom

FORMULA NUMBER 21: Cordyceps Power CS–4: cordyceps standardized extract, astragalus, codonopsis, adenophora, eucommia, Siberian ginseng, white atractylodes, ginger; use for chronic coughs with weakness, lower back pain, difficulty inhaling, and fatigue.

FORMULA NUMBER 22: Cramp Bark Comfort: vitex, cramp bark, *dong quai, fu ling,* partridgeberry, cyperus, ginger, *dong quai* extract; use for menstral cramps.

FORMULA NUMBER 23: Cranberry Bladder Defense: cranberry extract, uva ursi extract, *fu ling,* echinacea, coptis, polyporus, marshmallow, alisma; use for bladder infections from heat, with scanty, dark painful urination.

FORMULA NUMBER 24: Damiana Male Potential: ginseng, saw palmetto, epimedium, sarsaparilla, damiana, morinda, schisandra, ophiopogon, cinnamon bark, ginkgo

FORMULA NUMBER 25: Digestive Comfort: *fu ling,* coix, white atractylodes, angelica, kudzu, magnolia bark, agastache, saussurea, leavened wheat, sprouted rice, trichosanthes, chrysanthemum, citrus, gastrodia, mint; Removes food stagnation, harmonizes the stomach, subdues rebellious stomach Qi, transforms dampness, subdues yang, relieves pain; use for abdominal bloating, gas and cramps, belching, hiccups, nausea, abdominal distension and pain, hyperacidity, overeating, hangover, motion sickness, morning sickness, stomach flu and food poisoning.

FORMULA NUMBER 26: Digestive Grape Bitters: angelica, gentian, artemisia, astragalus, dill, goldenseal, juniper, magnolia, Oregon grape, yerba santa, cardamom, sarsaparilla, white atractylodes, pau d'arco, yarrow, coriander, galangal, ginger, cyperus, essential oils of anise and sweet orange, grape juice; use to promote good digestion and prevent gas, bloatedness, abdominal distension.

FORMULA 27: Echinacea Glycerite: *Echinacea pallida* root and *Echinacea purpurea* root, available in peppermint, lemon, and orange flavors, especially suitable for kids.

FORMULA NUMBER 28: Echinacea Full Spectrum Extract: *Echinacea angustifolia* root and *Echinacea purpurea* root, available in peppermint, lemon, and orange flavors, especially suitable for kids.

FORMULA NUMBER 29: Echinacea Root Tablets (pure)

FORMULA NUMBER 30: Echinacea-Elderberry Syrup: elderberry, echinacea, isatis, honeysuckle, forsythia, boneset, platycodon, licorice, apricot, gastrodia; antiviral and antibacterial for colds, flu, fever and cough.

FORMULA NUMBER 31: Echinacea Defense Force: echinacea root extract, schisandra, ligustrum, astragalus, pau d'arco extract, garlic, reishi, Siberian ginseng, pau d'arco bark, goldenseal, ginger, echinacea, suma; use to prevent colds and flu.

FORMULA NUMBER 32: Echinacea Elderberry Syrup: elderberry, *Echinacea purpurea* root, isatis, honeysuckle, forsythia, boneset, platycodon, licorice, apricot seed, gastrodia; antiviral and antibacterial for colds, flu, fever and cough.

FORMULA NUMBER 33: Echinacea–Goldenseal Liquid Extract: *Echinacea purpurea* root, goldenseal root, *Echinacea purpurea* seed; use for infections and inflammations.

FORMULA NUMBER 34: Echinacea–Goldenseal with Olive Leaf: echinacea, goldenseal, olive leaf, garlic, andrographis extract, isatis extract, dandelion extract, licorice extract, ginger extract; antiviral for acute and prolonged colds, flu, fever, infections and inflammations.

FORMULA NUMBER 35: Elderberry Fluid Extract, full spectrum

FORMULA NUMBER 36: Elderberry Syrup: elderberry, honey

FORMULA NUMBER 37: Feverfew Head Aid: willow bark extract, feverfew extract, schizonepeta leaf and stem, notopterygium root, green tea leaf, licorice root, ligusticum rhizome, angelica root, siler root, cyperus rhizome, ginger root; use for headaches due to liver heat with irritability, stress.

FORMULA NUMBER 38: Flex–Ability (Tablets or Liquid): *Angelica pubescent* root (*du huo*), chaneomales, gambir, achyranthes, ligusticum, teasel, angelica, tienchi ginseng, lycii, notopterygium, siler, *dong quai*

FORMULA NUMBER 39: GarliChol (Enteric-coated Garlic Extract) Full Spectrum and Standardized: 650 mg garlic clove tablet; lowers high cholesterol and blood pressure.

FORMULA NUMBER 40: Ginger Tablets: full spectrum and standardized extract

FORMULA NUMBER 41: Ginger Warming Compound: ginger, cinnamon bark, cayenne, white pine bark, cloves, bayberry, marshamllow, licorice; use for colds, flu, fever and sore throats due to Coldness, cough or runny nose with white mucus, cold hands and feet, poor circulation, coldness, menstrual cramps and pain due to coldness.

FORMULA NUMBER 42: Ginkgo Awareness: Indian valerian, dendrobium, polygala, calamus, eclipta, nutmeg, cardamom, gotu kola extract, ginkgo extract; use to improve memory, concentration and eyesight.

FORMULA NUMBER 43: Ginseng Classic (traditional Chinese formula: Four Gentleman): Asian ginseng, white atractylodes, *fu ling*, licorice; use for poor appetite, energy and digestion.

FORMULA NUMBER 44: Ginseng Elixir (traditional Chinese formula: *Bu Zhong Yi Qi Wan*): Asian ginseng, astragalus, licorice, molasses, white atractylodes, bupleurum, citrus, cimicifuga, jujube, *dong quai* extract, *dong quai* root, ginger; use for poor appetite, energy and digestion, prolapsed organs, frequent urination.

FORMULA NUMBER 45: Ginseng Revitalizer: angelica, white atractylodes, codonopsis, Asian ginseng, polygonum, licorice, astragalus, Siberian ginseng, American ginseng, ginger, tienchi ginseng, *fu ling,* Siberian ginseng extract, Asian ginseng extract; use for poor energy, fatigue, exhaustion, and weakness.

FORMULA NUMBER 46: Glucosamine–MSM Herbal: d–Glucosamine Sulfate, MSM, molybdenum aspartate citrate, rehmannia, wild yam, teasel, eucommia, boswellia, drynaria, calcium citrate, myrrh; use for painful joints.

FORMULA NUMBER 47: Guggul Cholesterol Compound: guggul, plumbago root, harada *(Terminalia chebula),* behada *(Terminalia belerica),* amla *(Emblica officinalis),* longan pepper, vidanga, cumin, cardamom, deodar cedar bark, tribulus, nut grass rhizome, ginger, cinnamon bark, vetiver grass, barley grain, Himalayan fir bark; use to lower cholesterol.

FORMULA NUMBER 48: Hawthorn Extract: full spectrum

FORMULA NUMBER 49: Hawthorn Extract, glycerin syrup

FORMULA NUMBER 50: Hawthorn Heart: hawthorn berry, hawthorn leaf and flower extract, tienchi ginseng, motherwort, Chinese salvia, polygala, *dong quai,* codonopsis, *dong quai* extract, juniper berry, longan; use for palpitations, arrhythmias, irregular heartbeat, chest pain, insomnia due to Deficient Heart Blood.

FORMULA NUMBER 51: Horny Goat Weed: epimidium; use for low sex drive and for peri/menopausal disorders with hot flashes, night sweats, dry throat at night, heat in palms and soles, malar flush, thirst, weakness, tiredness, low back pain.

FORMULA NUMBER 52: Horsechestnut Cream: horsechestnut seed and bark extract, butcher's broom extract, witch hazel extract, white oak bark extract, myrrh extract, rosemary oil, purified water, aloe vera gel, glyceryl stearate, caprylic/capric triglyceride, glycerin, stearic acid, beeswax, cetyl alcohol, cetearyl alcohol, methyl glucose, lecithin phospholipik, jojoba oil, vitamin E, xanthan gum, grapefruit seed extract, methylparaben, propylparaben, sorbic acid; use externally for hemorrhoids, bruises, and varicose veins.

FORMULA NUMBER 53: Horsechestnut Vein Strength: horsechestnut seed extract, witch hazel, butcher's broom, bitter orange, *dong quai,* ginkgo extract; use internally for hemorrhoids, bruises and varicose veins.

FORMULA NUMBER 54: Jiagulan Full Spectrum Tablets; use to regulate blood sugar.

FORMULA NUMBER 55: Kava Concentrate: full spectrum and standardized extract—liquid or tabs

FORMULA NUMBER 56: Super Kava 80: standardized to 80 percent or greater kavalactones in soft-gel capsules

FORMULA NUMBER 57: Kava Dreams: zizyphus, kava kava extract, *fu ling,* American ginseng, ligusticum, anemarrhena, licorice; use for insomnia, restlessness, and night sweats due to deficient yin.

FORMULA NUMBER 58: Kudzu Recovery: kudzu root and flower, havenia fruit, coptis, *fu ling,* grifola, white atractylodes, codonopsis, saussurea, *shen qu (Massa fermentata* extract), cardamom, ginger; use for quick recovery from hangovers.

FORMULA NUMBER 59: Lower Back Support: loranthes, achyranthes, eucommia, angelica (*du huo*), rehmannia, dioscorea, alisma, *fu ling* psoralea, moutan peony, cornus; use for low-back, hip, and knee pain.

FORMULA NUMBER 60: Maca Extract: full spectrum and standardized

FORMULA NUMBER 61: Maitake Beta-Factor: Dr. Nanba's (the Japanese scientist who pioneered the extraction of beta glucam from maitake mushrooms)

FORMULA NUMBER 62: Maitake Mushroom: full spectrum

FORMULA NUMBER 63: MenoChange (modified traditional Chinese formula): magnesium citrate, chaste tree berry, *dong quai* extract, wild yam extract, calcium citrate, anemarrhena, white atractylodes, bupleurum, epimidium, gardenia, moutan peony, phellodendron, *fu ling,* black cohosh extract, white peony, ginger, motherwort, licorice; effective for stiff and painful neck and shoulders, upper back pain, shoulder joint pain.

FORMULA NUMBER 64: Mullein Lung Complex: platycodon, ephedra, ophiopogon, elecampane, licorice, mullein, wild cherry, ginger, cinnamon twig, wild ginger; use for cough, asthma, wheezing, bronchitis, and all other upper respiratory complaints.

FORMULA NUMBER 65: Myelin Sheath Support: guggul, elderberry, ginseng, tienchi ginseng, hawthorn berry, shilafit mineral resin, bromelain, amla, boswellia, licorice, ashwagandha, salvia, vitamin B_{12}, pantothenic acid, calcium, kelp, magnesium citrate, malate, zinc picolinate, selenium, copper sebaceae, chromium picolinate, molybdenum chelate, potassium citrate, turmeric root extract, hericium erinaceus mycelium, astragalus, bacopa plant extract, black pepper, ginger root, longan pepper, boron chelate, black pepper extract; highly effective for MS when taken as prescribed over a long time.

FORMULA NUMBER 66: Narayana Muscle Oil (traditional Ayruvedic formula): sesame seed oil, ashwagandha, bael fruit, Indian nightshade herb, mallow, *trianthema monogyna* root, Chinese flower plant, asparagus root, saffron, musk, black pepper, valerian, catechu wood, natural fragrance; topical oil for sore and aching muscles and joints.

FORMULA NUMBER 67: Neck and Shoulders Support: kudzu root, notopterygium, ligusticum turmeric, *dong quai,* white peony root, kava kava root extract, astragalus root, cinnamon twig, milettiae stem, clematis root and stem extract; effective for stiff and painful neck and shoulders, upper back pain, shoulder joint pain.

FORMULA NUMBER 68: Old Indian Herbal Syrup: yerba santa, echinacea, osha, grindelia, wild ginger, elecampane, horehound, hyssop, platycodon, white pine bark, polypodii, wild cherry, mullein, Irish moss, marshmallow, nettle, loquat leaf, fritillaria, licorice, bitter almond seed, angelica root; fabulous for all sorts of coughs.

FORMULA NUMBER 69: Olive Leaf: full spectrum extract

FORMULA NUMBER 70: Pau D'Arco Deep Cleansing: burdock root, pau d'arco bark, red clover, echinacea, *fu ling,* astragalus, licorice, ginger, American ginseng, kelp, reishi mushroom

FORMULA NUMBER 71: Prosta Palmetto concentrate: full spectrum and standardized

FORMULA NUMBER 72: Pumpkin Seed Oil: full spectrum

FORMULA NUMBER 73: Red Clover Cleanser: honeysuckle, forsythia, red clover, echinacea, sarsaparilla, yellow dock, echinacea extract, ginger, goldenseal, licorice, cinnamon twig, American ginseng; clears heat and toxins; use to cleanse the blood and skin eruptions.

FORMULA NUMBER 74: Rehmannia Endurance (modified traditional Chinese formula): rehmannia, cornus, lycii, alisma, dioscorea, *fu ling,* tree peony, *ho shou wou,* chrysanthemum, ligustrum, saw palmetto; use for dry eyes, mouth, throat or vagina, weak lower back, headache, dizziness, tinnitus, hypertension, insomnia, night sweats, anxiety, fatigue and peri/menopausal disorders, all due to Deficient Kidney Yin.

FORMULA NUMBER 75: Rehmannia Vitalizer (modified traditional Chinese formula): morinda, cistanche, cuscuta, rehmannia, psoralea, cornus, dioscorea, moutan peony, alisma, Asian ginseng, *dong quai,* epimidium, *fu ling,* schisandra, saw palmetto, cinnamon bark, lycii; use for low back pain or weakness, weak knees, frequent urination, impotence, infertility, cold limbs, edema (especially of ankles), chronic nephritis, chronic prostatitis, geriatric tonic.

FORMULA NUMBER 76: Reishi Mushroom: full spectrum extract: reishi mushroom body and mycelia biomass

FORMULA NUMBER 77: Reishi Mushroom Supreme: reishi, shiitake, Siberian ginseng, schisandra, astragalus, atractylodes, grifola, ligustrum, poria cocos, reishi extract, polygala, ginger, cyperus; use for poor energy, lowered resistance to colds and flu, weakness, low immunity in general.

FORMULA NUMBER 78: Rhodiola Rosea: full spectrum extract and standardized: *rhodolia rosea* root

FORMULA NUMBER 79: Saw Palmetto Classic: saw palmetto berry extract, pygeum bark extract, pumpkin seed oil extract, echinacea root, gardenia, alisma, salvia, gravel root, codonopsis, cuscuta, ligustrum, plantain seed, *dong quai;* use for prostate issues, including swollen prostate and frequent urination.

FORMULA NUMBER 80: Schisandra Adrenal Complex: schisandra, dioscorea, cornus, *fu ling,* alisma, rehmannia, cuscuta, plantain, rubus, lycii; astringes and holds yin and fluids.

FORMULA NUMBER 81: Shiitake Mushroom: full spectrum extract: mature shiitake fruiting body and mycelia biomass

FORMULA NUMBER 82: Shiitake Mushroom Supreme: shiitake, reishi, schisandra, angelica, lycii, salvia, turmeric, milk thistle extract, ligustrum, rehmannia, cyperus, shiitake extract, reishi extract, *Letinus edodes* mycelium extract; use to tonify immunity, particularly of liver in cirrhosis and hepatitis.

FORMULA NUMBER 83: Silymarin 80: full spectrum extract and standardized: milk thistle seed extract and whole milk thistle seed

FORMULA NUMBER 84: Sinus Free: horseradish, thyme, yarrow, eyebright; use for sinus infections.

FORMULA NUMBER 85: Soy Genistein Isoflavone 1000: isoflavone-rich soybean powder Soylife yielding genistein, glycitein, daidzein

FORMULA NUMBER 86: Stevia Powder: full spectrum

FORMULA NUMBER 87: Stinging Nettles Freeze Dried

FORMULA NUMBER 88: St. Johnswort Junior Syrup: St. Johnswort leaf and flower, lemon balm, hawthorn berry, elder, zizyphus, passionflower, chamomile, jujube; use for hyperactivity, insomnia, and crying.

FORMULA NUMBER 89: St. Johnswort Full Spectrum and Standardized Extract: St. Johnswort extract and St. Johnswort extract prepared from flowering tops

FORMULA NUMBER 90: St. Johnswort–Kava Compound: St. Johnswort extract, kava kava extract, bupleurum, moutan peony, atractylodes, *dong quai, fu ling,* lemon balm, licorice, cyperus, ginger; treats depression from liver heat.

FORMULA NUMBER 91: Stone Free: turmeric, gravel root, dandelion extract, ginger, lemon balm, marshmallow, parsley, dandelion root, licorice; effective for gallbladder or kidney stones.

FORMULA NUMBER 92: Stress Free: zizyphus, skullcap, valerian, American ginseng, hawthorn, black cohosh, ginger, licorice, valerian extract, wood betony, chamomile, hops, magnesium citrate and oxide, Siberian ginseng, Siberian ginseng extract, calcium carbonate; very effective in relieving and helping one handle stress without inducing sleep.

FORMULA NUMBER 93: Suma: 500 mg suma per tablet

FORMULA NUMBER 94: Three Spices Sinus Complex: ginger, longan pepper, black pepper, dehydrated honey; use for sinus infections, coughs with white mucus.

FORMULA NUMBER 95: Tri-Cleanse Internal Cleanser with Triphala (modified traditional Ayurvedic formula): psyllium husk, triphala, flaxseed (partially defatted to prevent rancidity), guar gum, oat bran, wild yam, anise, stevia, cyperus, ginger, natural licorice flavor; use for constipation.

FORMULA NUMBER 96: Triphala-Garcinia Program: spirulina, garcinia berry extract, triphala compound (amla, behada, harada fruits), kelp, guar gum fiber, atractylodes root, L-tyrosine, cleavers leaf and stem, fennel seed, bladderwrack, astragalus, echinacea, ginger, licorice, watercress leaf and stem, lecithin, apple cider vinegar, vitamin B₆, burdock root, zizyphus seed

FORMULA NUMBER 97: Triphala Internal Cleanser (traditional Ayurvedic formula): harada fruit *(Terminalia chebula)*, amla fruit *(Emblica officinalis)*, behada fruit *(Terminalia beterica)*; use for constipation.

FORMULA NUMBER 98: Upper Back Support: pueraria (kudzu), notopterygium, ligusticum, turmeric, *dong quai*, white peony, kava kava, astragalus, cinnamon twigs, millettiae, clematis; use for pain in the upper back, neck and shoulders.

FORMULA NUMBER 99: Uva Ursi Diurite: cleavers, *fu ling*, dandelion extract, dandelion root, ginger, marshmallow, parsley, uva ursi extract, uva ursi leaf; use for bladder and kidney infections.

FORMULA NUMBER 100: Valerian Easy Sleep: zizyphus, valerian, skullcap, passionflower, chamomile, hops, wood betony, calcium citrate, magnesium taurinate, amber, American ginseng, *dong quai,* ginger, licorice, pinellia, *fu ling,* valerian root extract; use for insomnia.

FORMULA NUMBER 101: Valerian: full spectrum and standardized extract: valerian root

FORMULA NUMBER 102: Vitex: full spectrum and standardized extract: vitex extract, vitex whole berry

FORMULA NUMBER 103: Well Child Echinacea Elderberry Herbal Syrup: honeysuckle, elder, lemon balm, chamomile, catnip, echinacea root and leaf, cinnamon twig, licorice root; use for colds, flu, fever.

FORMULA NUMBER 104: Wild Yam–Black Cohosh Complex: American ginseng, black cohosh, *dong quai* extract, *dong quai,* licorice, sarsaparilla, wild yam extract, kelp, wild yam root, ginger, saw palmetto extract, saw palmetto berry, goldenseal; use for hormonal imbalances to ease menstrual and peri/menopausal phases.

FORMULA NUMBER 105: Willow Aid: willow bark extract, corydalis, *dong quai,* valerian, guggul, boswellia extract; relieves pain from headaches, painful joints, and general pain.

FORMULA NUMBER 106: Women's Dong Quai Tonifier: *dong quai* extract, white peony, white atractylodes, codonopsis, rehmannia, *fu ling,* molasses, ligusticum, licorice; tonifies blood and Qi; use for pale complexion, tiredness, dizziness, vertigo, tinnitus, amenorrhea, threatened miscarriage, post-partum anemia, a pale tongue, and a thready and weak pulse. This is the main formula to tonify deficient blood and Qi.

FORMULA NUMBER 107: Women's Dong Quai Treasure (modified traditional Chinese formula): *dong quai* extract, cramp bark, false unicorn root, cooked rehmannia, *dong quai,* white atractylodes, white peony, ligusticum, tree peony, blue cohosh, ginger, *fu ling*

FORMULA NUMBER 108: Yellow Dock Skin Cleanse: yellow dock, bupleurum, echinacea extract, echinacea root, gentian, myrrh, Oregon grape, *fu ling,* wild yam, wild yam extract, marshmallow

FORMULA NUMBER 109: Yin Chiao Classic (traditional Chinese formula): forsythia, honeysuckle, mint, phragmites, burdock seed, platycodon, soybean, licorice, schizonepeta, bamboo

FORMULA NUMBER 110: Yin Chiao–Echinacea Complex (modified traditional Chinese formula): forsythia, honeysuckle, phragmites, notopterygium, bamboo leaf, burdock root, echinacea, horehound, schizonepeta, boneset, elecampane, isatis root and leaf, platycodon, soybean, licorice, mint

APPENDIX 2

*Sources for
Quality Nutritional Supplements*

The complete line of Planetary products is available at the herb store and online at the following Web site. Personal e-mail health consultations are also available for a fee. http://www.planetherbs.com

Threshold Enterprises

23 Janis Way
Scotts Valley, CA 95066
Tel: (408) 438-1700
Fax: (408) 438-7410

Manufacturer of Planetary formulas and Source Naturals nutritional supplements. Those interested in wholesale purchasing, or for the location of the nearest retailer of these and a wide range of other supplements, should contact them for information.

Source Naturals Nutritional Supplements

Check them out online at:
http://www.sourcenaturals.com/home.html

Rainbow Light Nutritional Supplements

Manufacturer of a complete line of quality nutritional supplements, including their Complete Nutritional Program, which is a unique food-based multivitamin supplement.
http://www.rainbowlight.com

ORGANIC WESTERN HERBS

Frontier Herbs and Nature's Herbs

P.O. Box 118, Dept. 34Q
Norway, IA 52318
Tel: (800) 365-4372

Trinity Herb Company

P.O. Box 199
Bodega Bay, CA 94222
Tel: (707) 874-3418

CHINESE HERBS

Bio Essence

5221 Central, Suite 105
Richmond, CA 94804
Tel: (800) 538-1333
Fax: (510) 873-8676

Great China Herb Company

857 Washington St.
San Francisco, CA 94108
Tel: (415) 982-2195
Fax: (415) 982-5138

Mayway Chinese Herb Company

1338 Mandela Parkway
Oakland, CA 94607
Tel: (800) 262-9929

One of the largest wholesale and practitioner suppliers in
the country. They are the manufacturer of Plum Flower
Brand patent formulas. They do not sell direct to individuals but they will let you know who sells their products in
your area.

AYURVEDIC HERBS AND SUPPLEMENTS

Bazaar of India

Located in Berkeley, California, since 1971. They are one
of the biggest Indian import stores in the country and
carry a complete line of Ayurvedic herbal health supplements from India.
Tel: (510) 849-3329
Online: http://www.bazaarofindia.com

RETAIL SOURCES FOR HOMEOPATHIC REMEDIES

These companies can also provide kits of selected remedies that one would find most useful for everyday home
use as well as many of the conditions mentioned throughout this book.

Homeopathy Overnight

929 Shelburne Ave.
Absecon, NJ 08201
Tel: (800) ARNICA 30 (276-4223)

Bailey's Natural Pharmacy / Johnson Drugs

175 Harvard Ave.
Allston, MA 01234
Tel: (617) 782-7202
(800) 239-6206
Fax: (617) 782-4328

APPENDIX 3

Finding an Alternative Health Practitioner

The following represent sources to help you locate qualified alternative practitioners nearest to you. More can be
found on the Internet, but the sources marked with an as-
terisk (*) I would personally endorse.

ONLINE PERSONALIZED HERBAL CONSULTATIONS

With Michael Tierra or his staff of personally trained
herbalists of the East West Herbs and Acupuncture clinic
in Santa Cruz. Go to http://www.planetherbs.com and
click on Health and Herbal Consultations with Michael
and Lesley Tierra at the lower right corner of the screen *or
call* (831) 429-8066 for information.

HERBOLOGY

American Herbalists Guild
1931 Gaddis Rd.
Canton, GA 30115
Tel: (770) 751-6021
Fax: (770) 751-7472
E-mail: ahgoffice@earthlink.net

Call or check their Web site for a professional clinical herbalist closest to you.

ACUPUNCTURE AND TRADITIONAL CHINESE MEDICINE

Acupuncture and Oriental Medicine Alliance

14637 Starr Rd. SE
Olalla, WA 98359
Tel: (253) 851-6896
Fax: (253) 851-6883
www.AcupunctureAlliance.org

Contact them for a licensed clinical acupuncturist.

American Association of Acupuncture and Oriental Medicine (AAAOM)

433 Front St.
Catasqua, PA 18032-2526
Tel: (610) 266-1433
Fax: (610) 264-2768

NATUROPATHY

Naturopathic Directory
http://www.naturopathicdirectory.com/index.asp

American Association of Naturopathic Physicians (AANP)

601 Valley St., Suite 105
Seattle, WA 98109
Tel: (206) 298-0126
Fax: (206) 298-0129
For physician referrals: (206) 298-0129

HOMEOPATHY

*National Center for Homeopathy

http://www.homeopathic.org/NCHSearch.htm
In the UK:
*http://www.homeopath.co.uk/

NUTRITIONISTS

Find a Nutritionist is a Web site where you can find a nutritionist in your area.
http://www.findanutritionist.com/index.html

*American Dietetic Association

http://www.eatright.org/find.html
To locate a licensed medical dietician closest to you.

CHIROPRACTORS

*International Chiropractors Association

http://www.chiropractic.org/

AYURVEDIC PRACTICTIONERS

International Ayurvedic Practitioner Listing

http://www.ayurvedahc.com/community/Family/
VaidaFind.htm

HOLISTIC MEDICINE

American Holistic Medical Association

4104 Lake Boone Trail, Suite 201
Raleigh, NC 27607
Tel: (919) 787-5146

National Institute of Medical Herbalists (NIMH)

56 Long Brook St.
Exeter, Devon EX 4 6AH England
Tel: 011-44-39-242-6022
Fax: 011-44-39-249-8963

The Holistic Resource Center offers a directory of homeopathic and alternative practitioners around the world and it would be a good place to search on the Internet at http://www.holisticmed.com/www/directory.html.

The National Center for Homeopathy

1500 Massachusetts Ave., NW
Washington, DC 20005
http://www.homeopathic.org/NCHSearch.htm/
In the UK:
http://www.homeopath.co.uk

North American Society of Homeopathy (NASH)

Offers an online directory of homeopathic physicians from around the country.
http://www.homeopathy.org/

Homeopathy Home

A complete online listing of homeopathic practitioners, associations, and other matters related to homeopathy.
http://www.homeopathyhome.com/directory/usa/organizations.html

British Homeopathic Association

For homeopathic practitioners in the UK.
http://trusthomeopathy.org/trust/tru_su02.html

APPENDIX 4

Educational Resources

EAST WEST SCHOOL OF HERBAL MEDICINE

By Michael Tierra, L.Ac., OMD, ND, and Lesley Tierra, L.Ac., both founding members of the American Herbalists Guild (AHG)
P.O. Box 275
Santa Cruz, CA 95005
Tel: (831) 336-5010 or (800) 717-5010
Fax: (831) 336-4548
www.planetherbs.com

A distance-learning (correspondence) course that offers a thorough, guided training in herbal medicine in thirty-six lessons that you can do at your own pace. It is unique in its integration of the world's major systems, with a special emphasis on the integration of Western, Chinese, and Ayurvedic herbal medicine. Each year it offers a fun-filled, inspirational, weeklong training, usually in April, where its students have the opportunity to study directly with Michael and Lesley Tierra and some of the finest teachers in the country. The East West Herb Seminar is offered each year in the spring in one of the most beautiful areas of the country, amid the giant redwood forests of the Santa Cruz Mountains. Santa Cruz itself, located no more than thirty minutes away, has wonderful beaches and adjoins the beautiful Monterey Bay and Big Sur wilderness areas. Space is limited, so those who are interested should plan to register early.

PLANETHERBS ONLINE

A highly informative source for information on herbal medicine, including Western, Chinese, and Ayurvedic herbal medicine. There is an online forum for questions, answers, and comments relating to herbal medicine, updated regularly.
www.planetherbs.com

AMERICAN HERBALISTS GUILD

E-mail: ahgoffice@earthlink.net

They offer an informative Web site with an online forum as well as yearly herbal symposiums throughout the country.

OTHER ORGANIZATIONS

American Botanical Council

P.O. Box 201660
Austin, TX 78720-1660
Tel: (512) 331-8868
Publishers of *HerbalGram* magazine
http://www.herbalgram.org/browse.php/defaulthome

Herb Research Foundation (HRF)

1007 Pearl St., Suite 200
Boulder, CO 80302
Tel: (303) 449-2265
Fax: (303) 449-7849

United Plant Savers

P.O. Box 420
East Barre, VT 05649
Tel: (802) 479-9825
Fax: (802) 476-3722

UPS is devoted to preserving and replanting endangered and threatened medicinal plant species for nonharvestable purposes.

BIBLIOGRAPHY

By Michael Tierra

Planetary Herbology, published by Lotus Press
The Way of Herbs, published by Pocket Books
The Way of Chinese Herbs, published by Pocket Books
Biomagnetic and Herbal Therapy, published by Lotus Press
(This book is the simplest description of the most ef-
fective use of magnets for pain, inflammation, and
many other conditions.)
Chinese Traditional Herbal Medicine, Vols. 1 and 2 by
Michael and Lesley Tierra
(A complete text for the study of Chinese herbal
medicine.)
The Herbal Treatment of Cancer, published by Lotus Press

By Lesley Tierra

Herbs of Life, published by Crossing or Ten-speed Press
A Children's Herbal, published by Crossing or Ten-speed Press
(This is a beautiful book to be used by parents for
teaching children about the wonderful uses of herbs,
complete with a guide to herb uses, preparations,
identification, fun projects, and wonderful herb stories.)

Other Authors

This list is by no means complete but represents a few books by a few fine herbalists.

Herbal Healing Secrets of the Orient by Darlena L'Orange, published by Prentice Hall

Ancient Roots, Many Branches by Darlena L'Orange, L.Ac., and Gary Dolowich, M.D., Prentice Hall
(Energetics of healing across cultures and through time, with many practical remedies from diverse cultures of the world.)

The One Earth Herbal Sourcebook by Alan Keith Tillotson, Ph.D., AHD, published by Twin Streams Press (Kensington Publishers)
Another book that offers a practical source for the use of Chinese, Western, and Ayurvedic herbal treatments.

Herbal Healing for Women by Amanda McQuade, AHG, MNIMH, published by Prima

By Aviva Jill Romm, AHG, CPM

Natural Healing for Babies and Children, published by Crossing Press

The Natural Pregnancy Book, published by Crossing Press

The Pocket Guide to Midwifery Care, published by Crossing Press

ADHD Alternatives, published by Storey Communications
(These outstanding books come from the diverse and practical experience of an herbalist, currently executive director of the AHG, from her many years of mothering and midwifery.)

Herbal Medicine by Sharol Tilgner, N.D., published by Wise Acres Press

Ayurvedic Healing by David Frawley, published by Passage Press

Green Pharmacy by James Duke, Ph.D., published by Rodale

Beating Cancer with Nutrition by Patrick Quillin with Noreen Quillin, published by Nutrition Times Press

Healing with Whole Foods by Paul Pitchford, published by North Atlantic

Between Heaven and Earth by Harriet and Efrem Korngold, published by Ballantine

INDEX

Visit the
Simon & Schuster Web site:
www.SimonSays.com

and sign up for our
mystery e-mail updates!

Keep up on the latest
new releases, author appearances,
news, chats, special offers, and more!
We'll deliver the information
right to your inbox — if it's new,
you'll know about it.

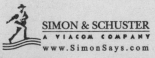